ENVIRONMENTAL ASTHMA

LUNG BIOLOGY IN HEALTH AND DISEASE

Executive Editor

Claude Lenfant
Director, National Heart, Lung and Blood Institute
National Institutes of Health
Bethesda, Maryland

ADDITIONAL VOLUMES IN PREPARATION

The opinions expressed in these volumes do not necessarily represent the views of the National Institutes of Health.

ENVIRONMENTAL ASTHMA

Edited by

Robert K. Bush

*University of Wisconsin–Madison Medical School
and William S. Middleton Memorial Veterans Hospital
Madison, Wisconsin*

MARCEL DEKKER, INC.   NEW YORK · BASEL

Library of Congress Cataloging-in-Publication Data

Environmental asthma / edited by Robert K. Bush.
    p. cm. — (Lung biology in health and disease ; v. 153)
    Includes bibliographical references and indexes.
    ISBN: 0-8247-0301-4 (alk. paper)
    1. Asthma—Environmental aspects.   2. Asthma—Etiology. I. Bush, Robert K. II.
Series.
    RC591 .E585 2000
    616.2′38071—dc21

                                      00-060191

This book is printed on acid-free paper.

Headquarters
Marcel Dekker, Inc.
270 Madison Avenue, New York, NY 10016
tel: 212-696-9000; fax: 212-685-4540

Eastern Hemisphere Distribution
Marcel Dekker AG
Hutgasse 4, Postfach 812, CH-4001 Basel, Switzerland
tel: 41-61-261-8482; fax: 41-61-261-8896

World Wide Web
http://www.dekker.com

The publisher offers discounts on this book when ordered in bulk quantities. For more
information, write to Special Sales/Professional Marketing at the headquarters address
above.

Current printing (last digit):
10 9 8 7 6 5 4 3 2 1

PRINTED IN THE UNITED STATES OF AMERICA

INTRODUCTION

"Nature or nurture?"—this topic has been, and is, the subject of debates that, of course, have only limited rationale because it is now well recognized that both nature *and* nurture are the determining factors in most complex (and chronic) conditions. Asthma is certainly one of the best examples of this dual origin. Furthermore, in reality it is not a matter of one factor competing against the other but, rather, a synergetic action that results from an "alliance" between the environment and the genes to cause asthma and to determine its severity.

In practical terms, genetic determinants cannot be modified. Identification of the environmental factors, however, offers the possibility of breaking the alliance and developing strategies for prevention.

The worldwide increase in the incidence and prevalence of asthma has been noted and studied, but it remains largely unexplained. In the last two decades, we have witnessed intense and very successful basic and clinical research on asthma. Significant therapeutic benefit has resulted from this effort.

The Lung Biology in Health and Disease series has presented many volumes on various aspects of asthma. Progress has been reported and questions raised that are the subject of continued investigations. This volume is one more step in the search to minimize, if not eliminate, the impact of asthma in the United States and elsewhere. Environment, with regard to asthma, is complex and multifaceted, whether at home or at work, indoors or outdoors, seasonal or continuous.

This volume, conceived and developed by Dr. Robert Bush and the authors, is a significant and important contribution to the breadth and scope of the series. Physicians caring for asthmatics will use it to help their patients.

As the executive editor of the series, I am grateful to all the contributors to this volume for the opportunity to present it.

Claude Lenfant, M.D.
Bethesda, Maryland

PREFACE

Asthma prevalence and mortality have been increasing in the past two decades. Children and young adults seem to be most susceptible to the increase in asthma prevalence and children residing in inner city environments have a greater risk for asthma mortality. Although the exact cause of the increase in asthma prevalence and mortality is not known, environmental factors are felt to play an important role.

Sensitization to indoor allergens, such as house dust mites, animal dander, cockroaches, and fungi, is recognized as an important risk factor for the development of asthma in children. Since people are spending more time indoors, exposure to these allergens is likely to continue to contribute to the pathogenesis of asthma. In addition to indoor allergens, air pollutants, in both the indoor and outdoor environment, can cause airway inflammation. Second-hand tobacco smoke exposure may be a contributing factor in childhood asthma. Occupational exposures play a significant role in asthma arising in adulthood.

The contributors to this volume of the Lung Biology in Health and Disease series have prepared state-of-the-art reviews on important aspects of environmental exposures that are felt to play a role in the development and severity of chronic asthma in children and adults. The immunological mechanisms involved in allergic airway inflammation are explored, and approaches to the identification, quantitation of exposure, and remedial methods for exposure reduction to aeroallergens are discusssed. Diagnostic algorithms for environmentally induced asthma both at home and in the workplace are presented. The role of indoor and outdoor air pollutants on the airway is addressed. Albeit controversial, the use of immunotherapy as an adjunct to proper environmental control measures and appropriate medical treatment is discussed. These topics will provide the treating physician with a comprehensive appreciation of the influence of the environment on asthma prevalence, morbidity, and mortality, as well as practical methods for controlling exposure and improving patient quality of life.

For physicians caring for patients with asthma, an understanding of the contribution of environmental exposures to the pathogenesis and treatment of the disease is essential. Complete exposure avoidance of the offending agent can be curative in some instances. Although environmental control measures to reduce exposure to pollutants and allergens may not achieve complete elimination of symptoms or the need for medication, these efforts may have significant benefits. Patients with asthma should receive an assessment of environmental exposures and of the presence of sensitization, and recommendations for exposure reduction in order to achieve maximum benefits from their care.

Robert K. Bush

CONTRIBUTORS

Rebecca Bascom, M.D., M.P.H.   Professor and Chief, Division of Pulmonary, Allergy, and Critical Care Medicine, Department of Medicine, Penn State College of Medicine, Hershey, Pennsylvania

David I. Bernstein, M.D.   Professor, Division of Immunology, Department of Internal Medicine, University of Cincinnati College of Medicine, Cincinnati, Ohio

Jonathan A. Bernstein, M.D.   Associate Professor, Division of Immunology, Department of Internal Medicine, University of Cincinnati College of Medicine, Cincinnati, Ohio

Jean Bousquet, M.D.   Professor, Department of Respiratory Diseases, University Medical School, and Hôpital Arnaud de Villeneuve, Montpellier, France

Robert K. Bush, M.D.   Professor, Department of Medicine, University of Wisconsin–Madison Medical School, and Chief of Allergy, William S. Middleton Memorial Veterans Hospital, Madison, Wisconsin

André Cartier, M.D.   Department of Medicine, Sacré-Coeur Hospital, Montreal, Quebec, Canada

Pascal Demoly, M.D., Ph.D.   Associate Professor, Department of Respiratory Diseases, University Medical School, and Hôpital Arnaud de Villeneuve, Montpellier, France

Peyton A. Eggleston, M.D.   Professor, Department of Pediatrics, Johns Hopkins University School of Medicine, Baltimore, Maryland

Joanne K. Fagan, Ph.D.   Research Associate, School of Public Health, The Harlem Lung Center, Harlem Hospital Center, Columbia University College of Physicians and Surgeons, New York, New York

Enrique Fernández-Caldas, Ph.D.   Director, Research and Development, C.B.F. LETI, S.A., Madrid, Spain

Jean G. Ford, M.D.   Florence Irving Assistant Professor, Department of Medicine, Assistant Professor, School of Public Health, and Director, The Harlem Lung Center, Harlem Hospital Center, Columbia University College of Physicians and Surgeons, New York, New York

Denyse Gautrin, Ph.D.   Department of Medicine, University of Montreal, Sacré Coeur Hospital, Montreal, Quebec, Canada

Leslie C. Grammer, M.D.   Professor, Department of Medicine, Northwestern University Medical School, and Northwestern Memorial Hospital, Chicago, Illinois

Javed Iqbal, M.D., M.P.H.   Research Assistant, School of Public Health, The Harlem Lung Center, Harlem Hospital Center, Columbia University College of Physicians and Surgeons, New York, New York

Nizar N. Jarjour, M.D.   Associate Professor, Department of Medicine, University of Wisconsin–Madison Medical School, Madison, Wisconsin

Elizabeth A. Becky Kelly, Ph.D.   Associate Scientist, Department of Medicine, University of Wisconsin–Madison Medical School, Madison, Wisconsin

Carol A. Kiekhaefer, M.D.   Clinical Research Scholar, Laboratory of Genetics, University of Wisconsin–Madison Medical School, Madison, Wisconsin

Jean-Luc Malo, M.D.   Professor, Department of Medicine, University of Montreal, and Department of Medicine, Sacré-Coeur Hospital, Montreal, Quebec, Canada

François-Bernard Michel, M.D.   Professor, Department of Respiratory Diseases, University Medical School, and Hôpital Arnaud de Villeneuve, Montpellier, France

John J. Ouellette, M.D., F.A.C.P., F.A.A.A.I.   Associate Clinical Professor, Department of Medicine, University of Wisconsin Health Physicians Plus, University of Wisconsin Medical School, Madison, Wisconsin

David B. Peden, M.S., M.D.   Associate Professor, Department of Pediatrics, and Center for Environmental Medicine and Lung Biology, University of North Carolina School of Medicine, Chapel Hill, North Carolina

William R. Solomon, M.S.(Int.Med.), M.D.   Professor, Division of Allergy and Clinical Immunology, Department of Internal Medicine, University of Michigan Medical School, Ann Arbor, Michigan

Jeffrey R. Stokes, M.D.   The Asthma & Allergy Center, Papillion, Nebraska

Robert A. Wood, M.D.   Associate Professor, Department of Pediatrics, Johns Hopkins University School of Medicine, Baltimore, Maryland

CONTENTS

15. Future Directions   **321**
  Robert K. Bush

ENVIRONMENTAL ASTHMA

1

Introduction

ROBERT K. BUSH

University of Wisconsin–Madison Medical School and
William S. Middleton Memorial Veterans Hospital
Madison, Wisconsin

I. Increasing Asthma Prevalence and the Environment

The prevalence of asthma and asthma mortality have been increasing in the last
two decades (1–3). The increase in prevalence has been noted particularly in
industrialized countries with market economies, especially in urban areas compared to rural areas. Increases are more obvious in children and young adults.
Children residing in inner cities seem to be particularly at risk for asthma mortality (4). Although the exact cause of the rise in asthma prevalence and mortality is not known, environmental factors are felt to play an increasingly
important role. Environmental risk factors, which include exposure to indoor
allergens such as house dust mites, pet dander, cockroaches, and possibly
fungi, appear to be important in the pathogenesis of asthma. Children and
adults are spending increasing amounts of time indoors (5), which may account
for the rise in asthma prevalence.

   Although exposure to pollens certainly can produce attacks of asthma in sensitive individuals, their contribution to the pathogenesis of asthma has not been as clearly defined as has exposure to indoor allergens. In addition, air pollutants may be important triggers in precipitating acute episodes of asthma and the need for emergency therapy (6). Not to be neglected is the role of environmental tobacco smoke, particularly second-hand exposure of infants and children.

In adulthood, the role of allergen exposure may have less impact than in childhood. Nonetheless, up to 50% of asthmatic individuals may exhibit positive skin tests (5). In the adult population attention must also be paid to occupational exposures. The prevalence of occupational asthma is not known; however, up to 15% of all cases of asthma in adults may be due to workplace exposure (7). Therefore, environmental factors in the home, the outdoor environment, and the workplace need to be considered in the overall evaluation and treatment of patients with asthma (8).

II. Immune Mechanisms in Allergic Asthma

Asthma is characterized by inflammation of the airways, which can be induced by a variety of stimuli including respiratory infections, exposure to pollutants and other irritants, and exposure to allergens. The recognition that exposure to inhaled allergens can result in immediate and late-phase responses in sensitive individuals has led to the development of this model as an important tool in the investigation of chronic asthma. The simple model of allergen binding to IgE on the surface of mast cells with subsequent release of histamine and other chemical mediators that cause bronchoconstriction has given way to a much more complex paradigm. An interplay of mast cells, antigen-presenting cells such as macrophages, T-lymphocytes, epithelial cells, fibroblasts, and eosinophils is involved in the production of the condition known as asthma. It is recognized that a variety of chemical mediators, cytokines, and other inflammatory factors are important in the generation of the inflammatory responses that lead to bronchoconstriction, mucous secretion, airway hyperresponsiveness, and airway remodeling. The central role of the T-lymphocyte in orchestrating the allergic response has become apparent. Antigens (allergens) are taken up by antigen-presenting cells such as dendritic cells and macrophages. These cells present antigens to Th0 cells, which can lead to the development of either Th1 or Th2 helper lymphocytes. Th1 cells produce interferon-γ, while the Th2 cytokine profile includes IL-4, IL-5, IL-10, and IL-13, which are important in the pathogenesis of allergic reactions. Under the influence of cytokine IL-4, B-lymphocytes produce IgE antibodies to specific allergens. IL-5 is important in the chemotaxis, maturation, and homing of eosinophils to the airway.

In addition, the epithelial cells are sources of cytokines and chemokines that can enhance the development of allergic inflammation in the airway. These factors include GM-CSF, IL-8, RANTES, and eotaxin (9). Further, release of cytokines can upregulate the appearance of adhesion molecules that allow for the chemotaxis and passage of inflammatory cells such as eosinophils into the airway. Particularly important in the transmigration of eosinophils into sites of allergic inflammation are the adhesion molecules ICAM and VCAM-1 (10).

The response of the host in the generation of allergic inflammation is dependent upon the interplay of genetic and environmental factors. Although the genetic factors are not completely understood, research in this regard is increasing and may allow the identification of the population most at risk. An understanding of the interactions between genetic and environmental factors is critical for the discovery of new approaches for asthma therapy.

III. Diagnostic Approaches

The role of environmental exposures in asthma should be defined as part as the overall assessment of any patient presenting with asthma. Asthma is characterized by the presence of variable airway flow. Patients with asthma should have assessment of pulmonary function to determine the degree of airway obstruction and to assess improvement with appropriate therapy. In cases where pulmonary functions are normal and the diagnosis is in question, the use of methacholine, histamine challenge, or exercise challenge may be appropriate to demonstrate the presence of airway hyperresponsiveness. These measures, however, do not establish a cause-and-effect relationship between environmental exposure and the presence of asthma.

The medical history, of course, remains the mainstay in determining the role of environmental factors in asthma. The history should include assessment of the home environment such as the presence of pets, smoking, and avocational pursuits such as woodworking. In adults, an occupational history is also critical to establish the role of occupational exposures. Seasonal variability in symptoms is important in establishing the role of pollen exposure and fungal allergen exposure in the production of symptoms. The presence of cockroach infestation is particularly relevant in patients dwelling in urban areas.

Ultimately, the role of allergen exposure needs to be demonstrated by appropriate skin testing or in vitro testing. Skin testing offers immediate results; however, it is limited to physicians who have had experience in this type of testing. As an alternative, the demonstration of specific IgE antibodies by in vitro tests such as the radioallergorsorbent tests (RAST) or by enzyme-linked immunoassay (ELISA) may be appropriate where skin testing is not available. These methods are less sensitive and may be more expensive than skin testing, however.

In the case of occupational asthma, a major part of the evaluation is the medical history. Changes in airflow while the individual is exposed to the work environment must be demonstrated in order to establish the diagnosis. In some instances, skin testing or in vitro testing for high molecular weight allergens may be available to demonstrate sensitivity. For low molecular weight compounds, either skin testing or in vitro testing is not available or the reaction may be through non-IgE-dependent mechanisms. In some instances a bronchoprovocation challenge may be necessary to establish the diagnosis. Objective assessment of lung function is critical not only for the diagnosis but also for the management of asthma. Likewise, evaluation of the patient for sensitization to environmental allergens is a significant consideration in asthma therapy.

IV. House Dust Mite Allergens

Sensitivities to several allergens have been identified as risk factors for asthma. The house dust mite has been recognized as an important source of indoor allergen exposure. In susceptible populations, exposure and sensitization to house dust mite allergen is a risk factor for the development of asthma. Quantitative measures to assess exposure levels in settled dust samples have been developed. A threshold level of 2 µg per gram of dust has been shown to lead to sensitization, and a level of 10 µg/g dust has been shown to be associated with the development of asthma symptoms (11).

The principal reservoirs for exposure include bedding and carpeting. A number of environmental control measures have been suggested to reduce house dust mite exposure (12,13) (Table 1). However, a recent meta-analysis of 23 studies that used either chemical or physical means to reduce mite exposure

Table 1   House Dust Mite Control Measures

---

1. Maintain relative humidity at ≤50%.
2. Encase pillows and mattresses.
3. Launder bedding in hot water (≥130°F) weekly.
4. Remove carpeting.
5. If removal is not possible, treat carpet with acaricide.
6. Vacuum with vacuum cleaner fitted with a HEPA filter and double-thickness bag.
7. Minimize stuffed toys.

---

showed no significant benefit in either symptoms or morning peak flow rates (14). Nevertheless, descriptive analyses have indicated that reduction in house dust mite exposure may alter asthma symptoms (15).

V. Animal Allergens

Pets and dogs are kept in up to 50% of homes in many countries (16). Sensitization appears to be more common to cats than to dogs, perhaps due to greater intimacy between the owner and the pet. A threshold level of 1–8 µg per gram of dust of Fel d 1 has been associated with sensitization (17); however, it should be noted that individuals who have not been exposed to cats directly in their home may become sensitized. Therefore, the threshold level for sensitization may be less than previously reported (17).

Approximately 20–30% of airborne Fel d 1 is carried on particles ≤5 µm in aerodynamic size. In addition, Fel d 1 is a highly charged protein, which allows it to stick surfaces and clothing. In contrast to house dust mite allergen, some Fel d 1 is amenable to air filtration because of the smaller size of the particles and their ability to remain suspended in the air.

The threshold for dog allergens are not as well established as for cat allergens. Can f 1 has been shown to produce significant sensitization at a level of 10 µ g per gram of settled dust. The reservoirs and control measures for reducing exposure to the major dog allergen have not been as fully elucidated as for cat allergen.

Ideally, pets should be removed from the home. It has been shown, however, that it requires at least 6 months after the cat is removed from the environment for the levels to reach the same level as when no cat was present. Recommendations for reducing cat allergen exposure are shown in Table 2. It should be noted that in spite of these measures showing a reduction in allergen exposure, no clinical correlation with asthma symptoms has been reported.

Table 2 Animal Allergen Control Measures

Remove animal from home. If that is not possible, then
1. Keep animal out of bedroom and main living areas.
2. Bathe cat/dog once a week.
3. Remove carpets, if possible.
4. Use HEPA-filtered and double-thickness bag vacuum cleaner.
5. Use HEPA-filtered air cleaner in bedroom and main living areas.

Table 3   Fungal Allergen Control Measures

Indoors
1. Maintain relative humidity at ≤50%.
2. Clean washable surfaces with 5% bleach and detergent solution.
3. Remove contaminated carpets.
4. Warm surfaces on exterior walls (closets).
5. Keep windows closed in warm months; use air conditioning.

Outdoors
1. Avoid heavy exposure to moldy vegetation.
2. Wear dust-mist respirator when working with moldy material.
3. Use air-conditioned vehicles.

VI.   Fungal Allergens

Sensitivity to fungal allergens, particularly *Alternaria* and basidiomycetes, are recognized as important risk factors for asthma (18). During warm weather months in northern climates, most fungal exposure occurs in the outdoor environment; however, indoor levels generally reflect the outdoor environment. The effect of dampness and mold growth in homes on respiratory health was recently reviewed (19,20). Examination of data collected from a variety of studies seems to indicate that the presence of mold growth within the home may be a source of exposure and therefore a risk factor for asthma.

Because quantitative relationships between exposure and asthma symptoms have been difficult to establish, the role of fungal allergen exposure in the indoor environment has not been as well characterized as that of house dust mite, cockroach, and animal danders. The methodologies employed to assess fungal allergen exposure include spore counts, cultures of viable material, and quantitative methods for major allergens. However, these techniques are not as well developed as they are for other indoor allergens. As a consequence, no exposure level or threshold levels for sensitization have appeared. Suggested methods for reducing fungal allergen exposure are given in Table 3.

VII.   Inner City Problems

Children with asthma residing in inner city environments are at an increased risk for morbidity and mortality from asthma (4). A number of factors may be

Table 4 Cockroach Allergen Control Measures

1. Remove food sources (waste).
2. Remove water sources (leaking pipes).
3. Seal access areas: cracks in flooring and walls.
4. Spray contaminated areas with diazinon, chlorpyritos, or boric acid.
5. Bait traps with hydramethylanon or abermictin.

involved in this increase in asthma morbidity and mortality. Poverty can reduce the access to medical care and the use of appropriate medications. Environmental factors may also play a significant role. Environmental tobacco smoke is more common in homes in inner cities than in suburban areas (4). Indoor pollution with nitrogen dioxide is also an important pollutant in the inner city environment.

Recently, cockroach allergy was recognized as a major contributing risk factor to asthma morbidity in the inner city population (21). Sensitization was associated with indoor levels of 2 U per gram of dust of the major cockroach allergen Bla g 1 (21).

Not only is cockroach allergy associated with the risk for developing asthma in children, it may also have a significant role in asthma in adults. Weiss et al. (22) demonstrated that cockroach allergen exposure in adult men, aged 21–80, living in inner city areas had significant declines in FEV_1 on an annual basis compared to unexposed individuals.

Suggested control measures to reduce cockroach allergen exposure are listed in Table 4. Decreasing the ability of the insects to find food supplies and access to water are very important control measures. Entryways such as cracks in walls should be sealed. Treatment of infested areas with chemicals such as diazinon, chlorpyritos, and boric acid may be successful. Bait stations containing hydramethylnon or abermictin may also be useful.

VIII. Pollen Allergens

Exposure to pollen allergens has long been recognized as a cause of asthma symptoms. The association of sensitivity to pollens from grasses, ragweed, and trees with risk factors for the development of asthma is not as apparent as that of exposure to indoor allergens. This may be attributable in part to the fact that exposure to pollens occurs over relatively brief periods of time up to 6–8 weeks, compared to indoor allergens, which are perennial in nature.

Natural exposure to pollen allergens does result in increased asthma symptoms and airway hyperresponsiveness to nonspecific stimuli. This may be due to the generation of inflammatory changes in airways as a consequence of the late-phase allergic response.

It has also been shown that exposure to grass pollen during the spring season in California is associated with increased frequency of emergency room visits. Recently, epidemics of asthma have been ascribed to pollen allergen exposure. Reports from Australia and England suggested that during the course of thunderstorms many patients present to emergency rooms. These individuals have the common factor of being allergic to grass pollen, and these epidemics occur during the pollen season. It was subsequently shown that these episodes were associated with the release of starch granules from the grass pollen that carried the allergen (23). Thus, pollen exposure can be a contributing factor in asthma severity.

Avoidance of exposure to pollen is more problematic than to indoor allergens, since, other than wearing masks, little can be done to reduce outdoor exposures. Indoors, running air conditioning is useful; however, air filtration systems added to air conditioning have little if any benefit.

IX. Air Pollutants

As previously mentioned, exposure to cigarette smoke, either actively or passively, is a major factor in asthma. Relevant outdoor pollutant exposures that have been associated with increased frequency or exacerbation of asthma include ozone and sulfuric acid (6). Indoor exposure to nitrogen dioxide has been shown to be associated with problems of increased asthma symptoms in inner city populations (4). The recent identification of diesel exhaust particles as being potential adjuvants in the development of allergic reactions to pollens has also been described. Public health policies to address these issues need further investigation and recommendations.

X. Occupational Asthma

In adults, up to 15% of cases of asthma may be attributable to workplace exposures (7). Typically, symptoms are worse while the individual is exposed at the workplace and resolve after a period of absence such as a weekend or while the employee is on vacation. However, persistent symptoms may occur, which can make the diagnosis difficult. Establishment of the diagnosis requires evidence that impairment of airflow occurs while the individual is exposed to the workplace environment. Peak expiratory flow measurements made at work and while away from work may give some helpful information, but these measurements are subject to significant error. Spirometric studies before and during work shifts may prove helpful but are cumbersome to perform.

To demonstrate sensitivity to high molecular weight agents, which often are organic dusts, skin testing may be available for some agents. However, standardized diagnostic reagents are not universally available. For low molecular weight agents, IgE mechanisms may only occasionally be involved. In the case of isocyanates, an IgE mechanism has been proposed and in vitro testing is available in some centers. Nonetheless, for the majority of low molecular weight agents no specific testing is available short of bronchoprovocation studies. Bronchoprovocation may be necessary in some instances to establish the diagnosis, but the general availability of this procedure is limited to specialized centers.

Accumulating evidence indicates that early removal from occupational exposure is important in terms of the overall prognosis. Individuals who are removed shortly after the onset of symptoms have better prognosis than those who continue to work. Therefore, prompt recognition is necessary to prevent potential long-term disability.

XI. Immunotherapy

The role of immunotherapy in the treatment of asthma remains controversial. A number of placebo-controlled, double-blind trials have been conducted that indicate that appropriate immunotherapy with pollen extracts and house dust mite and cat dander allergens has improved individuals symptomatically, reduced the need for medication, and improved lung function. However, in many instances the improvement is small. Immunotherapy also has the risk of adverse reactions, particularly in asthmatic individuals.

For many allergens, appropriate reagents for treatment either are not standardized or are not commercially available. Nonetheless, advances have been made in the standardization of allergenic extracts, including ragweed, grass pollen, house dust mite, and cat dander. Immunotherapy may be indicated for individuals who continue to have symptoms despite appropriate avoidance techniques and the use of pharmacological agents.

When immunotherapy is considered for treatment of environment-related asthma, appropriate precautions need to be taken. Individuals undergoing therapy should be informed of the risks and benefits of the treatment. They should be under observation in a setting that offers emergency resuscitation for at least 30 min following the injection. Individuals should be given self-administered epinephrine to have available should they encounter an untoward event after leaving the physician's office. Individuals on beta-blocker therapy are not considered to be appropriate candidates for immunotherapy. Immunotherapy can be continued at maintenance levels that are tolerated in pregnant asthmatic women, but initiation of therapy should be avoided during pregnancy.

New approaches to conventional immunotherapy are being evaluated. These include T-cell peptide based treatments and DNA-based vaccines. Potentially, these approaches will confer improvement in symptoms with less risk of adverse reactions than conventional treatment.

XII. Summary

Asthma prevalence is increasing and may be due in part to environmental exposure (24). A number of allergens have been identified as risk factors for the development of asthma; these include house dust mite allergens, pet dander allergens, cockroaches, and fungi, particularly *Alternaria* and basidiomycetes.

Many exposures to these environmental allergens occur indoors. Appropriate control measures have been identified. Reduction of exposure, in theory, should reduce the need for pharmacological intervention, but unless total exposure avoidance is practiced, such treatment may continue to be necessary.

Exposure to air pollutants, particularly cigarette smoke, should be strongly discouraged. Public health policies may be necessary to reduce industrial pollutants. Occupational settings are important in adult populations and need to be considered in the overall evaluation of patients.

Avoidance of exposure to allergens is a significant principle of asthma management. When avoidance and pharmacological measures are not effective, individuals with allergen-induced asthma may be considered as potential candidates for immunotherapy, although this type of treatment should be considered only as adjunctive and not curative.

Continued investigation into the epidemiological factors and exposure reduction methods will be important in primary prevention of asthma and in controlling the symptoms.

References

1. Peat JK, Li J. Reversing the trend: Reducing the prevalence of asthma. J Allergy Clin Immunol 1999; 103:1–10.

2. The International Study of Asthma and Allergies in Childhood (ISAAC) Steering Committee. Worldwide variation in prevalence of symptoms of asthma, allergic rhino conjunctivitis; and atopic eczema. Lancet 1998; 351:1225–1230.

3. Björnstein B. Environmental risk factors for atopy. Clin Rev Allergy Immunol 1997; 15:125–143.

4. Eggleston PA. Urban children and asthma. Immunol Allergy Clin No Amer 1998; 18:75–83.

5. Pope AM, Patterson R, Burge H, eds. Indoor Allergens. Washington, DC: National Academy Press, 1993.

6. Koenig JQ. The role of air pollutants in adolescent asthma. Immunol Allergy Clin No Amer 1998; 18:61–74.

7. Quirce S, Sustre J. Occupational asthma. Allergy 1998; 53:633–641.

8. National Institutes of Health. National Heart, Lung, and Blood Institute. Practical Guide for the Diagnosis and Management of Asthma. NIH Publication No. 97-4053. Bethesda, MD: NIH, 1997.

9. Barnes PJ. Pathophysiology of allergic inflammation. In: Middleton E Jr., Reed CE, Ellis EF, Adkinson NF Jr, Yunginger JW, Busse WW, eds. Allergy Principles and Practice. 5th ed. St. Louis: Mosby, 1998:356–365.

10. Bochner BS. Cellular adhesion in inflammation. In: Middleton E Jr., Reed CE, Ellis EF, Adkinson NF Jr., Yunginger JW, Busse WW, eds. Allergy Principles and Practice. 5th ed. St. Louis: Mosby, 1998:94–107.

11. Sporik R, Holgate ST, Platts-Mills TAE, Cogswell J. Exposure to home-dust mite allergen (Der p 1) and the development of asthma in childhood: a prospective study. N Engl J Med 1990; 323:502–507.

12. Platts-Mills TAE, Vervloet D, Thomas WR, Aalberge RC, Chapman MJ. Indoor allergens and asthma: report of Third International Workshop. J Allergy Clin Immunol 1997, 100:S2–S24.

13. Custovic A, Simpson A, Chapman MD, Woodcock A. Allergen avoidance in the treatment of asthma and atopic disorders. Thorax 1998; 53:63–72.

14. Gøtzsche PC, Hammarquist C, Burr M. House dust mite control measures in the management of asthma: meta-analysis. BMJ 1998; 317:1105–1110.

15. Peat J, Björkstein B. Primary and secondary prevention of allergic asthma. Eur Respir J 1998; 12(Suppl 27):28s–34s.

16. Noertjojo K, Dimich-Ward H, Obata H, Manfreda J, Chan-Yeung M. Exposure and sensitization to cat dander: asthma and asthma-like symptoms among adults. J Allergy Clin Immunol 1999; 103:60–65.

17. Munir AKM, Kjellman M, Bjorksten B. Exposure to indoor allergens in early infancy and sensitization. J Allergy Clin Immunol 1997; 100:177–181.

18. Horner WE, Lehrer SB, Salvaggio JE. Fungi. Immunol Allergy Clin No. Amer 1994; 14:551–566.

19. Verhoff AP, Burge HA. Health risk assessment of fungi in home environments. Am Allergy Asthma Immunol 1997; 78:544–554.

20. Peat JK, Dickerson J, Li J. Effect of damp and mold in the home on respiratory health: a review of the literature. Allergy 1998; 53:120–128.

21. Eggleston PA, Rosenstreich D, Lynn H, Gergen P, Baker D, Kattan M, Mortimer KM, Mitchell H, Ownbyy D, Slavin R, Malveaux F. Relationship of indoor allergen exposure to skin test sensitivity in inner-city children with asthma. J Allergy Clin Immunol 1998; 102:563–570.

22. Weiss ST, O'Connor GT, DeMolles D, Platts-Mills T, Sparrow D. Indoor allergens and longitudinal FEV_1 decline in older adults: the Normative Aging Study. J Allergy Clin Immunol 1998; 101:720–725.

23. Suphioglu C. Thunderstorm asthma due to grass pollen. Int Arch Allergy Immunol 1998; 116:253–260.

24. Sears MR. Descriptive epidemiology of asthma. Lancet 1997; 350(suppl 11):1–4.

2

Antigen-Induced Airway Disease

CAROL A. KIEKHAEFER, ELIZABETH A. BECKY KELLY, and NIZAR N. JARJOUR

University of Wisconsin–Madison Medical School
Madison, Wisconsin

I. Introduction

All forms of asthma, including atopic (extrinsic) asthma, nonatopic (intrinsic) asthma, and occupational asthma, have many similar immunological features, in particular, eosinophilic airway inflammation. The potential for eosinophilic airway inflammation is initiated upon the first exposure to antigen (sensitization). Subsequent exposure triggers a complex cascade of events, which can be divided into two phases, the immediate (within minutes) and the late-phase (within hours) responses. The pathophysiological features attributed to chronic airway inflammation include airway obstruction, bronchial hyperresponsiveness, and tissue injury. Furthermore, recent evidence suggests that chronic airway inflammation in asthma leads to structural changes in the airway that are characterized by subepithelial fibrosis (1,2).

In this chapter, we briefly outline the general immunological features associated with allergen-induced asthma, highlight key cellular and chemical mediators that occur during the immediate and late-phase response (LPR), and discuss how these components contribute to persistent eosinophilic airway inflammation, to airway hyperresponsiveness, and ultimately to airway remodeling. (For a more detailed description of this complex cascade of events, the reader is referred to Ref. 3.)

II. Antigen Sensitization

The CD4[+] T helper (h) cell is a central player in the allergic airway response to antigen (AG). However, in order for the AG to be recognized by T cells, it must be processed into small peptide fragments and presented on the surface of an AG-presenting cell (APC) in association with major histocompatibility (MHC) class II proteins. A number of airway cells, including airway monocytes, alveolar macrophages, and dendritic cells, have the necessary machinery to process and present AG. However, the major APC, at least in initiating the primary immune response, appears to be the dendritic cell (reviewed in Ref. 4).

The number of dendritic cells is increased in the bronchial mucosa of asthmatic subjects compared to that of normal individuals (5). Dendritic cells are also increased in the lungs of guinea pigs following intratracheal challenge with toluene diisocyanate (6). These cells form an extensive network above the basement membrane of the airway epithelium that allows continuous immunosurveillance of the epithelial surface.

Upon initial exposure to a sensitizing AG, dendritic cells capture and internalize the AG, then migrate to the draining lymph node, where the processed peptides are displayed on the cell surface in association with MHC class II. This complex of AG and MHC is recognized by naive T cells through a T-cell receptor with specificity for a particular antigenic peptide. To become activated, the naive T cell must also receive costimulatory signals, the most common of which is the interaction between the B7 molecule (B7.1 or B7.2) on the APC and its counter receptor, CD28, on the T cell (Fig. 1). (See Ref. 7 for a review of AG presentation.) Once activated, the T cell undergoes multiple rounds of replication, which require autologous production of IL-2 and cell surface expression of the IL-2 receptor, CD25. The resulting multipotential population (Th0) has the capacity to differentiate into two types of effector cells, each with the potential to generate a selective, mutually exclusive array of cytokines. The Th1-type cells preferentially secrete IL-2, IFN-γ, and TNF-β, while Th2-type cells produce IL-4, IL-5, IL-9, and IL-13 (8) (Fig. 2). (For a detailed review, see Ref. 9.) T-cell polarization is affected by the type and dose

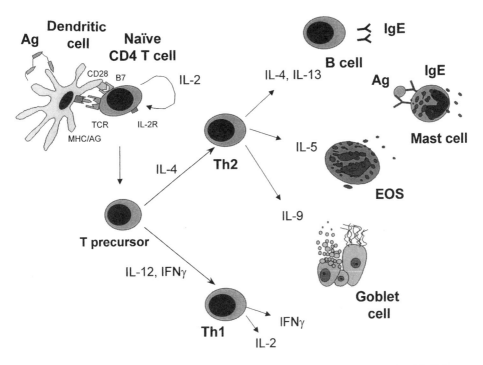

Figure 1 Antigen presentation to naive T cells requires (1) recognition of AG/MHC complex by T-cell receptor (TCR) and (2) costimulatory signals provided through the interaction of CD28 and B7. Differentiation of T precursor cells into Th1 or Th2 effector cells is influenced by the presence of IL-4 and IL-12. Th2-type cells contribute to AG-induced airway inflammation through the generation of IL-4, IL-5, IL-9, and IL-13.

of AG, differential expression of B7.2 versus B7.1 costimulatory molecules on APC (10,11), and the cytokine milieu present during initial priming. The most important factor appears to be the presence of particular cytokines. The Th2 cells are induced in the presence of IL-4, while the Th1 cells are induced in the presence of IL-12. Elicitation of a Th2-type response [and in some cases, a deficiency in Th1-type responses (12)] is a key feature of all forms of asthma, including occupational asthma (13). After expansion in the draining lymph node, the resulting T-cell population responds to chemotactic signals that direct

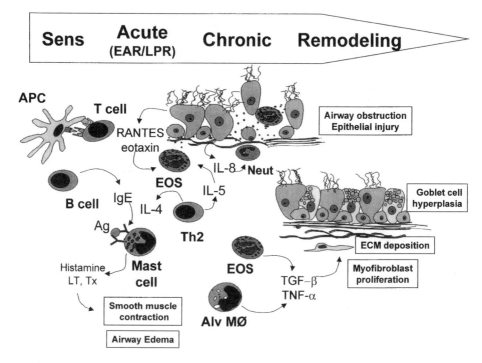

Figure 2 Asthma is a continuum of cellular responses that are influenced by antigens and occupational sensitizers. During sensitization, dendritic cells are the key antigen-presenting cell. This initial step sets the stage for subsequent Th2-mediated responses. The EAR is characterized by IgE-mediated mast cell release of preformed mediators that trigger bronchial constriction and airway edema. The CD4+ Th2 cell plays a key role in the LPR. IL-5 release by Th2-type cells is essential for EOS recruitment and activation. EOS, as well as neutrophils (Neut) and alveolar macrophages (Alv Mφ) contribute to airway obstruction and damage of airway epithelium. Chronic airway inflammation and resulting repair mechanisms lead to airway remodeling. Generation of profibrogenic cytokines such as TGF-β and TNF-α by EOS and Alv Mφ stimulate myofibroblast proliferation and generation of ECM proteins. Thus, asthma severity, progression, and ultimately airway remodeling are influenced by airway inflammation.

their recruitment to the airway (i.e., the site of inflammation). AG-driven activation of the T cell initiates molecular events that will eventually lead to programmed cell death, or apoptosis, and thus will limit the immune response. A small proportion of T cells do not undergo apoptosis but rather develop into memory T cells that can recirculate for a long period of time (potentially years). Subsequent exposure to the initial sensitizing AG elicits a rapid and vigorous response by these memory T cells.

Although recent studies in mice implicate dendritic cells as the major APCs during a secondary immune response (14), other cells may serve in this capacity as well. Previously activated T cells have less stringent requirements for costimulatory signals than naive T cells; thus any cell [including alveolar macrophages, eosinophil (EOS), epithelial cells, fibroblasts, and even airway T cells] that expresses MHC class II and can take up and process AG can potentially serve as an APC. Although it was thought that AG presentation can take place only in the draining lymph node, a recent study demonstrated Ag presentation in situ in tissue transplants from asthmatic patients (11). In the next sections we discuss the airway response to subsequent AG exposure. The contributions of various cells and mediators are summarized in Table 1.

III. The Early-Phase Response

Within minutes of exposure to an appropriate antigen, patients with allergic asthma develop asthma symptoms including cough, wheezing, and dyspnea, provided that an adequate dose of AG was inhaled. Typically the early allergic response (EAR) resolves within 30–60 min. The immediate response is mediated by preformed mediators, of which histamine and leukotrienes (LTs) are probably the most important. The mast cell is a key player in the EAR. AG binds to surface-bound IgE and triggers mast cell release of histamine, LTs, prostaglandin (PGs) D_2, thromboxane (Tx) B_2, platelet-activating factor (PAF), and potentially a vast array of cytokines, including TNF-α, IL-1, -4, -5, -6, -8, -16, and chemokines (MIP-1α, MIP-1β, MCP-1, and RANTES) (15). The preformed chemical mediators result in contraction of airway smooth muscle (ASM), airway edema, and increased mucus secretions, all of which contribute to the symptoms of acute asthma.

Studies of AG challenge with direct sampling of the airway 5–10 min after local airway challenge (LAC) have shown a dramatic rise in bronchoalveolar lavage (BAL) fluid levels of histamine, LTs, tryptase, PGs, and Tx within a few minutes of challenge (16–19). Histamine is a major contributor to the upper airway allergic response. Levels of histamine have been found to correlate with the degree of airway obstruction and responsiveness (20,21). The source of histamine in BAL is not entirely clear. Histamine can be produced by either basophils or mast cells, whereas tryptase, another mediator of allergic response, is restricted to mast cells. The levels of tryptase in BAL fluid of stable asthmatic patients did not correlate with histamine levels, suggesting that

Table 1   Cells and Mediators Involved in Airway Response to Allergens

Phase	Cellular response	Mediators	Function
Sensitization	Dendritic cells		AG presentation
	T cells (Th0, Th2)	Cytokines	Memory
	?	IL-4	Differential of Th2-type cells, mast cell maturation, expression of adhesion molecules
Immediate phase	Mast cells	Lipid mediators (LT, PGE_2, PAF, TX)	ASM contraction, edema, mucus secretion, chemotactic or inflammatory cells
		Cytokines (TNF-α, IL-1, 4, 5, 6, 8, 16)	
		Chemokines (MIP-1a and b, MCP-1, RANTES)	Chemotactic for inflammatory cells
	B cells	IgE	Mast cell triggering
LPR	T cells	Cytokines	
		IL-4	Differential of Th2-type cells, mast cell maturation, expression of adhesion molecules
		IL-5	EOS differentiation, migration, and activation
	EOS	Granule proteins (MBP, ECP, EDN)	Cytotoxic to airway epithelium
		ROS	Cytotoxic to airway epithelium
		Lipid mediators (LT, PGE_2, PAF)	Directly induce bronchial hyperreactivity, chemotactic for inflammatory cells
		Cytokines (IL-2, 3, 4, 5, 6, 8, 10, 12, GM-CSF, IFN-γ, TGF-β)	Perpetuate EOS response, initiate remodeling
		MMPs	Remodeling
	Neutrophils	Proteolytic enzymes	Cytotoxic to airway epithelium, matrix turnover and remodeling

Table 1 *Continued*

Phase	Cellular response	Mediators	Function
		ROS	Cytotoxic to airway epithelium
		MMPs	Matrix turnover and remodeling
	Mast cells	Cytokines (IL-4, 5, 6 TNF-α)	
	Macrophages	Proteolytic enzymes	Cytotoxic to airway epithelium, matrix turnover and remodeling
		ROS	Cytotoxic to airway epithelium
		MMPs	Matrix turnover and remodeling
		Cytokines (IL-6, GM-CSF, IL-1, TGF-β)	
	Epithelial cells	Cytokines (IL-5, 6, 8, GM-CSF)	
		Chemokines (RANTES, eotaxin, MCP-1, MCP-4, MIP-1α)	Chemotactic for inflammatory cells
		MMPs	Matrix turnover and remodeling
Remodeling	EOS	Profibrogenic factors (TGF-β, TNF-α, IL-4)	
	Mast cells	Tryptase	Proliferation of ASM
	Epithelial cells	ECM proteins (FN) Cytokines (IL-11, TGF-β)	
	Fibroblasts	ECM proteins (FN, collagens)	
	Alveolar macrophages	ECM (FN)	Matrix turnover and remodeling
		MMPs	Matrix turnover and remodeling

the two mediators may have differences in cell source or release (17,20). Interestingly, following AG challenge the levels of histamine and tryptase show a dramatic increase and they do correlate (20). However, the increased airway responsiveness, which is a hallmark of asthma, may be the main reason for lower airway symptoms in asthmatic individuals and lack thereof in allergic nonasthmatic subjects despite similar patterns of mediator release in response to AG. The role of IgE-mediated events in EAR has recently been substantiated by studies showing that administration of monoclonal anti-IgE antibody attenuates AG-induced EAR (22).

IV. The Late Allergic Response

In approximately half of allergic subjects, the early-phase response is followed by a late-phase reaction (LPR), which begins 3–4 hr after exposure to AG, reaching a peak in 4–8 hr and resolving by 12–24 hr. The LPR is marked by airway obstructions with decreased peak expiratory flow (PEFR) or FEV_1 that is less responsive to inhaled bronchodilators than the early-phase response and is typically followed by a transient increase in nonspecific airway responsiveness. The symptoms of LPR are similar to those in the early phase and include cough, chest tightness, dyspnea, and wheezing. Nonallergic agents, such as occupational sensitizers (e.g., wood dust, diisocyanate), exercise, and challenge with inhaled distilled water, typically do not induce the IgE-mediated EAR; however, such agents have been reported to cause a pulmonary LPR. Although both allergic asthmatic and allergic nonasthmatic subjects can develop LPR, it is seen more frequently in asthmatic subjects. Other factors that influence the occurrence of LPR include AG type, dose, time of the day, and the presence of a recent viral respiratory tract infection. For example, when challenges are done at night, the occurrence, severity, and duration of LPR are increased (23,24), indicating circadian regulation of LPR. Experimental rhinoviral infections in allergic subjects also increase the frequency of LPR (25).

V. The Role of Inflammatory Mediators

Several mediators have been shown to contribute to bronchoconstriction in allergic asthma. Among these, LTs have received most of the attention. Various airway cells including mast cells and EOS can generate LTs. Anti-IgE stimulation of mast cells results in release of LTB_4, LTC_4, and LTD_4. LTB_4 is a potent neutrophil chemotactic factor, while LTC_4 and LTD_4 are potent inducers of bronchospasm, mucus secretion, and vascular permeability. Airway AG challenge leads to a significant rise in the LTC_4 level in BAL fluid (16,19). Emerging evidence suggests a close relationship between LTC_4 and eosinophilic airway inflammation. Treatment with an LT receptor blocker reduced eosinophilic airway inflammation as evaluated by BAL done 48 hr after LAC with AG (26). Furthermore, in a mouse model of allergen-induced airway inflammation, administration of eotaxin, an eosinophil-selective chemokine, resulted in increased levels of LTC_4 in BAL fluid. This phenomenon was attenuated by treatment with an LT antagonist (27).

Reactive oxygen species (ROS) can cause airway injury (28) and increase bronchial responsiveness (29). Multiple airway cells, including neutrophils, EOS, and macrophages can generate ROS. Increased generation of ROS has been demonstrated in patients with symptomatic asthma (30), following AG challenge (31), and in association with nocturnal exacerbations of asthma (32). Interestingly, the overnight rise in generation of superoxide anion correlated with the fall in FEV_1, suggesting a potential role for ROS in the pathogenesis of nocturnal asthma (32).

VI. The Role of Inflammatory Cells

T cells are key players in orchestrating the LPR. In asthma, the number of activated T cells [increased expression of IL-2 receptors (CD25), MHC class II (HLA-DR)] that are detected in peripheral blood (33), BAL (34), and bronchial mucosa (35) are increased. In particular, studies have shown increased numbers of cells expressing Th2-type cytokines including IL-4, IL-5, and IL-13 (36,37). The expression of these cytokines is further increased after AG challenge (16,20,34,38). Th2-type cells can contribute to airway hyperresponsiveness, mucus secretion, persistent inflammation, and airway remodeling. IL-9 and IL-4 contribute to mucus secretion, while IL-4 and IL-13 are necessary for isotype switching of B cells toward IgE production. In addition, IL-4 is a mast cell growth factor and potentiates eosinophilic inflammation by directing the differentiation of Th2 cells (which produce the EOS-selective cytokine IL-5) and by increasing the expression of VCAM-1 (an adhesion molecule with selectivity toward EOS). IL-5 is important for eosinophilopoeisis and is a terminal differentiation factor for eosinophil progenitor cells. IL-5 also prolongs EOS survival and primes EOS to respond to activating factors (for a review of EOS, see

Ref. 39). Studies of allergic subjects with and without asthma have confirmed increased release of IL-5 into BAL fluid 48 hr following the challenge (16,20,38). In addition, IL-5 protein has been localized to CD4+ cells by intracellular staining and flow cytometric studies (38). Finally, the levels of IL-5 correlate with the degree of BAL eosinophilia, confirming the key role of CD4+ cells and IL-5 in regulating allergic airway inflammation (16,20,38,40,41).

Topical instillation of recombinant IL-5 in mildly atopic asthmatic subjects induces significant eosinophilia in bronchial mucosa and BAL fluid (42). EOS recruitment to the airway involves a complex cascade of events that are not well defined. Secondary exposure to AG leads to the activation of Th2-type cells and the generation of IL-5. It is thought that IL-5 enters the circulation and triggers EOS differentiation, maturation, and release from the bone marrow. Although IL-5 results in increased numbers of circulating EOS, it is not sufficient to recruit EOS to the airway. A number of chemokines, including RANTES, MCP-1, MCP-4, and eotaxin, are chemotactic for EOS (for a comprehensive review see Ref. 43). Eotaxin may be of particular importance, as it is selective for EOS and has been shown to act in concert with IL-5 for EOS recruitment in a mouse model of airway inflammation (44).

The EOS, a hallmark of allergic inflammation, is probably the key effector cell in airway inflammation in asthma. EOS can release various mediators that contribute to airway damage and inflammation including granule proteins, LTs, cytokines, ROS, and matrix metalloproteinases (MMPs). Most studies have shown that the EOS numbers and/or activation are increased in the airways of asthmatic subjects. Airway EOS are increased during LPR to whole lung challenge. Studies of LAC have shown a dramatic increase in BAL EOS, which peaks 2–4 days following the challenge (45) and resolves over the following 1–3 weeks (46). This eosinophilic response is seen in allergic subjects regardless of the presence of asthma. Subjects with known LPR to allergen challenge generally show a more marked eosinophilic inflammation than single early-phase responders (47). Airway EOS have been shown to be upregulated in asthma, with increased expression of EG_2 (eosinophil cationic protein), release of granule proteins, enhanced survival, and marked increase in granule release in the airway (16).

Although neutrophils are not thought to be key players in the allergic response, they seem to play an important role in occupational asthma, in severe non-steroid-responsive asthma (48), and in acute asthma exacerbation leading to status asthmaticus. Neutrophils contribute to the pathogenesis presumably through the release of proteolytic enzymes, ROS, and MMPs. Studies of allergen challenge in asthmatics have shown an early rise in BAL neutrophils that precedes the influx of EOS (45). However, at 48 hr, the proportion of EOS is much greater than that of neutrophils. The increase in neutrophils seen 6 hr following LAC correlates with levels of IL-8 in BAL fluid (49). In most studies, saline-challenged airway segments demonstrate a degree of neutrophil influx similar to that seen following AG challenge when studied 48 hr after the challenge (16,50).

Macrophages are the predominant cells in the lower airway. They represent more than 90% of the cells recovered by BAL from normal and stable asthmatic subjects. Following allergen exposure, macrophages can function as effector cells by generating LTs, PGD_2, and ROS. Macrophages can upregulate the inflammatory response by generating cytokines such as IL-6, GM-CSF, and IL-1. On the other hand, they can downregulate this response by generating "anti-inflammatory" cytokines such as IL-10 and TGF-β. Alveolar macrophages inhibit T-cell proliferation (51); however, they may also perpetuate T-cell generation of Th2-type cytokines (52) and may contribute to airway remodeling by producing profibrogenic factors as well as fibronectin.

Epithelial cells are now viewed as more than a simple barrier in the airway. They are the first to encounter airborne particles. Cultured epithelial cells can generate various cytokines, including IL-6, IL-8, GM-CSF, RANTES, and eotaxin (53), that can play an important role in recruitment and activation of EOS, lymphocytes, and neutrophils to the airway.

VII. Airway Remodeling

Autopsy studies of asthma patients have demonstrated structural airway changes including increased bronchial smooth muscle mass, mucous gland hyperplasia, angiogenesis, and thickening of the lamina reticularis (reviewed in Refs. 54–56). Collectively these changes are known as airway remodeling. The subepithelial thickening associated with remodeling involves increased deposition of FN (57), collagen types I and III (57,58), $\alpha 2$ and $\beta 2$ laminin chains (2), and tenascin (58,59). Subepithelial fibrosis is characteristic of all forms of asthma but may be more accentuated in occupational asthma (1). Although these striking airway changes were thought principally to represent severe asthma, studies have shown that features of airway remodeling are present even in subjects with mild asymptomatic asthma (56) and in children with mild asthma, suggesting that such structural changes begin very early in the disease process (60). However, the association between disease severity and features of airway remodeling continues to be controversial, with one recent study showing no significant correlation between thickness of subbasement membrane and clinical parameters of disease severity (61).

Chronic airway inflammation contributes to remodeling by causing damage to airway epithelium, promoting turnover of extracellular matrix, and producing profibrogenic factors. Injury to airway epithelium and degradation of matrix is due at least in part to EOS granule proteins (62) and MMPs and other proteolytic enzymes released by a variety of inflammatory cells. Tissue repair is triggered and maintained by a variety of mediators including transforming growth factor (TGF)-β1, IL-4, platelet-derived growth factor (PDGF), epidermal growth factor (EGF), fibroblast growth factor (FGF), IL-1, tumor necrosis factor (TNF)-α, IL-11, endothelin (ET), insulin growth factor (IGF), tissue inhibitor of metalloproteinase (TIMP)-1, and histamine (63). Of these factors, TGF-β1 has emerged as a particularly potent stimulus for the synthesis of extracellular matrix (ECM) proteins including collagens, FN, vitronectin, and proteoglycans (64). In addition, TGF-β1 reduces matrix breakdown by decreasing production of MMPs and inducing TIMPs (65). Increased expression of TGF-β1 mRNA in bronchial biopsies (66) and elevated levels of TGF-β1 in BAL fluid (67) have been observed in atopic asthmatic patients compared to normal subjects. Finally, TGF-β1 expression relates to disease severity and extent of airway fibrosis (68), and the level of TGF-β1 in BAL fluid increases in response to AG challenge (67).

TGF-β1 is a potent stimulant of fibroblast function, including generation of FN and a number of EOS-active cytokines/chemokines (RANTES, GM-CSF, eotaxin). Gizycki et al. (69) recently reported that an AG-induced LPR in asthma is associated with increased numbers of fibroblasts (Fb's), Electron microscopy confirmed the presence of myofibroblast, i.e., "activated" Fb, in the bronchial mucosa 24 hr following inhaled AG challenge. These data suggest that short-term exposure to AG can initiate both an inflammatory response and early markers of remodeling.

A number of cytokines known for their proinflammatory effects may also have fibrogenic activity, either directly or indirectly. Among these, IL-4 and TNF-α stimulate fibroblast proliferation (70), expression of α-smooth muscle actin (SMA) (71), generation of cytokines (70,72–76), and, under certain conditions, ECM protein synthesis (77–79). As noted with TGF-β1, TNF-α and IL-4 are also elevated in airways of atopic asthmatic subjects and are further increased following exposure to AG (80,81). Potential cell sources of these proinflammatory/profibrogenic cytokines include T cells, macrophages, epithelial cells, EOS, and mast cells (63). It is of particular importance that TGF-β1, IL-4, and TNF-α are each expressed by EOS (82). Furthermore, EOS are associated with several conditions that are marked by prominent fibrosis (83,84), such as idiopathic pulmonary fibrosis (85), endomyocardial fibrosis (86), eosinophilic fasciitis (87) and adult respiratory distress syndrome (88). These associations raise the possibility that EOS can contribute not only to acute airway inflammation but also to the initiation and persistence of tissue fibrosis.

In summary, airway inflammation in asthma is a very complex and dynamic process that is influenced by factors that provoke asthma such as AG and occupational sensitizers (Fig. 2). Asthma severity and progression are probably influenced by ongoing inflammation. Recently the potential contribution of structural airway changes, i.e., remodeling, to disease severity, progression, and lack of reversibility has been emphasized. Yet to be identified are factors that contribute to the initiation and persistence of airway remodeling and whether it can be prevented or reversed by currently available asthma therapies or allergen avoidance measures.

References

1. Boulet LP, Laviolette M, Tucotte H, Cartier A, Dugas M, Malo JL, Boutet M. Bronchial subepithelial fibrosis correlates with airway responsiveness to methacholine. Chest 1997; 112:45–52.
2. Altraja A, Laitinen A, Virtanen I, Kämpe M, Simonsson BG, Karlsson S-E, Håkansson L, Venge P, Sillastu H, Laitinen LA. Expression of laminins in the airways of various types of asthmatic patients: a morphometric study. Am J Respir Crit Care Med 1996; 15:482–488.
3. Wills-Karp M. Immunological basis of antigen-induced airway hyperresponsiveness. Annu Rev Immunol 1999; 17:255–281.
4. McWilliam AS, Holt PG. Immunobiology of dendritic cells in the respiratory tract: steady-state and inflammatory sentinels? [Review] Toxicol Lett 1998; 102/103:323–329.
5. Moller GM, Overbeek SE, Van Helden-Meeuwsen CG, Van HJ, Prens EP, Mulder PG, Postma DS, Hoogsteden HC. Increased numbers of dendritic cells in the bronchial mucosa of atopic asthmatic patients: downregulation by inhaled corticosteroids. Clin Exp Allergy 1996; 26:517–524.
6. Ban M, Hettich D, Goutet M, Bonnet P. TDI inhalation in guinea-pigs involves migration of dendritic cells. Toxicol Lett 1997; 93:185–194.
7. Whitton JL. An overview of antigen presention and its central role in the immune response. Curr Topics Microbiol Immunol 1998; 232:1–13.
8. Mosmann TR, Cherwinski H, Bond MW, Giedlin MA, Coffman RH. Two types of murine helper T cell clone. Definition according to profiles of lymphokine activities and secreted proteins. J Immunol 1986; 136:2348–2357.

9. Swain SL. Helper T cell differentiation. [Review] Curr Opin Immunol 1999; 11: 180–185.

10. Tsuyuki S, Tsuyuki J, Einsle K, Kopf M, Coyle AJ. Costimulation through B7-2 (CD86) is required for the induction of a lung mucosal T helper cell 2 (TH2) immune response and altered airway responsiveness. J Exp Med 1997; 185:1671–1679.

11. Jaffar Z, Roberts K, Pandit A, Linsley P, Djukanovic R, Holgate S. B7 costimulation is required for IL-5 and IL-13 secretion by bronchial biopsy tissue of atopic asthmatic subjects in response to allergen stimulation. Am J Respir Cell Mol Biol 1999; 20:153–162.

12. Holt PG. Development of T-cell memory against inhalant allergens: risks for the future. [Review] Clin Exp Allergy 1999; 29(suppl 2):8–13.

13. Mapp CE, Balboni A, Baricordi R, Fabbri LM. Human leukocyte antigen associations in occupational asthma induced by isocyanates. [Review] Am J Respir Crit Care Med 1997; 156:S139–S143.

14. Lambrecht BN, Salomon B, Klatzmann D, Pauwels RA. Dendritic cells are required for the development of chronic eosinophilic airway inflammation in response to inhaled antigen in sensitized mice. J Immunol 1998; 160:4090–4097.

15. Bissonnette EY, Befus AD. Mast cells in asthma. [Review] [11 refs]. Can Respir J 1998; 5:23–24.

16. Sedgwick JB, Calhoun WJ, Gleich GJ, Kita H, Abrams JS, Schwartz LB, Volovitz B, Ben-Yaakov M, Busse WW. Immediate and late airway response of allergic rhinitis patients to segmental antigen challenge. Characterization of eosinophil and mast cell mediators. Am Rev Respir Dis 1991; 144:1274–1281.

17. Wenzel SE, Fowler AA, Schwartz LB. Activation of pulmonary mast cells by bronchoalveolar allergen challenge: in vivo release of histamine and tryptase in atopic subjects with and without asthma. Am Rev Respir Dis 1988; 137:1002–1008.

18. Wenzel SE, Westcott JY, Smith HR, Larsen GL. Spectrum of prostanoid release after bronchoalveolar allergen challenge in atopic asthmatics and in control groups. An alteration in the ratio of bronchoconstrictive to bronchoprotective mediators. Am Rev Respir Dis 1989; 139:450–457.

19. Wenzel SE, Larsen GL, Johnston K, Voelkel NF, Westcott JY. Elevated levels of leukotriene C4 in bronchoalveolar lavage fluid from atopic asthmatics after endobronchial allergen challenge. Am Rev Respir Dis 142:112–119.

20. Jarjour NN, Sedgwick JB, Swensen CA, Busse WW. Late allergic airway response to segmental bronchopulmonary provocation in allergic subjects is related to peripheral blood basophil histamine release. J Allergy Clin Immunol 1997; 99:87–93.

21. Casale TB, Wood D, Richerson HB, Zehr B, Zavala D, Hunninghake GW. Direct evidence of a role for mast cells in the pathogenesis of antigen-induced bronchoconstriction. J Clin Invest 1987; 80:1507–1511.

22. Frew AJ. Effects of anti-IgE in asthmatic subjects. [Review] Thorax 1998; 53(suppl 2):S52–S57.

23. Mohiuddin AA, Martin RJ. Circadian basis of the late phase asthmatic response. Am Rev Respir Dis 1990; 142:1153–1157.
24. Jarjour NN, Lacouture PG, Busse WW. Theophylline inhibits the late asthmatic response to nighttime antigen challenge in patients with mild atopic asthma. Ann Allergy Asthma Immunol 1998; 81:231–236.
25. Page CP, Coyle AJ. The interaction between PAF, platelets and eosinophils in bronchial asthma. Eur Respir J 1989; 6(suppl):483s–487s.
26. Calhoun WJ, Lavins BJ, Minkwitz MC, Evans R, Gleich GJ, Cohn J. Effect of zafirlukast (Accolate) on cellular mediators of inflammation: bronchoalveolar lavage fluid findings after segmental antigen challenge. Am J Respir Crit Care Med 1998; 157:1381–1389.
27. Hisada T, Salmon M, Nasuhara Y, Chung KF. Cysteinyl-leukotrienes partly mediate eotaxin-induced bronchial hyperresponsiveness and eosinophilia in IL-5 transgenic mice. Am J Respir Crit Care Med 1999; 160:571–575.
28. Freeman BA, Crapo JD. Biology of disease: free radicals and tissue injury. [Review]. Lab Invest 1982; 47:412–426.
29. Katsumata U, Miura M, Ichinose M, Kimura K, Takahashi T, Inoue H, Takishima T. Oxygen radicals produce airway constriction and hyperresponsiveness in anesthetized cats. Am Rev Respir Dis 1990; 141:1158–1161.
30. Jarjour NN, Calhoun WJ. Oxygen radical production by airspace cells is increased in active asthma. J Lab Clin Med 1994, 123:131–137.
31. Calhoun WJ, Bush RK. Enhanced reactive oxygen species metabolism of airspace cells and airway inflammation follow antigen challenge in human asthma. J Allergy Clin Immunol 1990; 86:306–313.
32. Jarjour NN, Busse WW, Calhoun WJ. Enhanced production of oxygen radicals in nocturnal asthma. Am Rev Respir Dis 1992; 146:905–911.
33. Corrigan CJ, Haczku A, Gemou-Engesaeth V, Doi S, Kikuchi Y, Takatsu K, Durham SR, Kay AB. CD4 T-lymphocyte activation in asthma is accompanied by increased serum concentrations of interleukin-5. Effect of glucocorticoid therapy. Am Rev Respir Dis 1993; 147:540–547.
34. Robinson D, Hamid Q, Bentley A, Ying S, Kay AB, Durham SR. Activation of CD4 T cells, increased TH2-type cytokine mRNA expression, and eosinophil recruitment in bronchoalveolar lavage after allergen challenge in patients with atopic asthma. J Allergy Clin Immunol 1993; 92:313–324.
35. Azzawi M, Bradley B, Jeffery PK, Frew AJ, Wardlaw AJ, Knowles G, Assoufi B, Collins JV, Durham S, Kay AB. Identification of activated T lymphocytes and eosinophils in bronchial biopsies in stable atopic asthma. Am Rev Respir Dis 1990; 142:1407–1413.
36. Robinson DS, Hamid Q, Ying S, Tsicopoulos A, Barkans J, Bentley AM, Corrigan C, Durham SR, Kay AB. Predominant TH2-like bronchoalveolar T-lymphocyte population in atopic asthma. N Engl J Med 1992; 326:298–304.
37. Humbert M, Durham SR, Kimmitt P, Powell N, Assoufi B, Pfister R, Menz G, Kay AB, Corrigan CJ. Elevated expression of messenger ribonucleic acid encoding IL-

13 in the bronchial mucosa of atopic and nonatopic subjects with asthma. J Allergy Clin Immunol 1997; 99:657–665.

38. Kelly EA, Rodriguez RR, Busse WW, Jarjour NN. The effect of segmental bronchoprovocation with allergen on airway lymphocyte function. Am J Respir Crit Care Med 1997; 156:1421–1428.

39. Elsner J, Kapp A. Regulation and modulation of eosinophil effector functions. [Review] Allergy 1999; 54:15–26.

40. Sur S, Gleich GJ, Offord KP, Swanson MC, Ohnishi T, Martin LB, Wagner JM, Weiler DA, Hunt LW. Allergen challenge in asthma: association of eosinophils and lymphocytes with interleukin-5. Allergy 1995; 50:891–898.

41. Sur S, Kita H, Gleich GJ, Chenier T, Hunt LW. Eosinophil recruitment is associated with IL-5, but not RANTES, twenty-four hours after allergen challenge. J Allergy Clin Immunol 1996; 97:1272–1278.

42. Shi H, Qin S, Huang G, Chen Y, Xiao C, Xu H, Liang G, Xie Z, Qin X, Wu J, Li G, Zhang C. Infiltration of eosinophils into the asthmatic airways caused by interleukin 5. Am J Respir Cell Mol Biol 1997; 16:220–224.

43. Nickel R, Beck LA, Stellato C, Schleimer RP. Chemokines and allergic disease. J Allergy Clin Immunol 1999; 104:723–742.

44. Mould AW, Matthaei KI, Young IG, Foster PS. Relationship between interleukin-5 and eotaxin in regulating blood and tissue eosinophilia in mice. J Clin Invest 1997; 99:1064–1071.

45. Metzger WJ, Zavala D, Richerson HB, Moseley P, Iwamota P, Monick M, Sjoerdsma K, Hunninghake GW. Local allergen challenge and bronchoalveolar lavage of allergic asthmatic lungs. Am Rev Respir Dis 1987; 135:433–440.

46. Shaver J, O'Connor J, Pollice M, Cho SK, Kane G, Fish J, Peters S. Pulmonary inflammation after segmental ragweed challenge in allergic asthmatic and nonasthmatic subjects. Am J Respir Crit Care Med 1995; 152:1189–1197.

47. Zangrilli JG, Shaver JR, Cirelli RA, Cho SK, Garlisi CG, Falcone A, Cuss FM, Fish JE, Peters SP. sVCAM-1 levels after segmental antigen challenge correlate with eosinophil influx, IL-4 and IL-5 production, and the late phase response. Am J Respir Crit Care Med 1995; 151:1346–1353.

48. Wenzel SE, Szefler SJ, Leung DY, Sloan SI, Rex MD, Martin RJ. Bronchoscopic evaluation of severe asthma. Persistent inflammation associated with high dose glucocorticoids. Am J Respir Crit Care Med 1997; 156:737–743.

49. Teran LM, Carroll MP, Frew AJ, Redington AE, Davies DE, Lindley I, Howarth PH, Church MK, Holgate ST. Leukocyte recruitment after local endobronchial allergen challenge in asthma. Relationship to procedure and to airway interleukin-8 release. Am J Respir Crit Care Med 1996; 154:469–476.

50. Jarjour NN, Calhoun WJ, Kelly EA, Gleich GJ, Schwartz LB, Busse WW. The immediate and late allergic response to segmental bronchopulmonary provocation in asthma. Am J Respir Crit Care Med 1997; 155:1421–1428.

51. Holt PG, Oliver J, Bilyk N, McMenamin C, McMenamin PG, Kraal G, Thepen T. Downregulation of the antigen presenting cell function(s) of pulmonary dendritic cells in vivo by resident alveolar macrophages. J Exp Med 1993; 177:397–407.

52. Tang C, Rolland JM, Li X, Ward C, Bish R, Walters EH. Alveolar macrophages from atopic asthmatics, but not atopic nonasthmatics, enhance interleukin-5 production by CD4⁺ T cells. Am J Respir Crit Care Med 1998; 157:1120–1126.
53. Polito AJ, Proud D. Epithelia cells as regulators of airway inflammation. [Review] J Allergy Clin Immunol 1998; 102:714–718.
54. Bousquet J, Chanez P, Lacoste JY, White R, Vic P, Godard P, Michel FB. Asthma: a disease remodeling the airways. Allergy 1992; 47:3–11.
55. Roberts CR. Is asthma a fibrotic disease? Chest 1995; 107(3):111S–117S.
56. Redington AE, Howarth PH. Airway wall remodelling in asthma. Thorax 1997; 52:310–312.
57. Roche WR, Beasley R, Williams JH, Holgate ST. Subepithelial fibrosis in the bronchi of asthmatics. Lancet 1989; 1:520–523.
58. Hoshino M, Nakamura Y, Sim JJ, Shimojo J, Isogai S. Bronchial subepithelial fibrosis and expression of matrix metalloproteinase-9 in asthmatic airway inflammation. J Allergy Clin Immunol 1998; 102:783–788.
59. Laitinen A, Altraja A, Kämpe M, Linden M, Virtanen I, Laitinen LA. Tenascin is increased in airway basement membrane of asthmatics and decreased by an inhaled steroid. Am J Respir Crit Care Med 1997; 156:951–958.
60. Cutz E, Levison H, Cooper DM. Ultrastructure of airways in children with asthma. Histopathology 1978; 2:407–421.
61. Chu HW, Halliday JL, Martin RJ, Leung DW, Szefler SJ, Wenzel SE. Collagen deposition in large airways may not differentiate severe asthma from milder forms of the disease. Am J Respir Crit Care Med 1998; 158:1936–1944.
62. Gleich GJ, Loegering DA, Fujisawa T, Vanhoutte PM. The eosinophil as a mediator of damage to respiratory epithelium: a model for bronchial hyperreactivity. J Allergy Clin Immunol 1998; 81:776–781.
63. Redington AE, Sime PJ, Howarth PH, Holgate ST. Fibroblasts and the extracellular matrix in asthma. In: Holgate ST, Busse WW, eds. Inflammatory Mechanisms in Asthma. New York: Marcel Dekker, 1998:443–467.
64. Roman J. Extracellular matrix and lung inflammation. Immunol Res 1996; 15:163–178.
65. Edwards RE, Murphy G, Reynolds JJ, Whitham SE, Docherty AJ, Angel P, Heath JK. Transforming growth factor β modulates the expression of collagenase and metalloproteinase inhibitor. EMBO J 1987; 6:1899–1904.
66. Minshall EM, Leung DY, Martin RJ, Song Y, Cameron L, Ernst P, Hamid Q. Eosinophil-associated TGF-β1 mRNA expression and airways fibrosis in bronchial asthma. Am J Respir Cell Mol Biol 1997; 17:326–333.
67. Redington AE, Madden J, Frew AJ, Djukanovic R, Roche WR, Holgate ST, Howarth PH. Transforming growth factor-β1 in asthma. Measurement in bronchoalveolar lavage fluid. Am J Respir Crit Care Med 1997; 156:642–647.
68. Vignola AM, Chanez P, Chiappara G, Merendino A, Pace E, Rizzo A, IaRocca AM, Bellia V, Bonsignore G, Bousquet J. Transforming growth factor-β expression in mucosal biopsies in asthma and chronic bronchitis. Am J Respir Crit Care Med 1997; 156:591–599.

69. Gizycki MJ, Ädelroth E, Rogers AV, O'Byrne PM, Jeffery PK. Myofibroblast involvement in the allergen-induced late response in mild atopic asthma. Am J Respir Cell Mol Biol 1997; 16:664–673.

70. Doucet C, Brouty-Boyé D, Pottin-Clémenceau C, Canonica GW, Jasmin C, Azzarone B. Interleukin (IL)-4 and IL-13 act on human lung fibroblasts. J Clin Invest 1998; 101:2129–2139.

71. Mattey DL, Dawes PT, Nixon NB, Slater H. Transforming growth factor beta 1 and interleukin 4 induced alpha smooth muscle actin expression and myofibro-blast-like differentiation in human synovial fibroblasts in vitro: modulation by basic fibroblast growth factor. Ann Rheum Dis 1997; 56:426–431.

72. Elias JA, Zheng T, Whiting NL, Trow TK, Merrill WW, Zitnik R, Ray P, Alder-man EM. IL-1 and TGF-β regulation of fibroblast-derived IL-11. J Immunol 1994; 152:2421–2429.

73. Bartels J, Schluter C, Richter E, Noso N, Kulke R, Christophers E, Schroder JM. Human dermal fibroblasts express eotaxin: molecular cloning, mRNA expression, and identification of eotaxin sequence variants. Biochem Biophys Res Commun 1996; 225:1045–1051.

74. Mochizuki M, Bartels J, Mallet AI, Christopher E, Schroder JM. IL-4 induces eotaxin: a possible mechanism of selective eosinophil recruitment in helminth infection and atopy. J Immunol 1998; 160:60–68.

75. Hogaboam CM, Lukacs NW, Chensue SW, Strieter RM, Kunkel SL. Monocyte chemoattractant protein-1 synthesis by murine lung fibroblasts modulates CD4[+] T cell activation. J Immunol 1998; 160:4606–4614.

76. Maune S, Berner I, Sticherling M, Kulke R, Bartels J, Schroder JM. Fibroblasts but not epithelial cells obtained from human nasal mucosa produce the chemokine RANTES. Rhinology 1996; 34:210–214.

77. Postlethwaite AE, Holness MA, Katai H, Raghow R. Human fibroblasts synthe-size elevated levels of extracellular matrix proteins in response to interleukin 4. J Clin Invest 1992; 90:1479–1485.

78. Makhluf HA, Stepniakowska J, Hoffman S, Smith E, LeRoy EC, Trojanowska M. IL-4 upregulates tenascin synthesis in scleroderma and healthy skin fibroblasts. J Invest Dermatol 1996; 107:856–859.

79. Sato M, Ishikawa O, Abe M, Miyachi Y. Opposite effects of tumour necrosis fac-tor-alpha on type I and III collagen gene expression by human dermal fibroblasts in monolayer and three-dimensional cultures. Br J Dermatol 1998; 138:118–121.

80. Vignola AM, Chiappara G, Chanez P, Merendino AM, Pace E, Spatafora M, Bous-quet J, Bonsignore G. Growth factors in asthma. Monaldi Arch Chest Dis 1997; 52:159–169.

81. Shah A, Church MK, Holgate ST. Tumor necrosis factor alpha: a potential medi-ator of asthma. Clin Exp Allergy 1995; 25:1038–1044.

82. Moqbel R, Levi-Schaffer F, Kay AB. Cytokine generation by eosinophils. J Allergy Clin Immunol 1994; 94:1183–1188.

83. Levi-Schaffer F, Weg VB. Mast cells, eosinophils and fibrosis. Clin Exp Allergy 1997; 27(suppl 1):64–70.
84. Gharaee-Kermani M, Phan SH. The role of eosinophils in pulmonary fibrosis. [Review] Int J Mol Med 1998; 1:43–53.
85. Fujimoto K, Yamaguchi S, Honda T, Matsuzawa Y. Eosinophil activation in patients with pulmonary fibrosis. Chest 1995; 108:48–54.
86. Tai PC, Ackerman SJ, Spry CF, Dunnette S, Olson E, Gleich GJ. Deposits of eosinophil granule protein in cardiac tissues of patients with eosinophilic endomyocardial disease. Lancet 1987; 1:643–647.
87. Martin RW, Duffy J, Engel AG, Lie JT, Bowles CA, Moyer TP, Gleich GJ. The clinical spectrum of the eosinophilia-myalgia syndrome associated with L-tryptophan ingestion. Clinical features in 20 patients and aspects of pathophysiology. Ann Intern Med 1990; 113:124–134.
88. Hallgren R, Samuelsson T, Venge P, Modig J. Eosinophil activation in the lung is related to lung damage in adult respiratory distress syndrome. Am Rev Respir Dis 1987; 135:639–642.

The order Astigmata is divided into two suborders, Acaridia and Soroptidia (parasitic mites). Generally, all the Astigmata mites, which in the adult stage live in association with insects, vertebrates, or other animals, are included in the suborder Acaridia. Free-living Astigmata commonly occur in decaying organic matter and in nests of birds, insects, and mammals. Many of these mites infest stored foods, and certain species are of economic importance because of the serious damage they inflict to stored grains. Several species in this group are capable of producing respiratory allergic disease and contact dermatitis. It has been estimated that 34 genera of 10 families of the order Astigmata can be found in stored products and/or house dust (16).

Although there is some variation in the life cycle of various species, the usual life cycle consists of an egg, a six-legged larva, one to three nymphal stages, and adult males and females. Their digestive system is completely developed and produces spherical fecal pellets measuring 10–40 μm in diameter. Their respiration is cutaneous, with the skin serving as a barrier through which both gas and water vapor are exchanged. Most mites require for the completion of their life cycle a relative humidity ranging from approximately 70% to 90% and a temperature of approximately 25°C.

The water loss of the mite body conditions colonization and population growth. House dust mites are able to extract water vapor from unsaturated air by means of a hygroscopic salt solution in the supracoxal gland. If the humidity falls below a critical level (50%), the salt crystallizes and blocks the entrance of the gland and the mite slows down the rate of dehydration. The process of water uptake also depends of the temperature. *Dermatophagoides farinae* maintains water balance and survives at relative humidities of about 45% at 25°C and 65% at 30°C. This ability to survive at relative humidities below saturation accounts for their successful colonization of human dwellings. Since house dust mites cannot regulate their internal body temperature, egg production and population growth decline and mortality rates and the duration of the life cycle increase at low temperatures.

Since 1964, mites of the genus *Dermatophagoides* have been recognized as the most important sources of allergens in house dust. Therefore the name house dust mite was used to refer to members of the family Pyroglyphidae, especially *Dermatophagoides pteronyssinus* and *D. farinae* (17). *Euroglyphus maynei* and *Blomia tropicalis* are also regularly found in house dust; the latter species is mainly present in tropical and subtropical regions of the world. Mites belonging to the families Acaridae, Glycyphagidae, Chortoglyphidae, Tarsonemidae, and Carpoglyphidae, commonly found in silos, granaries, warehouses, bakeries, and barns, are known as "storage mites." These mites can also be found in house dust in rural and urban areas, especially in homes with high relative humidities. Other mites commonly inhabiting house dust are predator mites belonging to the genus *Cheyletus*. The term "domestic mites" has been coined to refer to all mite species that are present in house dust and may elicit an allergic response (18).

III. Assessment of Mite Allergens

New technologies and sensitive immunoassays have been developed to detect and measure minimal concentrations of mite allergens in indoor, outdoor, and occupational settings: ELISA, RIA, RAST-inhibition, and guanine detection are used for the determination of allergens from the main mite species. A two-site monoclonal antibody based enzyme-linked immunoassay, which is commercially available, is the most popular method to quantitate levels of mite allergens. The assay uses a monoclonal antibody on a plastic microtiter well to bind to the allergen present in a dust extract. Bound allergens are detected using a second antibody, either enzyme or ^{125}I-labeled, directed against a different epitope on the molecule. The assays are quantitated using reference preparations containing known amounts of a given allergen. Der p 1, Der f 1, Der p 2, and Der f 2 can be quantitated using this method. The total allergenic content in a house dust sample can be quantitated by RAST inhibition. This method is used when monoclonal antibodies are not available against specific allergenic components. The results are expressed in allergenic or arbitrary units.

Der p 1 and Der f 1 levels normally range between 100 ng/g and 100 μg/g, depending on the geographical area where the samples are collected. More than 10 μg/g can be considered a high level, and levels greater than 100 ng/g can be considered a risk for sensitization. Group 2 allergen levels are generally lower than those of group 1 and tend to correlate better with mite counts.

Dust samples can also be used to quantify and identify mite species. Samples of 10–25 mg of sieved dust are suspended in approximately 5 cm^3 of saturated saline in a small petri dish. After a few minutes, the whole petri dish is examined under a stereomicroscope. Mites are carefully removed with a fine needle and placed in two drops of Hoyer's solution on a microscope slide, where they can be morphologically identified and counted under the microscope. Results are expressed as mites per gram of sieved dust (15). It has been suggested that a count of more than 100 mites per gram is associated with allergic sensitization and that more than 500 could be associated with the clinical manifestations of asthma (18).

IV. Molecular Characteristics of Mite Allergens

In recent years, several mite allergens have been purified by conventional methods or produced as recombinant proteins. Molecular cloning is an efficient tool to produce pure polypeptides that, in their native source, form complex mixtures and are often represented in very small quantities. Sequence similarity searches have identified the biological function of many cloned allergens. Mite allergens are grouped according to their chronological characterization or homology with *Dermatophagoides* allergens. A list of these allergens is shown in Table 1.

Group 1. Group 1 allergens are 25 kDa glycoproteins with sequence homology and thiol protease function similar to those of the enzymes papain, bromelain, ficin, actinidin, and cathepsin H and B (19–21). *Der p* 1 and *Der f* 1 have a 81% sequence homology. Group 1 allergens are cysteine proteases, which can cleave the low affinity IgE receptor (CD23) from the surface of human B cell lymphocytes (22). This receptor is also present on eosinophils, follicular dendritic cells, macrophages and platelets. Because soluble CD23 promotes IgE production. It is hypothesized that fragments of CD23 released

Table 1 Purified Allergens from Domestic Mites[a]

Source	Allergen	MW (kDa)
Group 1	Der p 1, Der f 1, Eur m 1, Der m 1	25
Group 2	Der p 2, Der f 2, Eur m 2, Tyr p 2	14
Group 3	Der p 3, Der f 3, Eur m 3	28–30
Group 4	Der p 4	56–63
Group 5	Der p 5, Blo t 5	14
Group 6	Der p 6	25
Group 7	Der p 7, Der f 7	22
Group 8	Der p 8	25
Group 9	Der p 9	24–28
Group 10	Der p 10, Der f 10	37
Group 11	Der f 11	98
Group 12	Blo t 12	14
Group 12	Blo t 13	14.8

[a]All these allergens have a recognition rate by mite-allergic patients that varies from 10 to 90%.

by Der p 1 may enhance IgE synthesis. It has also been suggested that Der p 1 also cleaves the α subunit of the IL-2 receptor (IL-2R or CD25) from the surface of human peripheral blood T cells, and as a result these cells show markedly diminished proliferation and interferon γ secretion in response to potent stimulation by anti-CD3 antibody (23). The authors conclude that since IL-2R is pivotal for the propagation of Th1 cells, its cleavage by Der p 1 may consequently bias the immune response toward Th2 cells. The cleavage of CD23 and CD25 by Der p 1 enhances its allergenicity by creating an allergic microenvironment (24).

Other group 1 allergens that have been purified include Eur m 1 from *E. maynei*, Der s 1 from *D. siboney*, and Der m 1 from *D. microceras.*

Group 2. Der p 2 and Der f 2 are proteins of 14 kDa (25–29). These allergens have an 88% homology in their sequences. Der p 2, when expressed as a fusion protein, shows very high IgE reactivity. A major allergen of *L. destructor*, formerly known as Lep d 1, has been renamed Lep d 2 on the basis of its amino acid sequence homology with Der p 2 (30). Der p 2 and Led p 2 have 28% and 26.4% sequence identity with the epididymis-specific human HE1 gene product and chimpanzee EPI-1, respectively. These proteins seem to arise from secretions of the male mite reproductive tract (31). Anti group 2 monoclonal antibodies and confocal laser scanning microscopy have shown reactivity associated with the gut and other structures of the mite *L. destructor*, including the sebaceous glands (32). Der p 2 and Der f 2 show a significant degree of sequence polymorphism, similar to that found in group 1 allergens. The polymorphic residues are found in regions containing T-cell epitopes (33). The significance of these polymorphisms, in terms of antibody and T-cell recognition, might have some important implications if peptides were to be used as immunotherapeutic agents to modify T-cell function. Eur m 2 from *E. maynei* and Tyr p 2 from *T. putrescentiae* have also been described.

Group 3. Der p 3 and Der f 3 are 25–30 kDa proteins with trypsin-like serine proteinase activity and 50% homology with other serine proteases (34). Der p 3 is encoded by a single gene, and most cDNA clones constructed from commercial mites show minor sequence variations (35). Der p 3 has 81% homology with Der f 3 and Eur m 3 from *E. maynei*. Group 3 allergens are recognized by approximately 80% of mite-allergic individuals.

Group 4. Group 4 allergens have molecular weights of 56–63 kDa. IgE binding ranges from 46% in adults to 25% in children. Their N-terminal amino acid sequence shows homology with amylase (36).

Group 5. Der p 5 is a 14–15 kDa allergen that has a specific IgE binding frequency of 14% (37,38). Blo t 5 from *B. tropicalis* has a 43% sequence similarity with Der p 5 (39,40) and is recognized by 45–60% of the sera of *B. tropicalis*-allergic asthmatic individuals. Der p 5 seems to exhibit less polymorphism than other mite allergens.

Group 6. Der p 6 and Der f 6 are 25 kDa chymotrypsin-like serine proteases produced by *D. pteronyssinus* and *D. farinae*, respectively. They show a 40–60% frequency of IgE reactivity in mite-allergic patients. It has been shown that Der p 6 has 37% homology with the trypsin-like allergen Der p 3 (41).

Group 7. Der p 7 and Der f 7 have 86% sequence similarity and a significant serological cross-reactivity. Der p 7 obtained from a *D. pteronyssinus* cDNA library was recognized by RAST and/or skin testing in about 50% of mite-allergic patients. Antibodies to this allergen react with multiple bands in mite extracts, corresponding to components of 29, 27, and 24 kDa by Western blotting. Absorption of sera from allergic patients removed IgE reactivity to bands of 29, 27, 13, and 11 kDa. Six isoforms of Der p 7 have been identified (42).

Group 8. Der p 8 is a 25–26 kDa allergen characterized from a *D. pteronyssinus* lambda cDNA library. It is recognized by approximately 40% of mite-allergic sera and has a strong homology with the rat and mouse glutathione-*S*-transferase (43). It has a 25% homology with Bla g 5, an important allergen of the German cockroach, *Blatella germanica*. Apparently there is no cross-reactivity between these two allergens.

Group 9. Der p 9 is a 24–29 kDa allergen with three isoforms (pI 4.8, 7.8, and 10.5) from *D. pteronyssinus*. It is recognized by approximately 80% of mite-allergic individuals and has collagenolytic activity (44). Der p 9 shows some cross-reactivity with Der p 3 and Der p 6 by RAST inhibition.

Group 10. Correspond to the mite tropomyosin identified in *D. farinae* and *D. pteronyssinus* (45,46). It is a 33–37 kDa allergen that has 76.1%, 58.8%, and 58.1% identity with *Drosophila melanogaster* and rabbit and human alfa-tropomyosin, respectively, and a fairly high (> 60%) IgE binding frequency. This allergen seems to be involved in the cross-reactivity between mites, shrimp, and insects in shrimp-allergic patients (47).

Group 11. This group comprises allergens that have sequence homology with paramyosin, a structural muscle protein of invertebrates. Der f 11 has a molecular weight of 98 kDa and binds IgE at high frequency and intensity (48).

Groups 12 and 13. Groups 12 and 13 were created to include allergens purified from *B. tropicalis*. Blo t 12 has a molecular weight of 14 kDa and an IgE recognition frequency of 50% (49). Blo t 13 has a molecular weight of 14.8 kDa, an IgE recognition frequency of 10%, and high sequence homology to cytosolic fatty acid binding proteins (50).

V. Relationship of Allergen Exposure to Airway Disease Chronic Exposure

The relationship between exposure to indoor allergens and disease has been examined carefully in the case of chronic asthma. At the initial meeting of the newly formed Section of Occupational Medicine of the Royal Society of Medicine in 1965, Sir Austin Bradford Hill suggested that the members should organize evidence demonstrating association between some environmental feature and an illness, so that their colleagues could "pass from this observed *association* to a verdict of *causation*" (51). He suggested that the aspects listed in Table 2 should be considered. As reviewed by others (10,52–54), the evidence linking indoor aeroallergens and asthma meets all of these criteria.

In terms of plausibility, the first criterion in Table 2, IgE-mediated hypersensitivity presents a compelling mechanism. Sixty to eighty percent of asthmatic patients are sensitized to indoor allergens, as indicated by either skin tests or RAST (54–56); this figure is three times as high as in a population without asthma (55,57). The association is specific for asthma and is not seen with other chronic pulmonary diseases such as chronic bronchitis or cystic fibrosis. Sensitization and exposure to excessive environmental allergen concentrations is associated with a relative risk of 5–10 for diagnosed asthma as well as severe attacks of asthma requiring emergency room treatment (58–60). Experimentally, acute exposure of sensitized individuals can lead to inflammation with the same characteristic eosinophilia as that seen in chronic asthma (61).

Table 2 Essential Steps to Assign Causality to Association Between Environmental Exposures and Disease

Strength	The strength of the association is large.
Consistency	Repeated observations in different populations have consistent findings.
Specificity	A cause leads to a specific effect.
Temporality	A cause precedes an effect.
Biological gradient	There is a dose–response gradient.
Plausibility	The mechanism is biologically plausible.
Coherence	The mechanism should not conflict with facts of the natural history and biology of the disease.
Experiment	There is experimental evidence.
Analogy	There are analogous explanations.

Source: Adapted from Ref. 51.

Evidence associating allergen exposure, sensitization, and asthma has been found consistently in various settings, summarized in Table 3. Sporik et al. (62) surveyed school children in Los Alamos, New Mexico, and identified 19 with symptomatic asthma; the frequency of sensitization and exposure to indoor allergens among these children was significantly higher than in asymptomatic children. Gelber et al. (59) and call et al. (60) conducted case-control studies in urban emergency rooms and found a similarly strong association between sensitization, exposure, and symptomatic asthma. Pollart et al. (56) studied emergency room admissions for acute asthma at a U.S. Air Force base during several intense grass pollen seasons; although both asthma admissions and controls were exposed to the same seasonal pollens, the relative risk of sensitization to grass allergens in patients presenting with asthma was 69 compared to nonasthmatic controls. The effect of exposure to another indoor allergen, cockroach, on the chronic severity of asthma was examined in a multicenter study of risk factors for asthma among asthmatic children in U.S. inner cities (63). Among 476 children who had skin tests and a home visit to

Table 3 The Relation of Sensitization and Exposure to Indoor Allergens to Acute Severe Asthma

1. Sensitization rates to airborne allergens

Investigator	Asthma cases			Controls			
	n	Sensitized	%	n	Sensitized	%	p-Value
Sporik et al. (62)	19	16	84	101	37	36	<0.001
Gelber et al. (59)	114	44	39	114	5	4	<0.001
Call et al. (60)	40	29	73	40	11	27	<0.001
Pollart et al. (56)	59	54	92	59	8	14	OR = 69

2. Percent both sensitized and exposed to indoor allergens

Investigator	Asthma cases			Controls			
	n	Sensitized and exposed	%	n	Sensitized and exposed	%	OR[a]
Sporik et al. (62)	16	10	63	90	19	21	6.2
Gelber et al. (59)	35	93	38	93	7	8	7.4
Call et al. (60)	35	21	60	22	3	14	9.5

[a]OR = odds ratio for sensitization cases vs. controls.

measure allergens in settled dust, those who were both sensitized and exposed to cockroach allergen in their bedroom had over three times as many hospitalizations as children who were not sensitized or were sensitized but not exposed. These data suggest that a combination of exposure and sensitization markedly increases the frequency of asthma and the risk of morbidity from asthma.

The specific environmental exposures driving these relationships differ. Pollart and colleagues found a relationship to grass pollen allergens, while in urban emergency rooms and inner city populations the association was to house dust mite, cat, and cockroach allergens. In all of these studies, the asthmatic patients and controls were exposed to similar environmental allergen concentrations. This would suggest that individual genetic differences in persons with allergic asthma are an even more important determinant of sensitization; without the appropriate genetic background, exposure would not have been associated with asthma.

Sensitization is the first step in the pathogenesis of allergic asthma. Specific IgE antibody to allergens is rarely demonstrated in normal humans. However, specific IgE defines the atopic state (55) and has been shown to increase after environmental exposures such as pollen seasons (64). Atopic persons but not normal individuals have measurable concentrations of IgE antibody to house dust mites (65,66). Persons in animal care facilities produce IgG antibody to rat allergens, but only those with symptoms have specific IgE antibody (67). It appears that, in general, only IgE antibody is associated with disease.

Sensitization offers clear examples of Hill's biological gradient. Children living at high altitude in Briançon (68) or Los Alamos, New Mexico (62) or in dry climates in Lismore, Australia (55) have sensitization rates to mite allergens of no more than 20%. Coastal Australian towns have a higher mite population, higher rates of sensitization, and higher rates of symptomatic asthma (55). It has been shown that the frequency of measurable IgE antibody and symptomatic asthma in school-age children could be related directly to the exposure to house dust mites as infants, as measured by levels of antigen in settled dust (12). Cockroach sensitivity correlates with current reported levels of exposure (69). Lau et al. (13) demonstrated that the serum concentrations of IgE antibody to Der p 1 and Der f 1 in atopic children correlated with current exposure to these allergens ($Rs = 0.46$, $p < 0.0001$), Kuehr et al. (14) found similar relationships between mite skin test results and settled dust allergen levels.

The experimental evidence supporting this relationship comes both from acute bronchoprovocation studies and from allergen avoidance trials. Allergen avoidance trials have been conducted almost entirely with patients who are allergic to house dust mites. The most consistently positive trials have involved moving patients to isolated environments with very low mite allergen exposure (70–72). The results of trials involving the modification of home environments have been less consistent; over 50 trials have been reviewed elsewhere (73,74). These trials differ so much in methodology that it is difficult to group them to allow a given strategy to be tested reproducibly. In Table 4, we summarize a number of well-described trials. In five trials (75–79), mites or mite allergen reduction was demonstrated, and either asthma symptoms or airway hyperresponsiveness were improved in all five of them. In the other trials, mite aller-

Table 4 House Dust Mite Control: Clinical Trials

Trial	N	Age (yr)	Duration (mo)	Treatment[a]	Control[a]	Significance
Mites reduced						
Ehnert et al. (75)	24	10	10	HCT 300% decrease	HCT 20% increase	$p < 0.05$
Gillies et al. (76)	26	10	3	HCT 25% decrease	HCT 17% decrease	NS
Walshaw and Evans (77)	39	34	18	Meds 90% decrease; HCT 400% decrease	meds 11% decrease; HCT no change	$p < 0.05$ $p < 0.01$
Kneist et al. (78)	20	20	12	syx 47% decrease	syx no change	$p < 0.01$
Carswell et al. (79)	49	49	6	syx 32% decrease	syx no change	$p < 0.05$ $p < 0.05$
Mites unchanged						
Burr et al. (80)	53	9	24	syx no change	syx no change	NS
Korsgaard (81)	46	30	6	syx 67% decrease	syx 17% decrease	NS
Frederick et al. (82)	31	9	3	syx 33% decrease	syx 50% decrease	NS
Marks et al. (84)	35	25	6	syx 4% decrease	syx 3% decrease	NS
Dietmann et al. (83)	23	10	12	syx 41% decrease	syx 45% decrease	NS

[a]HCT = histamine challenge test (results expressed as dose causing 20% fall in FEV_1); meds = adrenergic medication doses; syx = symptom score.

gen levels were not reduced significantly and symptoms were unchanged (80–84). The evidence from controlled clinical trials is supported by uncontrolled trials showing similar effects (85,86) as well as a controlled trial showing that the incidence of asthma in children can be reduced with indoor allergen avoidance measures (87). Since avoidance measures for other allergens were not mentioned, it must be concluded that reducing exposure to a single important allergen can modify disease without other exposure changes.

VI. Acute Airway Response

The other experimental evidence supporting the relationship between environmental allergens and asthma comes from bronchoprovocation studies. Bronchoprovocation challenges have been conducted by administering aqueous extracts of various allergen vectors in increasing doses until a 20% change in FEV_1 is achieved; results are expressed as the $PD_{20}FEV_1$ or alternatively as the extract concentration causing a 20% change (88,89). Nasal challenges with nebulized solutions cause increased concentrations of proinflammatory mediators, such as histamine, prostaglandin (PGD2), leukotrienes (LTC/D/E), and mast cells with esterase activity for a synthetic substrate tosyl arginine methyl ester (TAME esterase), in nasal lavages as well as acute nasal obstruction (90). Although the nebulized solutions bear little physical resemblance to environmental airborne allergen vectors, such as house dust mite allergens, these challenges have shown that the IgE-dependent airway response is characterized by an immediate response lasting 30–60 min and a late-phase response that begins within 2–4 hr and is maximal at 8 hr (91). Also, it has been shown that the airway response depends on the level of specific IgE antibody as measured by skin test (92,93), RAST, or the response of sensitized basophils (93). The asthmatic response also depends on nonspecific bronchial hyperresponsiveness (86). This hyperresponsiveness relates to the level of IgE (57) and to the number of positive skin tests to environmental allergens other than the challenge allergen (55). After a late-phase allergen-induced asthma response, airway hyperresponsiveness may increase for several days (92).

A disadvantage of these nebulized challenge procedures is that they are a poor model of environmental exposure to house dust mite allergens. An asthmatic response can be induced readily in persons who are sensitized but do not have chronic asthma (93,94). Another disadvantage of this system is that the doses administered in the test bear no relationship to naturally occurring vectors, so that they cannot be used to set symptomatic thresholds for workplace or home abatement strategies. While it is possible to reduce house dust mite allergen concentrations with vigorously applied environmental control measures, the allergens are not entirely eliminated. Further studies will be necessary to understand the significance of naturally occurring exposure to the residual low concentrations of house dust mite allergens found in homes after effective control measures have been instituted.

VII. Environmental Control Measures

Environmental control measures can reduce house dust mite allergen exposure (70–87). Environmental control measures can be divided into

1. Most important
2. Important but difficult to institute
3. Of questionable importance

The most important measures to control house dust mite allergen exposure include

1. Installing mattress- and pillow-encasings impervious to allergens.
2. Thoroughly vacuuming the mattress and the base of the bed and encasing the mattress, pillow, blanket, and box spring in plastic covers. (Remove dust from the plastic covers weekly using an effective vacuum cleaner.)
3. Washing the sheets and mattress pads in hot water (> 130°F) weekly.
4. Vacuuming carpets and stuffed furniture with a double-bagged, efficient vacuum cleaner once a week.
5. Removing objects from the bedroom that collect dust, such as stuffed animals, drapes, and toys.

Difficult-to-institute measures for controlling house dust mite allergen exposure include

1. Applying an acaricide such as benzyl benzoate and/or a denaturing agent such as tannic acid to carpets and upholstered furniture.
2. Dehumidifying the entire home or the bedroom to <50% relative humidity.
3. Keeping air conditioning set at the lowest level possible (about 70°F).
4. Removing carpets.

Measures of questionable or no importance include

1. Using room air cleaner device.
2. Using a central air filter system.
3. Cleaning air ducts.

These last three methods are usually not helpful because house dust mite allergens do not freely circulate in the air in quantity and therefore are not available to be filtered. Second, house dust mites do not reside in air ducts but rather are found in bedding and carpets.

Effective house dust mite allergen avoidance will never be achieved by using a single control measure: Various methods are required to affect the multiple factors that facilitate high indoor allergen levels.

References

1. Tovey ER, Chapman MD, Platts-Mills TAE. Mite faeces are a major source of house dust allergen. Nature 1981; 289:592–593.
2. Giesler W, Maasch HJ, Wahl R. Kinetics of allergen release from house dust mite allergen Dermatophagoides pteronyssinus. J Allergy Clin Immunol 1986; 77:24–31.
3. Platts-Mills TAE, Heymann PW, Longbottom JL, Wilkins SR. Airborne allergens associated with asthma: particle sizes measured with a cascade impactor. J Allergy Clin Immunol 1986; 77:850–857.
4. Price JA, Polock I, Little SA, Longbottom JL, Warner JO. Measurement of airborne mite antigen in homes of asthmatic children. Lancet 1990; 336:895–897.
5. Reed CE, Swanson MC, Agarwal MK, Yunginger JW. Allergens that cause asthma: identification and quantitation. Chest 1985; 87:40S–44S.
6. Swanson MC, Agarwal MK, Reed CE. An immunochemical approach to indoor aeroallergen quantitation with a new volumetric air sampler: studies with mite, roach, cat, mouse, and guinea pig antigens. J Allergy Clin Immunol 1985; 76:724–729.
7. Swanson MC, Campbell AR, Klauck MJ, Reed CE. Correlations between levels of mite and cat allergens in settled and airborne dust. J Allergy Clin Immunol 1989; 83:776–783.
8. de Blay F, Heymann PW, Chapman MD, Platts-Mills TAE. Airborne dust mite allergens: comparison of group II allergens with group I mite allergen and cat-allergen Fel d 1. J Allergy Clin Immunol. 1991; 88:919–926.
9. Sakaguchi M, Inouye S, Irie T, Miyazawa H, Watanabe M, Yasueda H, Shida T, Nitta H, Chapman MD, Schou C, Aalberse RC. Airborne cat (Fel d I), dog (Can f I), and mite (Der I and Der II) allergen levels in the homes of Japan. J Allergy Clin Immunol 1993; 92:797–802.

10. Platts-Mills TAE, Chapman MD. Dust mites: Immunology, allergic disease and environmental control. J Allergy Clin Immunol 1987; 80:755–775.
11. Ferguson P, Broide DH. Environmental and bronchoalveolar lavage *Dermatophagoides pteronyssinus* antigen levels in atopic asthmatics. Am J Resp Crit Care Med 1995; 151:71–74.
12. Sporik R, Holgate ST, Platts-Mills TAE, Cogswell JJ. Exposure to house-dust mite allergen (Der p I) and the development of asthma in childhood. A prospective study. N Engl J Med 1990; 323:502–507.
13. Lau S, Falkenhurst G, Weber A, Werthmann I, Lind P, Buettner-Goetz P, Wahn U. High mite-allergen exposure increases the risk of sensitization in atopic children and young adults. J Allergy Clin Immunol 1989; 84:718–725.
14. Kuehr J, Frischer T, Meinert R, Barth R, Forster J, Schraub S, Urbanek R, Karmouse W. Mite allergen exposure is a risk for the incidence of specific sensitization. J Allergy Clin Immunol 1994; 94:44–52.
15. Fernandez-Caldas E, Puerta L, Mercado D, Lockey R, Caraballo L. Mite fauna, *Der p* I, *Der f* I and *Blomia tropicalis* allergen levels in a tropical city. Clin Exp Allergy 1993; 23:292–297.
16. Hughes AM. The Mites of Stored Food. Tech Bull 9. London: Her Majesty's Stationery Office, Minister of Agriculture and Fisheries, 1961.
17. Voorhost, R, Spieksma, FTM, Varekamp, H. Is a mite (Dermatophagoides sp.) the producer of the house dust allergen? Allergie Asthma 1964; 10:329.
18. Platts-Mills TAE, Vervloet D, Thomas WR, Aalberse RC, Chapman MD. Indoor allergens and asthma: report of the Third International Workshop. J Allergy Clin Immunol 1997; 100:S1–S24.
19. Dilworth RJ, Chua KJ, Thomas WR. Sequence analysis of cDNA coding for a major house dust mite allergen, Der f 1. Clin Exp Allergy 1991; 21:25–32.
20. Chua KY, Stewart GA, Thomas WR, Simpson RJ, Dilworth RJ, Plozza TM, Turner KJ. Sequence analysis of cDNA coding for a major house dust mite allergen, Der p 1. J Exp Med 1988; 167:175–182.
21. Chua KY, Kehal PK, Thomas WR, Vaughan P, Macreadie IG. High-frequency binding of IgE to the Der p 1 allergen expressed in yeast. J Allergy Clin Immunol 1992; 89:95–102.
22. Schulz O, Laing P, Sewell HF, Shakib F. Der p 1, a major allergen of the house dust mite, proteolytically cleaves the low-affinity receptor for human IgE (CD23). Eur J Immunol 1995; 25:3191–3194.
23. Schulz O, Sewell HF, Shakib F. Proteolytic cleavage of CD25, the α subunit of the human T cell interleukin 2 receptor, by Der p 1, a major mite allergen with cystein protease activity. J Exp Med 1998; 187(2):271–275.
24. Shakib F, Schulz O, Sewell H. A mite subversive: cleavage of CD23 and CD25 by Der p 1 enhances allergenicity. Immunol Today 1998; 19(7):313–316.
25. Heymann PW, Chapman MD, Aalbarse RC, Fox JW, Platts-Mills TAE. Antigenic and structural analysis of group II allergens. Der f II and Der p II from house dust mite *Dermatophagoides spp.* J Allergy Clin Immunol 1989; 83:1055–1068.

26. Trudinger M, Chua KY, Thomas WR. cDNA encoding the major mite allergen *Der f* II. Clin Exp Allergy 1991; 21:33–37.

27. Chua KY, Doyle CR, Simpson RJ, Turner KJ, Stewart GA, Thomas WR. Isolation of cDNA coding for the major mite allergen *Der p* II by IgE plaque immunoassay. Int Arch Allergy Appl Immunol 1990; 91:118–123.

28. Chua KY, Dilworth RJ, Thomas WR. Expression of *Dermatophagoides pteronyssinus* allergen, Der p II, in *Escherichia coli* and the binding studies with human IgE. Int Arch Allergy Appl Immunol 1990; 91:124–129.

29. Chua KY, Greene WK, Kehal P, Thomas WR. IgE binding studies with large peptides expressed from *Der p* II cDNA constructs. Clin Exp Allergy 1991; 21:161–166.

30. Varela J, Ventas P, Carreira J, Barbas JA, Gimenez-Gallego G, Polo F. Primary structure of Lep d 1, the main Lepidoglyphus destructor allergen. Eur J Biochem 1994; 225:93–98.

31. Thomas WR, Smith W. House-dust-mite allergens. Allergy 1998; 53:821–832.

32. van Hage-Hamsten M, Olsson S, Emilson A, Härfast B, Svensson A, Scheynius A. Localisation of major allergens in the house dust mite Lepidoglyphus destructor with confocal laser scanning microscopy. Clin Exp Allergy 1995; 25:536–542.

33. Chua KY, Huang CH, Shen HD, Thomas WR. Analysis of sequence polymorphism of a major mite allergen, Der p 2. Clin Exp Allergy 1996; 26:829–837.

34. Stewart GA, Ward LD, Simpson RJ, Thompson PJ. The group III allergen from the house dust mite *Dermatophagoides pteronyssinus* is a trypsin-like enzyme. J Immunol 1992; 75:29–35.

35. Smith WA, Thomas W. Sequence polymorphism of the *Der p* 3 house dust mite allergen. Clin Exp Allergy 1996; 26:571–579.

36. Lake FR, Ward LD, Simpson RJ, Thompson PJ, Stewart GA. House dust mite derived amylase: allergenicity and physicochemical characterization. J Allergy Clin Immunol 1991; 87:1035–1042.

37. Tovey ER, Johnson MC, Roche AL, Cobon GS, Baldo BA. Cloning and sequencing of a cDNA expressing a recombinant house dust mite protein that binds human IgE and corresponds to an important low molecular weight allergen. J Exp Med 1989; 170:1457–1462.

38. Lin KL, Hsieh KH, Thomas W, Chiang BL, Chua KY. Characterisation of Der p V allergen, cDNA analysis, and IgE-mediated reactivity to the recombinant protein. J Allergy Clin Immunol 1994; 94:989–996.

39. Arruda K, Vailes LD, Platts-Mills AE, Fernandez-Caldas E, Montealegre F, Lin K, Chua KY, Rizzo MC, Naspitz CK, Chapman MD. Sensitization to *Blomia tropicalis* in patients with asthma and identification of allergen Blo t 5. Am J Resp Crit Care Med 1997; 155:343–350.

40. Caraballo LR, Avjioglu A, Marrugo J, Puerta L. Marsh D. Cloning and expression of DNA coding for an allergen with common antibody binding s specificities with three allergens of the house dust mite *Blomia tropicalis*. J Allergy Clin Immunol 1996; 98:573–579.

41. Yasueda H, Mita H, Shida T, Ando T, Dugiyama S, Yamakawa H. Allergens from *Dermatophagoides* with chymotryptic activity. Clin Exp Allergy 1993; 23:384–390.

42. Shen HD, Chua KY, Lin KL, Hsieh KH, Thomas WR. Molecular cloning of a house dust mite allergen with common antibody binding specificities with multiple components in mite extracts. Clin Exp Allergy 1993; 23:934–940.

43. O'Neill G, Donovan GR, Baldo BA. Identification of a major allergen of the house dust mite, *Dermatophagoides pteronyssinus*, homologous with glutathione-S-transferase. Biochim Biophys Acta 1994; 1219:521–524.

44. King C, Simpson RJ Moritz RL, Reed GL, Thompson PJ, Stewart GA. The isolation and characterisation of a novel collagenolytic serine protease allergen (Der p 9) from the dust mite Dermatophagoides pteronyssinus. J Allergy Clin Immunol 1996; 98:739–747.

45. Aki T, Kadoma T, Fujikawa A, et al. Immunochemical characterisation of recombinant and native tropomyosins a new allergen from the house dust mite, D. farinae. J Allergy Clin Immunol 1995; 96:74–83.

46. Asturias JA, Arrilla MC, Gómez-Bayón N, Martínez J, Martínez A, Palacios R. Sequencing and high level expression in E. coli of the tropomyosin allergen Der p 10 from *Dermatophagoides pteronyssinus*. Biochim Biophys Acta 1998; 1397:27–30.

47. Witteman A, Akkerdaas J, Leeuwen J, van der Zee J, Aalberse RC. Identification of a cross-reactive allergen (presumably tropomyosin) in shrimp, mite and insects. Int Arch Allergy Immunol 1994; 105:56–61.

48. Tsai L-C, Chao P-L, Shen H-D, et al. Isolation and characterisation of a novel 98-kDa *Dermatophagoides farinae* allergen. J Allergy Clin Immunol 1998.

49. Puerta L, Caraballo L, Fernández-Caldas E, et al. Nucleotide sequence analysis of a complementary DNA coding for a *Blomia tropicalis* allergen. J Allergy Clin Immunol 1997; 98:932–937.

50. Caraballo L, Puerta L, Jiménez S, et al. Cloning and IgE binding of a recombinant allergen from the mite *Blomia tropicalis*, homologous with fatty acid-binding proteins. Int Arch Allergy Immunol 1997; 112:341–347.

51. Bradford-Hill A. Environment and disease: association or causation? Proc Roy Soc Med 1965; 58:295–300.

52. Platts-Mills TAE, Thomas WR, Aalberse RC, Vervloet D, Chapman MD. Dust mite allergens and asthma: report of a second international workshop. J Allergy Clin Immunol 1992; 89:1046–1060.

53. Sporik R, Chapman MD, Platts-Mills TAE. Review: house dust mite exposure as a cause of asthma. Clin Exp Allergy 1992; 22:897–906.

54. Platts-Mills TAE. Allergen-specific treatment of asthma III. Am Rev Respir Dis 1993; 148:553–555.

55. Peat JK, Britton WJ, Salome CM, Woolcock AJ. Bronchial hyperresponsiveness in two populations of Australian school children. III. Effect of exposure to environmental allergens. Clin Allergy 1987; 17:291–300.

56. Pollart SM, Reid MJ, Fling JA, Chapman MD, Platts-Mills TAE. Epidemiology of emergency room asthma in northern California: association with IgE antibody to ryegrass pollen. J Allergy Clin Immunol 1988; 82:224–230.

57. Burrows B, Martinez FD, Halonen M, Barbee RA, Cline MG. Association of asthma with serum IgE levels and skin-test reactivity to allergens. N Engl J Med 1989; 320:271–277.

58. Friedhoff LR, Meyers DA, Marsh DG. A genetic-epidemiologic study of human immune responsiveness to allergens in an industrial population: II. The association of skin sensitivity, total serum IgE, age, sex, and the reporting of allergies in a stratified random sample. J Allergy Clin Immunol 1984; 73:490–499.

59. Gelber LE, Seltzer LH, Bouzoukis JK, Pollart SM, Chapman MD, Platts Mills TAE. Sensitization and exposure to indoor allergens as risk factors for asthma among patients presenting to hospital. Am Rev Respir Dis 1993; 147:573–578.

60. Call RS, Smith TF, Morris E, Chapman MD, Platts-Mills TAE. Risk factors for asthma in inner city children. J Ped 1993; 121:862–866.

61. Reid MJ, Moss RB, Hsu YP, Kwasnicki IM, Commerford TM, Nelson BL. Seasonal asthma in northern California: allergic causes and efficacy of immunotherapy. J Allergy Clin Immunol 1986; 78:590–600.

62. Sporik R, Ingram JM, Price W, Sussman JH, Honsinger RW, Platts-Mills TAE. Association of asthma with serum IgE and skin test reactivity to allergens among children living at high altitude: tickling the dragon's breath. J Resp Crit Care Med 1995; 151:1338–1392.

63. Rosenstreich DL, Eggleston, PA, Kattan M, Baker D, Slavin RG, Gergen P, Mitchell H, McNiff-Mortimer K, Lynn H, Ownby D, Malveaux F. Role of cockroach allergy and exposure to cockroach allergen in causing morbidity among inner-city children with asthma. N Engl J Med 1997; 336:1356–1363.

64. Gleich GJ, Jacob GL, Yunginger JW, Henderson LL. Measurement of the absolute levels of IgE antibodies in patients with ragweed hay fever: effect of immunotherapy on seasonal changes and relationship to IgG antibodies. J Allergy Clin Immunol 1977; 60:188–198.

65. Smith TF, Kelly LB, Heymann PW, Wilkins SR, Platts-Mills TAE. Natural exposure and serum antibodies to house dust mite of mite-allergic children with asthma in Atlanta. J Allergy Clin Immunol 1985; 76:782–788.

66. Soliman MY, Rosenstreich DL. Natural immunity to dust mites in adults with chronic asthma. Am Rev Respir Dis 1986; 134:962–968.

67. Platts-Mills TAE, Longbottom J, Edwards J, Cockcroft A, Wilkins S. Occupational asthma and rhinitis related to laboratory rats: serum IgG and IgE antibodies to the rat urinary allergen. J Allergy Clin Immunol 1987; 79:505–515.

68. Vervloet D, Penaud A, Razzouk H, Senft M, Arnaud A, Boutin C, Charpin J. Altitude and house dust mites. 1982; 69:290–294.

69. Eggleston PA, Rosenstreich D, Lynn H, Gergen P, Baker D, Kattan M, Mortimer KM, Mitchell H, Ownby D, Slavin R, Malveaux F. Relationship of indoor aller-

gen exposure to skin test sensitivity in inner city children with asthma. J Allergy Clin Immunol 1998; 102:563–570.

70. Platts-Mills TAE, Tovey ER, Mitchell EB, Moszoro H, Nock P, Wilkins SR. Reduction of bronchial hyperreactivity during prolonged allergen avoidance. Lancet 1982; 2:675–678.

71. Peroni D, Boner AL, Vallone G, Antolini I, Warner JO. Effective allergen avoidance at high altitude reduces allergen-induced bronchial hyperresponsiveness. Am J Resp Crit Care Med 1994; 149:1442–1446.

72. Boner AL, Peroni D, Sette L, Vallarte EA, Piacentini G. Effects of allergen-exposure avoidance on inflammation in asthmatic children. Allergy 1993; 48:119–124.

73. Colloff MJ, Ayres J, Carswell F, Howarth PH, Merrett TG, Mitchell EB, Walshaw MJ, Warner JO, Warner Jill A, Woodcock AA. The control of dust mites and domestic pets. A position paper. Clin Exp Allergy 1992; 22(Suppl):1–28.

74. Thompson PJ, Stewart GA. House-dust mite reduction strategies in the treatment of asthma. Med J Aust 1989; 151:408–411.

75. Ehnert B, Lau-Schadendorf SM, Weber A, Buettner P, Schou C, Wahn U. Reducing domestic exposure to dust mite allergen reduces bronchial hyperreactivity in sensitive children with asthma. J Allergy Clin Immunol 1992; 90:135–138.

76. Gillies DRN, Littlewood JM, Sarsfield JK. Controlled trial of house dust mite avoidance in children with mild to moderate asthma. Clin Allergy 1987; 17:105–111.

77. Walshaw MJ, Evans CC. Allergen avoidance in house dust mite sensitive adult asthma. Quart J Med 1986; 58:199–215.

78. Kneist FM, Young E, van Praag MCG, Helianthe HV, Kort SM, Koers WJ, Van Bronswijk F, Van Bronswijk JEMH. Clinical evaluation of a double-blind dust avoidance trial with mite-allergic rhinitic patients. Clin Exp Allergy 1991; 21:39–47.

79. Carswell F, Birmingham K, Olivier J, Crewes A, Weeks J. The respiratory effects of reduction of mite allergen in the bedrooms of asthmatic children—a double-blind controlled trial. Clin Exp Allergy. 1996; 26:386–396.

80. Burr ML, Dean BV, Merrett TG, Neale E, St Leger AS, Verrier-Jones ER. Effects of anti-mite measures on children with mite sensitive asthma: a controlled trial. Thorax 1980; 35:506–512.

81. Korsgaard J. Preventive measures in mite asthma: a controlled trial. Allergy 1983; 38:93–102.

82. Frederick JM, Warner JO, Jessop WJ, Enander I, Warner JA. Effect of a bed covering system in children with asthma and house dust mite hypersensitivity. Eur Resp J 1997; 10:361–368.

83. Dietemann A, Bessot J-C, Hoyet C, Ott M, Verot A, Pauli G. A double-blind, placebo controlled trial of solidified benzyl benzoate applied in dwellings of asthmatic patients sensitive to mites: clinical efficacy and effect on mite allergens. J Allergy Clin Immunol 1991; 91:738–746.

84. Marks G, Tovey ER, Green W, Shearer M, Aalome C, Woodcock AJ. House dust mite allergen avoidance: a randomized controlled trial of surface treatment and encasement of bedding. Clin Exp Allergy 1994; 24:1078–1083.

85. Murray AB, Ferguson AC. Dust-free bedrooms in the treatment of asthmatic children with house dust or house dust mite allergy: a clinical trial. Pediatrics 1983; 71:418–422.

86. Platts-Mills TAE, Tovey ER, Mitchell EB, Moszoro H, Nock P, Wilkins SR. Reduction of bronchial hyperreactivity during prolonged allergen avoidance. Lancet 1982; 2:675–678.

87. Hide DW, Matthews S, Matthews L, Stevens M, Ridout S, Twiselton R, Gant C, Arshad SH. Effect of allergen avoidance in infancy on allergic manifestations at age two years. J Allergy Clin Immunol 1994; 93:842–846.

88. Townley RG, Dennis M, Itkin IH. Comparative action of acetyl-beta-methyl choline, histamine, and pollen antigens in subjects with hay fever, and patients with bronchial asthma. J Allergy 1965; 35:121–137.

89. Cockcroft DW, Ruffin RE, Frith PA, Cartier A, Juniper EF, Dolovich J, Hargreave FE. Determinants of allergen-induced asthma: dose of allergen, circulating IgE antibody concentration, and bronchial responsiveness to inhaled histamine. Am Rev Respir Dis. 1979; 120:1053–1058.

90. Naclerio RM, Meier HL, Kagey-Sobotka A, Adkinson NF Jr, Meyers DA, Norman PS, Lichtenstein LM. Mediator release after nasal challenge with allergen. Am Rev Respir Dis 1983; 128:597–602.

91. O'Byrne PM, Dolovich J, Hargreave FE. Late asthmatic response. Am Rev Respir Dis 1987; 136:740–751.

92. Cockcroft DW, Ruffin RE, Dolovich J, Hargreave FE. Allergen-induced increase in nonallergic bronchial reactivity. Clin Allergy 1977; 7:503–513.

93. Bruce CA, Rosenthal RR, Lichtenstein LM, Norman PS. Diagnostic tests in ragweed-allergic asthma: a comparison of direct skin tests, leukocyte histamine release and quantitative bronchial challenge. J Allergy 1974; 53:230–239.

94. Permutt S, Rosenthal RR, Norman PS, Menkes HA. Bronchial challenge in ragweed-sensitive patients. In: Lichtenstein LM, Austen KF, eds. Asthma: Physiology, Immunopharmacology and Treatment: A Second International Symposium. New York: Academic Press, 1977:265–281.

4

The Role of Animal Allergens
Assessment and Control

ROBERT A. WOOD

Johns Hopkins University School of Medicine
Baltimore, Maryland

I. Introduction

Animal allergens are well-recognized triggers for acute and chronic asthma
symptoms in both home and work environments. However, although a considerable body of information exists regarding the allergens themselves and their
environmental distribution, less is known about their clinical effects and environmental control. In this chapter we review the animal allergens, what is
known regarding their role in allergic asthma, and strategies that may be incor-
porated to control their effects.

Animal allergens can be divided into two major categories and several
minor categories. The major categories include domestic pets, especially cats
and dogs, and laboratory animals, particularly rats and mice. The bulk of this
chapter deals with these categories. Other categories include farm animals,
birds, exotic pets and zoo animals, and a variety of other rodents that may be
encountered either as household pets or as laboratory animals.

53

II. The Allergens

The major allergens of most domestic and laboratory animals have now been identified and characterized (Table 1). In cats and dogs, hair, dander, and saliva are the major sources of allergen production. Rodents and rodentlike animals have persistent proteinuria, and their urine is the major source of allergen production, while hair, dander, and saliva are less important sources of rodent allergens. Hair and dander also appear to be the major sources of allergens in cows and horses.

At least 12 proteins of cat origin have been found to be allergenic, with one major cat allergen, Fel d 1, being by far the most important (1–4). It is a

Table 1 Major Allergens of Domestic and Laboratory Animals

Animal	Allergen	MW (kDa)	Source
Cat (*Felis domesticus*)	Fel d 1	17	Hair, dander, saliva
Dog (*Canis familiaris*)	Can f 1	25	Hair, dander, saliva
Mouse (*Mus musculus*)	Mus m 1 (prealbumin)	17	Hair, dander, urine
	Mus m 2	16	Hair, dander
Rat (*Rattus norvegicus*)	Rat n 1 A (prealbumin)	20	Hair, dander, urine, saliva
	Rat n 1 B (a-euglobulin)	16	Hair, dander, urine, saliva
Guinea pig (*Cavia porcellus*)	Cav p 1		Hair, dander, urine
	Cav p 2		Hair, dander, urine
Rabbit (*Oryctolagus cuniculus*)	Ory c 1	17	Hair, dander, saliva
	Ory c 2		Hair, dander, urine
Cow (*Bos domesticus*)	Bos d 1	25	Hair, dander
	Bos d 2	22	Hair, dander
	Bos d 3	22	Hair, dander
Horse (*Equus callabus*)	Equ c 1	19	Hair, dander
	Equ c 2	51	Hair, dander
	Equ c 3	31	Hair, dander

tetrameric polypeptide with a molecular weight of 17–18 kDa. Fel d 1 is produced in hair follicles and, to a lesser extent, in the salivary glands. Male cats produce more Fel d 1 than female cats, and the allergen production of male cats is reduced after castration (3,5,6).

Several dog-specific proteins have been shown to possess antigenic activity (7–10). The most important of these, Can f 1, is produced in hair, dander, and saliva. It is a polypeptide with a molecular weight of 25 kDa. Dog albumin is a minor allergen, and another immunologically distinct allergen with a molecular weight of 19 kDa has also been identified (10).

At least three relevant mouse allergens have been identified (11–14). The major allergen, Mus m 1, which was previously designated MUP (major urinary protein) or Ag 1, is a prealbumin with a molecular weight of 17 kDa. It is found in urine as well as in hair follicles and dander. Mus m 1 is produced by normal liver cells, and levels in serum and urine are about four times higher in male mice than in female mice. A second mouse allergen, Mus m 2, is a glycoprotein with a molecular weight of 16 kDa that originates from hair follicles. This allergen is not found in urine. A final mouse allergen is albumin, which has been shown to be allergenic in about 30% of mouse-allergic patients.

Rats produce two major allergens that are found in urine as well as in hair, dander, and saliva (14–16). Rat n 1A is a prealbumin with a molecular weight of 20–21 kDa, while Rat n 1B is an α-euglobulin with a molecular weight of 16–17 kDa. These two allergens have some cross-reactivity. Rat n 1B is primarily a male allergen. Like mouse albumin, rat albumin has been shown to have some antigenic activity, with 24% of rat-allergic patients exhibiting sensitivity to albumin.

Allergens from guinea pig have not been extensively characterized, although two antigenic fragments, Cav p 1 and Cav p 2, have been identified (17,18). Both of these allergens are found in urine, hair, and dander. Rabbit allergens have also not been well characterized, although two have been identified (19). Ory c 1 is found in the hair, dander, and saliva, while Ory c 2 is found in the hair, dander, and urine.

The allergens of both cows and horses have also been identified and characterized. All of their major allergens are found in hair and dander. The three major cow allergens, Bos d 1, Bos d 2, and Bos d 3, have molecular weights of approximately 25, 22, and 22 kDa respectively (20). Three major horse allergens have also been identified, Equ c 1 (19 kDa), Equ c 2 (51 kDa), and Equ c 3 (31 kDa) (21).

III. Environmental Distribution

Many of these allergens have also been characterized with regard to their environmental distribution and aerodynamic properties. Cat and dog allergens have been best characterized in home environments, although they have also been studied in schools and other settings. Rodent allergens can certainly be present in household environments, but they have been studied primarily in laboratory settings. Cows, horses, and other farm animals are sources of primarily occupational allergens, although they may be present in home environments in some settings (22).

A number of studies have investigated the distribution of cat and dog allergens in home environments (23–29). Using air and settled dust analysis, it has been shown that levels of cat and dog allergen are clearly highest in homes housing these animals. However, it is also clear from a number of studies that the vast majority of homes contain cat and dog allergens even if a pet has never lived there. While most of these non-animal-containing environments have relatively low allergen levels compared to those with a cat or dog, it is not uncommon to find rather high levels in some of these homes. This widespread distribution is presumed to occur primarily through passive transfer of allergen from one environment to another. These allergens appear to be very sticky and, unlike dust mite allergens, can be found in high levels on walls and other surfaces within homes (28).

The characteristics of airborne cat and dog allergens have also been extensively studied. Cat allergen has been shown to be carried on particles that range from less than 1 μm to greater than 20 μm in mean aerodynamic diameter (30,31). Although estimates have varied, studies agree that at least 15% of airborne cat allergen is carried on particles smaller than 5 μm. Airborne levels and particle size distribution for dog allergen appear to be very similar to those of cat allergen, with about 20% of airborne allergens being carried on particles less than 5 μm in diameter (29).

Cat and dog allergens can also be detected in air samples from all homes with cats and dogs and from many homes that do not house a cat or dog. Bollinger et al. (32) detected airborne cat allergen in 10 out of 40 air samples from homes without cats, and Custovic et al. (29) found airborne dog allergen in 11 of 36 homes without dogs. In addition, when a subset of those homes in the Bollinger study were reinvestigated on a weekly basis for 4 weeks, all of them had detectable airborne cat allergen on at least one occasion, and when the original 40 air samples were reanalyzed using a more sensitive assay, all 40 homes were found to contain airborne cat allergen (33).

In an attempt to determine the clinical significance of this unsuspected cat exposure, patients were challenged in an experimental cat exposure facility to varying levels of cat allergen (32). It was found that allergen levels of less than 100 ng/m^3 were capable of inducing upper and lower respiratory symptoms as well as significant pulmonary function changes. These levels are similar to those found in a subset of homes without cats as well as homes with cats, suggesting that even patients without known cat exposure may be exposed to clinically significant concentrations of airborne cat allergen on a regular basis.

The widespread distribution of cat and dog allergens is further demonstrated by several studies looking at allergen levels in schools and other public buildings (34–37). These studies have demonstrated moderately high levels of cat and dog allergen in schools and on the clothing of schoolchildren. A relationship between the number of cat owners in a classroom and the settled dust cat allergen level in that room has also been demonstrated. Most important, a strong case was made in a study of Swedish schools by Munir et al. (34) that the levels of cat and dog allergens in school classrooms are high enough to induce sensitization and cause perennial symptoms in children with asthma who are sensitized to cat and dog allergens.

Mouse and rat allergens have been best studied in laboratory settings. Airborne mouse allergen has been shown to reside on particles ranging from 3.3 to 10 μm in one study (38) and from 6 to 18 μm in another study (11). Ohman et al. (38) also found that the particle size distribution was different, ranging from 0.43 to 3.3 μm, in rooms that did not contain mice. Airborne mouse allergen levels in the Ohman study ranged from 16.6 to 563 ng/m^3 in rooms with mice and from 1.2 to 2.7 ng/m^3 in rooms without mice, with the highest levels being associated with direct mouse contact. In another study, levels ranged from 1.8 to 825 ng/m^3 and varied with both the number of mice and the degree of work activity in the rooms (39). A final study demonstrated higher allergen levels in rooms with male mice than in rooms with female mice (Mus m 1 3050 pg/m^3 versus 317 pg/m^3) (40).

Airborne rat allergens are carried on particles ranging from <1 μm to >20 μm, with the majority of allergen on particles less than 7 μm in diameter (41,42). Levels of airborne rat allergen have been studied in a variety of settings, and it is clear that exposure is highly dependent on the type of activity being performed, with cleaning and feeding being associated with the highest levels of exposure (43,44).

Studies have also been performed on rat-allergic individuals to determine the levels of exposure that would be expected to induce symptoms. In one study of 12 rat-allergic volunteers, all subjects experienced nasal symptoms and five experienced a decrease in FEV_1 of greater than 10% during a 1 hr exposure with airborne Rat n 1 levels ranging from <1.5 to >310 ng/m^3 (44). In a follow-up study, exposures to high allergen levels (cage cleaning, mean Rat n 1 166 ng/m^3) were compared to exposures to low allergen levels (quiet sitting in a rat vivarium, mean Rat n 1 9.6 ng/m^3) in 17 subjects (45). Although no firm cutoff for a "safe" allergen level could be determined, a clear dose response was demonstrated, with both upper and lower airway responses being highly dependent on airborne allergen levels.

Much less information is available about other laboratory animal allergens. Airborne guinea pig allergens have been measured using RAST inhibition, which demonstrated urine and pelt allergen levels of 17 and 90 ng/m^3, respectively (18). Forty percent of the guinea pig allergen particles were found to be less than 0.8 μm in diameter.

IV. Clinical Aspects

Sensitivity to cat and dog allergens has been shown to occur in 22–67% of asthmatic patients, and in some settings these are clearly the dominant indoor allergens (23,25,46,47). This fact was best demonstrated in the study by Ingram et al. (23) conducted in Los Alamos, New Mexico. In this environment, where cat and dog allergens are common but exposure to dust mite and cockroach allergens is rare, IgE antibody to cat and dog was detected in 62% and 67%, respectively, of asthmatic children. The presence of these IgE antibodies was highly associated with asthma, whereas sensitivity to mite or cockroach allergen was not associated with asthma.

It has also been shown that intense exposure to cat allergen early in life leads to an increased risk of developing cat sensitivity (48). Warner et al. (48) found that 88% of 21 asthmatic children who had had a cat in their home at the time of birth developed cat sensitivity, compared to 36% of children whose homes contained no cat through the first year of life. On the other hand, it is clear from that and other studies that cat sensitivity is common even in the absence of obvious exposure. This is most likely related to the widespread distribution of cat and dog allergens even in homes that do not contain pets.

It has also been demonstrated that cat sensitivity is associated with asthma in older men and that cat sensitization in that population may predict the development of airway hyperresponsiveness (49). In that study, Litonjua et al. (49) reported that cat sensitivity was much more common in a group of asthmatic men with a mean age of 61 years than in controls (23.9% versus 4.4%, p < 0.001). In addition, they found that the development of new-onset airway hyperresponsiveness to methacholine was more common is subjects with established cat sensitivity than in those without cat sensitivity (18.2% versus 6.1%, $p = 0.059$).

The best demonstrations of the relationship of acute asthma to animal allergens come from the cat and rat challenge studies noted above. These studies clearly demonstrate that asthma symptoms and substantial pulmonary changes are common, with acute allergen exposure in sensitized subjects (32,34,45,50–52). Airway hyperresponsiveness to methacholine has also been shown to be strong predictor of an asthmatic response. While dose responses have been demonstrated in both cat and rat challenges, specific thresholds for airborne allergen levels at which an asthmatic response will either occur or not occur have not been defined.

The specific relationship of cat and dog allergens to chronic asthma has been less well characterized. Clinically, it is clear that many patients with asthma and cat or dog sensitivity have more severe disease because of ongoing exposure to a family pet. However, it has also become clear from the studies noted above that many patients have significant cat and dog exposure that they are not even aware of. It is therefore likely that animal allergens are important causes of chronic airway inflammation even in patients without known exposure. Further study will be needed to clarify this issue.

It is also clear that individuals who are in regular contact with rats, mice, and other laboratory animals commonly develop sensitivity to those animals. As such, laboratory animal allergy represents a major occupational illness to the thousands of technicians, animal caretakers, physicians, and scientists whose work requires such exposure. Allergy to rats and mice is the most common clinical problem, with sensitivity to rats being reported in 12–31% of laboratory workers (53–56) and sensitivity to mice occurring in 10–32% of workers (55–57).

While allergy to other animals in the workplace is overall less common than allergy to rats and mice, this is primarily because these other animals are used less often, not because they are necessarily less allergenic. Allergy to guinea pigs, rabbits, hamsters, gerbils, dogs, cats, pigs, cows, horses, sheep, and monkeys will therefore occur in workers exposed to these animals. In a very large epidemiological study involving over 5000 laboratory animal workers in Japan, symptoms were reported in 26% of workers exposed to mice, compared to 25% for rats, 31% for guinea pigs, 30% for rabbits, 26% for hamsters, 25% for dogs, 30% for cats, and 24% for monkeys (56).

The onset of symptoms after beginning to work with laboratory animals can also range widely. Cullison et al. (55) prospectively followed a group of workers without previous rat exposure and found a range of less than 30 days to 1369 days from the time of employment to the onset of symptoms. The mean duration of employment before symptom onset was 365 days for chest symptoms, 214 days for nose and eye symptoms, and 335 days for skin symptoms.

Symptoms in laboratory animal allergy range from mild skin irritation to severe asthma. Overall, the most common symptom is allergic rhinoconjunctivitis with itchy, watery eyes and nasal congestion, rhinorrhea, and sneezing (55,56). These symptoms have been reported to occur in up to 80% of symptomatic workers. Skin reactions, most commonly contact urticaria or pruritic maculopapular rashes, are typically next most prevalent, occurring in about 40% of symptomatic individuals. Asthmatic symptoms are reported in 20–30% of symptomatic workers. It is also important to recognize, however, that the majority of symptomatic workers have more than one type of symptom. This is especially true of asthma, which rarely occurs in the absence of upper respiratory symptoms.

V. Environmental Control of Animal Allergens

At the present time, specific information on the control of animal allergens is still relatively limited, especially compared to what is known about the control of dust mite allergens. In particular, there are still no convincing studies on the clinical benefits of environmental control measures for animal allergens. While it is assumed that removing an animal from the home will lead to clinical improvement in patients who have disease related to their pet, even this has not been proven. Even fewer data are available regarding the potential benefits of methods that might be used in lieu of animal removal. Cat allergen is specifically discussed here because the most information is available regarding this important allergen. Most of the information should be applicable to other allergens, although a great deal of study will need to be done before that statement can be made conclusively.

To begin, it should be stated that in any asthmatic patient who is known to be cat-sensitive and whose asthma is believed to be related to any significant degree to a pet cat, the most appropriate recommendation is to remove the cat from the home. This is clearly the correct advice from a medical standpoint, and healthcare providers should not shy away from strenuously recommending it. A number of potential alternative measures are also discussed here, however, because of the high proportion of patients who are either reluctant or completely unwilling to remove a household pet.

Once a cat has been removed from the home, it is important to recognize that the clinical benefit may not be seen for a period of at least several months, since allergen levels fall quite slowly after cat removal (27). In most homes, levels in settled dust will have fallen to those seen in homes without cats within 4–6 months of cat removal. Levels may fall much more quickly if extensive environmental control measures are undertaken, such as removal of carpets, upholstered furniture, and other reservoirs from the home, while in other homes the process may be considerably slower. This information points to the fact that thorough and repeated cleaning will be required once the animal has been removed. It has also been shown that cat allergen may persist in mattresses for years after a cat has been removed from a home (58), so that new bedding or impermeable encasements must therefore also be recommended.

A number of studies have investigated other measures that might help to reduce cat allergen exposure without removing the animal from the home. De Blay et al. (59) demonstrated significant reductions in airborne Fel d 1 with a combination of air filtration, cat washing, vacuum cleaning, and removal of furnishings, although these results were based on a small sample size and did not include any measure of clinical effect. When cat washing was evaluated separately in that study, dramatic reductions in airborne Fel d 1 were seen after cat washes. Subsequent studies, however, have presented conflicting results. Klucka et al. (60) studied both cat washing and Allerpet/c (Allerpet, Inc., New York, NY) and found no benefit from either treatment. More recently, Avner et al. (61) studied three different methods of cat washing and found transient reductions in airborne cat allergens after each. There was no sustained benefit, however, with levels returning to baseline within 1 week of washing.

Information is limited as to the clinical benefits of these environmental control measures if one or more cats are allowed to remain in the home. Three fairly recent studies (62–64) evaluated different combinations of control measures, and although all showed reductions in allergen levels, clinical effects were less consistent. Of the first two studies, thus far only reported in abstract form, one showed a clear benefit while the second showed benefit only in the group in which environmental control was done along with intranasal steroid treatment. The third study (64) evaluated a combination of a HEPA air cleaner in the patient's bedroom, mattress and pillow covers, and restricting the cat from the bedroom. While airborne allergen levels were reduced, no significant differences were detected between the active and placebo filter groups in any clinical parameter, including symptom scores, peak flow rates, medication requirements, pulmonary function studies, or methacholine challenge. It therefore still remains to be seen whether allergen exposure can be sufficiently reduced by any combination of environmental control measures to produce a clinical effect in the absence of cat removal.

In families who insist on keeping their pets, the following should be recommended pending more definitive studies. The animals should be restricted to one area of the home and certainly kept out of the patient's bedroom. HEPA or electrostatic air cleaners should be used, especially in the patient's bedroom. Carpets and other reservoirs for allergen collection should be removed whenever possible, again focusing on the patient's bedroom. Finally, mattress and pillow covers should be routinely employed. Although tannic acid has been shown to reduce cat allergen levels (65,66), the effects are modest and short-lived when a cat is present so that this treatment should not be routinely recommended. Similarly, cat washing appears to be of such transient benefit that it is not likely to add significantly to the other avoidance measures.

VI. Immunotherapy

Immunotherapy with cat and dog allergens has been evaluated in a number of well-controlled studies over the past 20 years (67–74). Most of these studies have shown a positive effect, particularly for cat allergen, and animal allergy is typically included on the list of conditions for which immunotherapy has been proven effective (75–77). However, the outcome of most of these studies has been based on challenge studies, and there is still relatively little information regarding the benefits of animal allergen immunotherapy for the average patient with asthma.

The most useful data on animal dander immunotherapy have come from the series of studies by Hedlin, Sundin, and colleagues in Sweden (71–74). They have now had the opportunity to follow a group of subjects for 5 years after the completion of a 3 year course of cat or dog immunotherapy. In the initial 2 years of immunotherapy, significant reductions in specific bronchial reactivity to cat and dog were demonstrated, as were subjective reports of symptoms experienced upon exposure to cats and dogs. Possibly even more significant, nonspecific bronchial reactivity was significantly reduced in the subjects treated with cat immunotherapy. In the 5 year follow-up, all subjects still reported either no change in symptoms or increased tolerance on exposure to cats or dogs. In contrast, however, 17 of the 19 subjects who underwent bronchial allergen challenges had increased sensitivity compared to when treatment was stopped, and the results were no longer different than when the therapy was started.

Based on the available data, which have demonstrated at best a ten-fold improvement in bronchial challenge responses after immunotherapy, it is most likely that the benefits provided will not allow the average patient to live with a cat or dog more comfortably. However, with the emerging data about the widespread exposure that all patients have to both cats and dogs, there may be a greater role for immunotherapy in patients with less intense exposure.

VII. Summary

Animal allergens are widespread and antigenically potent. It is likely that their true contribution to asthma has been thus far underestimated. Further study will be required to more fully define their roles in airway inflammation and the strategies, either immunological or environmental, that will be most effective in combatting their effects.

References

1. Bartholome K, Kisler W, Baer H, et al. Where does cat allergen come from? J Allergy Clin Immunol 1985; 76:503–508.
2. Leitermann K, Ohman JL. Cat allergen 1: biochemical, antigenic, and allergenic properties. J Allergy Clin Immunol 1984; 74:147–154.
3. Charpin C, Mata P, Charpin D, Lavaut M, Allasia C, Vervloet D. Fed d 1 allergen distribution in cat fur and skin. J Allergy Clin Immunol 1991; 88:77–82.
4. Anderson MC, Baer H, Ohman JL. A comparative study of the allergens of cat, urine, serum, saliva, and pelt. J Allergy Clin Immunol 1985; 76:563–569.
5. Jalil-Colome J, Dornelas de Andrade A, Birnbaum J, Casanova D, Mege JL, Lanteaume A, Charpin D, Vervloet D. Sex differences in Fel d I allergen production. J Allergy Clin Immunol 1996; 98:165–168.
6. Wentz PE, Swanson MC, Reed CE. Variability of cat allergen shedding. J Allergy Clin Immunol 1990; 85:94–98.
7. Larsen JN, Ford A, Gjesing B, et al. The collaborative study of the international standard of dog, Canis domesticus, hair/dander extract. J Allergy Clin Immunol 1988; 82:318–325.
8. deGroot H, Goei KGH, VanSwieten P, Aalberse. Affinity purification of a major and a minor allergen from dog extract: serologic activity of affinity-purified Can f 1 and of Can f 1-depleted extracts. J Allergy Clin Immunol 1991; 87:1056–1065.
9. Schou C, Svendsen VG, Lowenstein H. Purification and characterization of the major dog allergen, Can f 1. Clin Exp Allergy 1991; 21:321–328.
10. Spitzauer S, Schwiger C, Anrather J Ebner C, Scheiner O, Kraft D, Rumpold H. Characterization of dog allergens by means of immunoblotting. Int Arch Allergy Immunol 1993; 100:60–67.
11. Price JA, Longbottom J. Allergy to mice. Further characterization of two major mouse allergens (Ag 1 and Ag 3) and immunohistochemical investigations of their sources. Clin Exp Allergy 1990; 20:71–77.

12.   Schumacher MJ. Characterization of allergens from urine and pelts of laboratory mice. Mol Immunol 1980; 17:1087–1095.
13.   Siraganian R, Sandberg A. Characterization of mouse allergens. J Allergy Clin Immunol 1979; 63:435–442.
14.   Longbottom J. Purification and characterization of allergens from the urines of mice and rats. In: Oehling A, ed. Advances in Allergology and Immunology. Oxford, UK: Pergamon, 1980:483–490.
15.   Newman Taylor A, Longbottom J, Pepys J. Respiratory allergy to urine proteins of rats and mice. Lancet 1977; 2:837–839.
16.   Walls A, Longbottom J. Comparison of rat fur, saliva, and other rat allergen extracts by skin testing, RAST and RAST inhibition. J Allergy Clin Immunol 1985; 75:242–251.
17.   Walls A, Taylor A, Longbottom J. Allergy to guinea pig: II. Identification of specific allergens in guinea pig dust by crossed radio-immunoelectrophoresis and investigation of the possible origin. Clin Allergy 1985; 15:535–546.
18.   Swanson M, Agarwal M, Yuninger J, Reed C. Guinea pig derived allergens. Clinicoimmunologic studies. Characterization, airborne quantification and size distribution. Am Rev Respir Dis 1984; 129:844–849.
19.   Warner JA, Longbottom J. Allergy to rabbits. Allergy 1991; 46:481–491.
20.   Prahl P, Bucher D, Plesner T, Weeke B, Lowenstein H. Isolation and partial characterization of three major allergens in an extract from cow hair and dander. Int Arch Allergy Appl Immunol 1982; 67:293–301.
21.   Lowenstein H, Markussen B, Weeke B. Isolation and partial characterization of three major allergens of horse hair and dandruff. Int Arch Allergy Appl Immunol 1976; 51:48–67.
22.   Lind P, Norman PS, Newton M, Lowenstein H, Schwartz B. The prevalence of indoor allergens in the Baltimore area: house dust mite and animal-dander allergens measured by immunochemical techniques. J Allergy Clin Immunol 1987; 80:541– 547.
23.   Ingram JM, Sporik R, Rose G, Honsinger R, Chapman MD, Platts-Mills TAE. Quantitative assessment of exposure to dog (Can f 1) and cat (Fel d 1) allergens: relationship to sensitization and asthma among children living in Los Alamos, New Mexico. J Allergy Clin Immunol 1995; 96:449–456.
24.   Munir AKM, Bjorksten B, Einarsson R, Schou C, Ekstrand-Tobin A, Warner A, Kjellman N-I. Cat (Fel d I), dog (Can f 1) and cockroach allergens in homes of asthmatic children from three climatic zones in Sweden. Allergy 1994; 49:508–516.
25.   Sporik R, Ingram JM, Price W, Sussman JH, Honsinger RW, Platts-Mills TAE. Association of asthma with serum IgE and skin-test reactivity to allergens among children living at high altitude: tickling the dragon's breath. Am J Res Crit Care Med 1995; 151:1388–1392.
26.   Wood RA, Eggleston PA, Ingemann L, Schwartz B, Graveson S, Terry D, Wheeler B, Adkinson NF Jr. Antigenic analysis of household dust samples. Am Rev Respir Dis 1998; 137:358–363.

27. Wood RA, Chapman MD, Adkinson NF, et al. The effect of cat removal on allergen content in household dust samples. J Allergy Clin Immunol 1989; 83:730–734.
28. Wood RA, Mudd KE, Eggleston PA. The distribution of cat and dust mite allergens on wall surfaces. J Allergy Clin Immunol 1992; 89:126–30.
29. Custovic A, Green R, Fletcher A, Smith A, Picjering CAC, Chapman MD, Woodcock A. Aerodynamic properties of the major dog allergen, Can f 1: distribution in homes, concentration, and particle size of allergen in air. Am J Resp Crit Care Med 1997; 155:94–98.
30. Luczynska CM, Li Y, Chapman MD, Platts-Mills TAE. Airborne concentrations and particle size distribution of allergen derived from domestic cats (*Felis domesticus*). Am Rev Respir Dis 1990; 141:361–367.
31. Wood RA, Laheri AN, Eggleston PA. The aerodynamic characteristics of cat allergen. Clin Exp Allergy 1993; 23:733–739.
32. Bollinger ME, Eggleston PA, Wood RA. Cat antigen in homes with and without cats may induce allergic symptoms. J Allergy Clin Immunol 1996; 97:907–914.
33. Bollinger ME, Wood RA, Chen P, Eggleston PA. Measurement of cat allergen levels in the home by use of an amplified ELISA. J Allergy Clin Immunol 1998; 101:124–125.
34. Munir AKM, Einarsson R, Schou C, Dreborg SKG. Allergens in school dust. J Allergy Clin Immunol 1993; 91:1067–1074.
35. Patchett K, Lewis S, Crane J, Fitzharris P. Cat allergen (Fel d 1) levels on school children's clothing and in primary school classrooms in Wellington, New Zealand. J Allergy Clin Immunol 1997; 100:755–759.
36. Dynbendal T, Elsayed S. Dust from carpeted and smooth floors. V. Cat (Fel d 1) and mite (Der p 1 and Der f 1) allergen levels in school dust. Demonstration of basophil histamine release induced by dust from classrooms. Clin Exp Allergy 1992; 22:1100–1106.
37. Custovic A, Taggart SC, Woodcock A. House dust mite and cat allergen in different indoor environments. Clin Exp Allergy 1994; 24:1164–1168.
38. Ohman JL, Hagberg K, MacDonald MR, Jones RR, Paigen BJ, Kacergis JB. Distribution of airborne mouse allergen in a major mouse breeding facility. J Allergy Clin Immunol 1994; 94:810–817.
39. Twiggs JT, Agarwal MK, Dahlberg MJE, Yuninger JW. Immunochemical measurement of airborne mouse allergens in a laboratory animal facility. J Allergy Clin Immunol 1982; 69:522–526.
40. Sakaguchi M, Inouye S, Miyazawa H, Kamimura H, Kimura M, Yamazaki S. Evaluation of countermeasures for reduction of airborne mouse allergens. Lab Animal Sci 1990; 40:613–615.
41. Platts-Mills TAE, Heymann PW, Longbottom JL, Wilkins SR. Airborne allergens associated with asthma: particle sizes carrying dust mite and rat allergens measured with a cascade impactor. J Allergy Clin Immunol 1986; 77:850.
42. Corn M, Koegel A, Hall T, Scott A, Newill A, Evans R. Characteristics of airborne

particles associated with animal allergy in laboratory workers. Ann Occup Hyg 1988; 32:435–446.

43. Eggleston PA, Newill CA, Ansari AA, Pustelnik A, Lou SR, Marsh DG, Longbottom JL, Corn M. Task related variation in airborne concentrations of laboratory animal allergens: studies with Rat n 1. J Allergy Clin Immunol 1989; 84:347–352.

44. Eggleston PA, Ansari AA, Zeimann B, Adkinson NF Jr. Occupational challenge studies with laboratory workers allergic to rats. J Allergy Clin Immunol 1990; 86:63–72.

45. Eggleston PA, Ansari AA, Adkinson NF, Wood RA. Environmental challenge studies in laboratory animal allergy. Am J Respir Crit Care Med 1995; 151:640–646.

46. Rosenstreich DL, Eggleston P, Kattan M, et al. The role of cockroach allergy and exposure to cockroach allergen in causing morbidity among inner-city children with asthma. N Engl J Med 1997; 336:1356–1363.

47. Ohman JL, Kendall S, Lowell FC. IgE antibodies to cat allergens in an allergic population. J Allergy Clin Immunol 1977; 60:317–321.

48. Warner JA, Little SA, Pollock I, et al. The influence of exposure to house dust mite, cat, pollen, and fungal allergens in the home on primary sensitization in asthma. Pediatr Allergy Immunol 1991; 1:79–86.

49. Litonjua AA, Sparrow D, Weiss ST, O'Connor GT, Long AA, Ohman JL. Sensitization to cat allergen is associated with asthma in older men and predicts new-onset airway hyperresponsiveness. Am J Respir Crit Care Med 1997; 156:23–27.

50. Sicherer SH, Wood RA, Eggleston PA. Determinants of airway responses to cat allergen: comparison of environmental challenge to quantitative nasal and bronchial allergen challenge. J Allergy Clin Immunol 1997; 99:798–805.

51. Wood RA, Eggleston PA. Environmental challenges to animal allergens. In: Spector S, ed. Provocation Testing in Clinical Practice. New York: Marcel Dekker, 1994.

52. Wood RA, Eggleston PA. Effects of intranasal steroids on nasal and pulmonary responses to cat exposure. Am J Respir Crit Care Med 1995; 151:315–320.

53. Bland SM, Levine MS, Wilson PD, Fox NL, Rivera JC. Occupational allergy to laboratory animals: an epidemiologic study. J Occup Med 1986; 28:1151–1157.

54. Venables KM, Upton JL, Hawkins ER, Tee RT, Longbottom JL, Newman Taylor AJ. Smoking, atopy, and laboratory animal allergy. Br J Ind Med 1988; 45:667–671.

55. Cullison P, Lowson D, Nieuwenhuijsen MJ, Gordon S, Tee RD, Venables KM, McDonald JC, Newman Taylor AJ. Work related symptoms, sensitization and estimated exposure in workers not previously exposed to laboratory rats. Occup Environ Med 1994; 51:589–592.

56. Aoyama K, Ueda A, Manda F, Matsushita T, Ueda T, Yamauchi C. Allergy to laboratory animals: an epidemiologic study. Br J Ind Med 1992; 49:41–47.

57. Schumacher MJ, Tait BD, Holmes MC. Allergy to murine antigens in a biological research institute. J Allergy Clin Immunol 1981; 68:310–318.
58. Van der Brempt X, Charpin D, Haddi E, da Mata P, Vervloet D. Cat removal and Fel d 1 levels in mattresses. J Allergy Clin Immunol 1991; 87:595–596.
59. De Blay F, Chapman MD, Platts-Mills TAE. Airborne cat allergen (Fel d 1): environmental control with the cat in situ. Am Rev Respir Dis 1991; 143:1334–1339.
60. Klucka CV, Ownby DR, Green J, Zoratti E. Cat shedding of Fel d 1 is not reduced by washings, Allerpet-c spray, or acepromazine. J Allergy Clin Immunol 1995; 95:1164–1171.
61. Avner DB, Perzanowski MS, Platts-Mills TAE, Woodfolk JA. Evaluation of different techniques for washing cats: quantitation of allergen removed from the cat and effect on airborne Fel d 1. J Allergy Clin Immunol 1997; 100:307–312.
62. Bjornsdottir US, Jakobinudottir S, Runarsdottir V, Blondal Th, Juliusson S. Environmental control with cat *in situ*, reduces cat allergen in house dust samples—but does it alter clinical symptoms? [Abstract]. J Allergy Clin Immunol 1997; 99(1):S389.
63. Soldatov D, De Blay F, Greiss P, Charles P, Charpentier C, Ott M, Pauli G. Effects of environmental control measures on patient status and airborne Fel d 1 levels with a cat in situ [Abstract]. J Allergy Clin Immunol 1995; 95(1):263.
64. Wood RA, Flanagan E, Van Natta M, Chen PH, Eggleston PA. A placebo-controlled trial of a HEPA air cleaner in the treatment of cat allergy. Am J Respir Crit Care Med. (In press).
65. Woodfolk JA, Hayden ML, Couture N, Platts-Mills TAE. Chemical treatment of carpets to remove allergen. J Allergy Clin Immunol 1996; 96:325–333.
66. Woodfolk J, Hayden M, Miller J, Rose G, Chapman M, Platts-Mills T. Chemical treatment of carpets to reduce allergen: a detailed study of the effects of tannic acid on indoor allergens. J Allergy Clin Immunol 1994; 94:19–26.
67. Taylor WW, Ohman JL, Lowell FG. Immunotherapy in cat-induced asthma: double blind trial with evauation of bronchial responses to cat allergen and histamine. J Allergy Clin Immunol 1978; 61:283–288.
68. Ohman JL, Findlay SR, Leitermann KM. Immunotherapy in cat-induced asthma: double blind trial with evaluation of in vivo and in vitro responses. J Allergy Clin Immunol 1984; 74:230–235.
69. Valovirta A, Koivikko A, Vanto T. Immunotherapy in allergy to dog: a double-blind clinical study. Ann Allergy 1984; 53:85–91.
70. Van Metre TE, Marsh DG, Adkinson NF, Norman PS. Immunotherapy for cat asthma. J Allergy Clin Immunol 1988; 82:1055–1062.
71. Sundin B, Lilja G, Graff-Lonnevig V, Hedlin G, Heilborn H, Norrlind K, Pagelow KO, Lowenstein H. Immunotherapy with partially purified and standardized animal dander extract: I. Clinical results of a double-blind study on patients with animal-dander asthma. J Allergy Clin Immunol 1986; 77:478–487.
72. Hedlin G, Graff-Lonnevig V, Heilborn H, Lilja G, Norrlind K, Pagelow KO,

Sundin B, Lowenstein H. Immunotherapy with cat- and dog-dander extracts: II. In vivo and in vitro immunologic effects observed in a 1-year double-blind placebo study. J Allergy Clin Immunol 1986; 77:488–496.

73. Lilja G, Sundin B, Graff-Lonnevig V, Hedlin G, Heilborn H, Norrlind K, Pagelow KO, Lowenstein H. Immunotherapy with cat- and dog-dander extracts: IV. Effects of 2 years of treatment. J Allergy Clin Immunol 1989; 83:37–44.

74. Hedlin G, Heilborn H, Lilja G, Norrlind K, Pagelow KO, Schou C, Lowenstein H. Long-term follow-up of patients treated with a three-year course of cat or dog immunotherapy. J Allergy Clin Immunol 1995; 96:879–885.

75. Ohman JL. Allergen immunotherapy in asthma: evidence for efficacy. J Allergy Clin Immunol 1989; 84:133–137.

76. Bousquet J, Hejjaoui A, Michel FB. Specific immunotherapy in asthma. J Allergy Clin Immunol 1990; 86:293–297.

77. Nicklas RA, Bernstein IL, Blessing-Moore J, Fineman SM, Gutman AA, Lee RE, Li JT, Berger WE, Spector SL. Practice parameters for allergen immunotherapy. J Allergy Clin Immunol 1996; 98:1001–1011.

5

The Role of Fungal Allergens
Assessment and Control

ROBERT K. BUSH

University of Wisconsin–Madison Medical School and
William S. Middleton Memorial Veterans Hospital
Madison, Wisconsin

I. Introduction

Fungi, commonly and erroneously referred to as "molds," are a significant cause
of allergic disease. Fungi belong to a separate kingdom of multicellular eukary-
otes. "True fungi" include zygomycetes, ascomycetes, and basidiomycetes (1).
A current classification of fungi is found in Figure 1. Fungi classified as Basid-
iomycotina and Ascomycotina comprise a group known as the dikaryomycota.
Zygomycota comprise the other major group of fungi. Fungi imperfecti, which
were earlier classified as deuteromycetes, are among the best studied fungal
allergens. It is now recognized that fungi imperfecti are asexual forms of
ascomycetes. Fungi are obligate parasites or saprophytic decomposers that grow
where carbon sources are available and sufficient moisture is present.

In the northern areas of the United States, seasonal patterns of fungal
spores are identified in the atmosphere. Typically, fungal spores appear as snow
cover leaves the ground and become more prevalent as the weather warms in
May and June. Peak spore counts can be found in the late summer months and

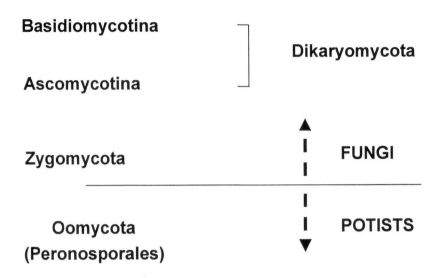

Figure 1 Current classification of fungi. (Adapted from Ref. 1.)

begin to recede as snow cover appears in October or November. In southern areas of the United States, fungal spores are present throughout the year, with peaks occurring in the summer or early fall. Spore prevalence is also dictated by local environmental conditions. During wet weather, recoveries of *Fusarium*, *Phoma*, ascospores, and basidiospores predominate (2). During dry weather, particularly on windy days, spores from *Cladosporium*, *Alternaria*, *Epicoccum*, and *Helminthosporium-Drechslera* will predominate (2).

Fungal allergen exposure is generally considered to arise from the outdoor environment, but indoor exposure to fungal allergens also occurs. Much of the indoor environmental exposure is a reflection of fungal spores emanating from the outdoor environment that invade interiors through open windows and cracks. Certain species such as *Penicillium* and *Aspergillus* may be recovered in indoor environments at rates higher than outdoors (2). The role of indoor fungal exposure in asthma is discussed more fully later. Clearly, homes and worksites that have been flooded or have excessive moisture problems are at risk for fungal contamination.

Fungi can cause a number of human diseases. They can act as pathogens and cause hypersensitivity pneumonitis, allergic bronchopulmonary mycoses, allergic fungal sinusitis, allergic rhinitis, and allergic asthma. This chapter focuses on the role of fungi as etiological agents in allergic asthma.

II. Prevalence of Fungal Sensitivity

Allergy to fungi mediated by IgE is demonstrated by skin testing with extracts prepared from fungi or by in vitro assays such as the radioallergosorbent test (RAST) or enzyme-linked immunoassays (ELISA). While sensitivity does not necessarily reflect disease, it is one way of determining the frequency of the sensitization and its relationship to respiratory symptoms. Unfortunately, many of the extracts available commercially for testing are of unstandardized materials and therefore give variable results. This has been demonstrated in studies from Scandinavia where positive skin tests to *Cladosporium herbarum* ranged from 12.5 to 86% in patients who had histories suggesting fungal allergy (3). Using a standardized *Cladosporium herbarum* extract, far larger numbers of individuals were identified than when less well characterized materials were used (3). Until such time as standardized extracts are available, estimates of the true prevalence of sensitivity to fungi in asthma will be difficult to establish. Some clinically relevant allergenic fungi are listed in Table 1.

Nevertheless, surveys conducted in various parts of the world indicate that fungal sensitivity is common, particularly among asthmatic individuals. In the general population of the United States, a large-scale epidemiological study indicated that 3.6% of the population are sensitized to the fungus *Alternaria alternata* (4). In a study of 981 children aged 4 years on the Isle of Wight, 0.5% of children reacted to *Alternaria* and 2.9% reacted to *Cladosporium* extracts (5). In one Scandinavian study, 4% showed positive skin tests, while in reports from the United States up to 80% of asthmatic patients demonstrated positive reactivity to one or more fungi (9).

As would be expected, in individuals presenting with respiratory symptoms of allergic rhinitis or asthma, the prevalence of skin test reactivity to fungi is increased. D'Amato et al. (6) studied the skin test reactivity to *Alternaria* and *Cladosporium* in patients throughout Europe presenting with suspected respiratory allergy. The frequency of positive skin test varied from country to country. Approximately 3% of the patients in Portugal had a positive skin test to either *Alternaria* or *Cladosporium*, while in Spain 20% demonstrated positive skin tests (6). Lehrer et al. (7) studied basidiomycete skin test reactivity in symptomatic patients residing in the United States and various European countries. Of these subjects 25–33% reacted to one or more basidiomycete species,

Table 1 Some Clinically Relevant Allergenic Fungi

DEUTEROMYCETES (IMPERFECT FUNGI)

Alternaria alternata

Alternaria tenuissima

Aspergillus flavus (var. *columnaris*)

Aspergillus fumigatus

Aspergillus niger

Aspergillus ornatus

Aspergillus repens/chevalieri/amsterdami

Aspergillus versicolor

Aspergillus wentii

Aureobasidium pululans

Botrytis cinerea

Cladosporium cladosporioides

Cladosporium herbarum

Curvularia lunata (or other common species)

Drechslera state of *Pyrenophora tritici-repentis* (= *Helminthosporium tritici repentis*)

Dreschslera state of *Cochliobolus heterostrophus* (= *Helminthosporium maydis*)

Epicoccum nigrum (= *Epicoccum purpurascens*)

Fusarium roseum

Fusarium moniliforme

Nigrospora sphaerica

Paecilomyces varioti

Paecilomyes lilacinum

Penicillium brevicompactum

Penicillium chrysogenum (= *Penicillium notatum*)

Penicillium giabrum

Penicillium oxalicum/citrinum

Penicillium purpurogenum

Phoma glomerata or *P. exiguia*

Rhodotorula rubrum

Scopulariopsis brevicaulis

Sporobolymyces roseus

Stemphylium botryosum

Ascomycetes (ascospore-producing stages)

Chaetomium globusum Didymella exitialis

BASIDIOMYCETES

A. Holobasidiomycetes (common fleshy fungi)

   Coprinus micaceus

   Ganoderma applantum

B. Heterobasidiomycetes (Teliomycetes)

   Puccinia graminis

   Ustilago nuda

   Ustilago zeae

Source: Ref. 77.

which suggested that there was a strong association between sensitivity to this fungus and the presence of allergic respiratory diseases (7).

In a large-scale epidemiological study of children with asthma residing in inner cities of the United States, the most common sensitizer was *Alternaria*; 38.3% of 1286 asthmatic children had positive skin test to this allergen (8). This was comparable to their sensitivities to cockroach (35.8%) and house dust mites (34.6%) (8).

III. Association of Fungal Sensitivity with Asthma

Sensitivities to house dust mite, cockroach, and animal dander allergens have been well established as risk factors for asthma. Epidemiological studies have now established a role for fungal sensitization in the development of symptomatic asthma. An accumulating body of evidence suggests that sensitization to fungi, particularly the fungus *Alternaria*, is associated with asthma. Gergen and Turkeltaub (10) reported that in individuals with *Alternaria* sensitivities the adjusted odds ratio for those having self-reported asthma was 2.3 (95% CI, 1.5–3.4).

Peat et al. (11) evaluated the roles of house dust mite allergen exposure and *Alternaria* in children living in different regions of Australia. Along the coastal areas of Australia where humidity is high, house dust mite antigen was highly correlated with the presence of asthma (11). In the inner part of the country, which is less humid, *Alternaria* was more likely to be associated with asthma with an adjusted odds ratio of 5.6 (95% CI, 3.1–10.1) (11).

In a study of children residing in the desert southwest of the United States, skin test responsiveness to *Alternaria* at age 6 was associated with persistent asthma and the onset of new asthma (12). At age 11 this correlation did not occur (12). This is consistent with the previous reports by Kaufmann et al. (13), who found an age-related decline in fungal sensitization in asthmatic patients. In a study of school-age children residing in North Carolina, Henderson et al. (14) demonstrated that *Alternaria* sensitivity was associated with recurrent wheezing in this population (adjusted odds ratio 6.8; 95% CI, 2.1–21.5). Perzanowski et al. (15) conducted a similar study in which serum antibodies to *Alternaria* were linked with the presence of asthma in school-age children residing in two cities in Virginia and one in New Mexico. A positive association between *Alternaria* sensitivity and asthma was demonstrated in Charlottesville, Virginia but not in Albemarle, Virginia (15). A linkage was also established between *Alternaria* sensitivity and asthma and school-age children residing in Los Alamos, New Mexico (15).

While skin test or evidence of IgE sensitivity by in vitro methods indicate a linkage between sensitization in asthma, it has been more difficult to directly correlate exposure to fungal spores and the development of asthma symptoms in sensitized individuals. Bruce et al. (16) indicated that asthma symptoms were correlated with the presence of *Alternaria* sensitivity by skin test in approximately 50% of their subjects. In a study of children aged 9–18 years conducted in San Diego, California, fungal exposure was significantly associated with asthma symptoms (17). Asthma symptoms scores were correlated with the total outdoor spore count; asthma symptoms scores increased by 0.1–0.3 for every 1000 spores per cubic meter of air (17). The need for inhaled bronchodilators also was correlated in a similar fashion (17). Interestingly, there was a better correlation with non-skin-tested fungi (basidiomycetes and ascospores) spore counts than with fungi to which the patients had a positive skin test (17).

These studies demonstrate the limitations in assessing exposure–response relationships. However, it does appear clear that fungal spores play a role in symptoms of asthma. The ability to test for sensitivity to many of the fungal spores is limited, and therefore exact assessments cannot be made at the present time.

A.   Role of Fungal Exposure in Emergency Room Visits for Asthma

Exposure to fungal spores has been associated with emergency room visits for asthma. Rosas et al. (18) found a correlation between asthma emergency room visits in children and the presence of high levels of the ascospore *Leptosphaeria.* Nelson et al. (19) reported that emergency room visits for asthma in children was associated with sensitivity to a variety of allergens, including *Alternaria alternata.*

B.   Role of Fungal Allergens in Epidemic Asthma

Epidemic asthma is defined as an excessive outbreak of symptomatic asthma requiring emergency medical care. Salvaggio et al. (20) indicated that a high volume of hospital admissions (40 over 24 hr) for asthma occurred during a period of time in which there were high total basidiomycete spore counts in the air in New Orleans. These epidemics occurred during the months of June through December, with peaks occurring in September and November. Similar outbreaks have occurred in England and New Zealand during periods of high fungal spore counts (21). Ascospores have been associated with epidemics of asthma in England (22).

Fungi may have played a secondary role as an etiological agent in the outbreaks of asthma in Barcelona, Spain, which were initially attributed to soybean hull sensitivity (23). The investigators demonstrated that the patients who developed asthma episodes on exposure to soybean hulls were sensitized not only to these proteins but also to *Aspergillus* and *Penicillium* species (23).

C. Role of Fungal Allergy in Severe and Fatal Asthma

Fungal sensitivity and exposure to airborne fungal spores have been associated with severe episodes of asthma. O'Hollaren et al. (24) reported on 11 patients aged 11–25 years who presented with respiratory arrest due to asthma. There were two fatalities in the group. Ten of the 11 patients were sensitized to *Alternaria*. These patients developed their difficulty during the peak of the *Alternaria* season, and there was a correlation between the *Alternaria* spore counts and the time of their presentation to the emergency room. The adjusted odds ratio (189; CI = 6.5–5535.8) for a severe and potentially fatal attack of asthma was highly correlated with *Alternaria* sensitivity (24). Thus, sensitivity to *Alternaria* was recognized as a major risk factor for severe and potentially fatal asthma.

The risk of death from asthma has also been correlated with the presence of fungal spores in the atmosphere. Based on death certificates from asthma in the Chicago, Illinois area, Targonski et al. (25) found that the adjusted odds ratio for death on a day when the fungal spore counts exceeded 1000 per cubic meter of air was 2.3 times as high as when the spore counts were less than 1000 per cubic meter of air (95% CI = 1.3–3.56). It was also found that for every increase in the fungal spore count by $1000/m^3$, there was an increased odds ratio for death of 1.2 (95% CI, 1.07–1.34) (25). These observations indicate that fungal sensitivity not only carries an increased risk for the development of asthma but also plays a role in epidemics of asthma, acute severe life-threatening episodes of asthma, and asthma deaths.

IV. Asthma and Fungi in the Indoor Environment

Indoor spores are usually from a mixture of indoor and outdoor sources. If outdoor air has access and there is no indoor source of fungal exposure, indoor air reflects the outdoor fungal concentration, albeit at a lower level. In northern climates, especially during cold weather or snow cover, little or no contribution occurs from the outdoor environment. If the rank order of fungal spores recovered from the indoor environment shows a high ratio of so-called indoor species such as *Aspergillus* or *Penicillium*, then an indoor source is most likely (26).

Concentrations of indoor fungal spores vary considerably even over a period of a few hours, ranging from 1000 to 60,000 per cubic meter of air (26).

Similarly, culture data from indoor environments shows that there is a considerable range of recoverable fungi, from 10 to 10,000 colony-forming units (CFU)/m^3 air. No threshold value for a "safe" level of fungal exposure has been established, although, generally, cultures showing less than 100–500 CFU/m^3 are described as "healthy" (26).

Most studies of fungal exposure in the indoor environment rely on air-sampling methods in which spores are counted using a Burkard trap. Another alternative is to conduct culturing of viable spore or fungal elements from the air or from dust samples. A single sampling method is prone to error, and several approaches may be required to fully assess the indoor exposure to fungal allergens (26). Since much of the indoor environment reflects the outdoor environmental levels, sampling must be done simultaneously in both outdoor and indoor environments. Since single samples of specimens are reflective of only that particular point in time, this approach may not adequately assess the overall exposure to fungal allergens in the environment. Therefore, time–exposure relationships are difficult to establish because of the enormous cost involved in studying both indoor and outdoor environments over long periods of time.

Peat et al. (27) extensively reviewed the literature for the previous 15 years regarding the relationship between dampness or mold in the home and respiratory health. Although the studies did not employ standardized methodology for measuring either exposure or health outcomes, a number of studies in children evaluated cough and wheeze in a more consistent fashion. Analysis of the data obtained from these studies indicates that the risk for children having respiratory symptoms in an home that is damp or has fungal growth has an odds ratio in the range of 1.5–3.5. This is similar to that observed in environments where children are exposed to environmental tobacco smoke or outdoor air pollutants (27). Figure 2 demonstrates the association between asthma in children and adults and their exposure to dampness or fungal growth in the home.

Although correlates between indoor fungal exposure and asthma are somewhat tenuous, damp conditions that would be conducive to fungal growth have also been shown to have significant health effects, at least in children (27). Allergic reactions to fungi as a cause of these symptoms have not been established by appropriate skin testing or in vitro IgE tests, however. Some symptoms that patients experience in indoor environments may be related to exposure to mycotoxins such as trichothecne (28) or to other agents such as $(1 \rightarrow 3)$ β-D-glucan (29).

Verhoeff and Burge (26) also reviewed the association between fungi in homes and health risks. These authors came to the same conclusions as Peat and coworkers concerning a positive association between damp homes and respiratory morbidity of the occupants (26). Dampness and fungal problems have

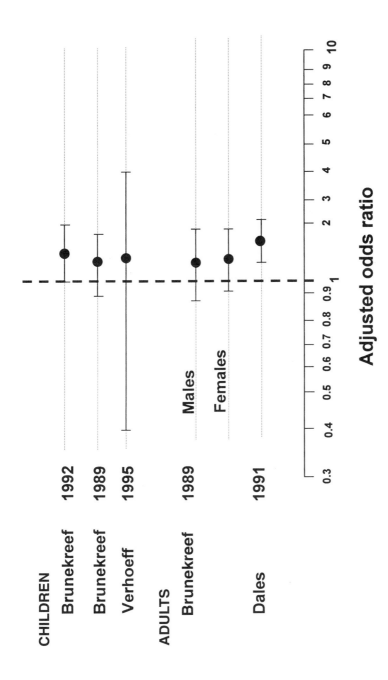

Figure 2 The association between asthma in children and adults exposed to fungal growth in the home. (Adapted from Ref. 27.)

been reported to occur in 20–50% of modern homes (26). Poorly maintained heating, ventilation, and air-conditioning systems are often sources of exposure to fungi. In seven of nine cross-sectional studies evaluated by Verhoeff and Burge (26), one or more positive associations were found between fungal levels and adverse health outcomes.

In addition to these literature reviews, Beaumont et al. (30) found that half the reported asthmatic symptoms of patients could be attributed to indoor or outdoor fungal spore peaks. Further, studies by Warburton et al. (31) indicated that there were larger effects from dampness or moldy housing in terms of respiratory symptoms in atopic versus nonatopic individuals.

V. Fungal Species Found in Indoor Environments

As previously mentioned, most of the indoor fungal exposure is the result of invasion from outdoor sources. However, some species are predominant in the winter months when outdoor fungal levels in northern climates are unmeasurable or at extremely low levels. Solomon (32) used cultures of air samples from homes in Michigan to detect fungi in the indoor environment. The major species of fungi found in the indoor environment during frost-free periods included *Cladosporium, Alternaria, Epicoccum, Fusarium, Penicillium,* and *Aspergillus* (32). The culturable levels were approximately 25% of those obtained from the outdoor environment during this time period. During the winter, the main recoverable fungal types were *Cladosporium, Penicillium, Aspergillus, Geotrichum,* pigmented yeasts, and miscellaneous filamentous genera (32).

Hirsh and Sosman (33) conducted culture studies on indoor air samples and dust samples collected by vacuum cleaners for fungal growth. They also measured outdoor spore counts over a 1 yr period of time in 12 homes in Wisconsin. The most commonly reported indoor organisms included *Cladosporium* species, *Alternaria, Penicillium,* and *Aspergillus fumigatus* (33). The latter two were present at the same level throughout most of the year, while *Cladosporium* and *Alternaria* fell significantly during the winter months (33).

Using an open petri dish culture method, Prahl (34) found that the major genera of indoor fungi in Denmark consisted of *Cladosporium, Penicillium,* mycelia sterilia (fungi that do not sporulate), yeasts, *Rhodotorula,* and *Aspergillus* species. Garrett et al. (35) found in their study of asthmatic children that common genera associated with indoor environments include *Cladosporium* and *Penicillium.* Asthma was associated with *Penicillium* exposure during the winter months with an adjusted odds ratio of 1.43 for each increase in CFUs/m^3 above 100. Measurements of specific fungal spore genera correlated better with predicted health outcomes such as asthma and respiratory symptoms than total fungal spore counts (35).

Using cultures from dust samples obtained from homes in the Netherlands, *Aspergillus repens*, *Aspergillus penicilloides*, and *Wallemia sebi* were found to occur in these Dutch homes (36). These organisms typically are reflective of dry indoor environments rather than humid conditions. Beaumont et al. (37) also studied Dutch homes. Using cultures of the airborne fungi obtained by Anderson samplers, *Penicillium* was found to be dominant in indoor environments throughout the year. *Cladosporium*, on the other hand, was virtually found only in the outdoor environment, with little if any in the indoor environment. *Aspergillus* species were present year-round and found in greater concentrations in the inside than the outside environment. *Alternaria* was predominantly found in the outdoor environment during the fall months, while mycelia sterilia were present indoors and outdoors in equal amounts throughout the year (37).

Dust samples from homes in the Baltimore, Maryland area indicated that species of *Penicillium* and *Aspergillus*, *Rhodotorula rubra*, *Alternaria*, *Cladosporium* species, and *Chaetomium* predominated in the winter and spring months (38). Cultures of airborne samples from English and Scottish homes in the winter months also indicated the presence of *Penicillium* and *Cladosporium* species but also identified *Sistotrema brinkmannii* and *Aspergillus versicolor* as prevalent species (39). Similar results were obtained by Strachen et al. (40) in homes in the United Kingdom.

Surveys from Canada (41) indicated that the *Cladosporium cladosporioides* and *Cladosporium sphaerospermum* predominated. Cultures of dust samples collected from Swedish homes during the winter indicated predominance of *Penicillium* species, *Alternaria alternata*, *Cladosporium* species, mycelia sterilia, and *Rhodotorula rubra* (42).

Surveys from Taiwan indicate that *Penicillium*, *Aspergillus*, and yeast species are common (43). In further analysis of the specific types of *Penicillium* species, *Penicillium citrinum* predominated (44). In Kansas, *Penicillium brevicompactum*, *P. citrinum*, and *P. chrysogenum* were the predominant species (45).

Two studies in the Netherlands showed somewhat different results depending on the time of year and the area of the home that was sampled (46). During September and October, *Aspergillus* species, *Cladosporium*, *Penicillium*, *Wallemia*, and *Alternaria* were present in over 85–100% of the homes (46). In contrast, during May, *Cladosporium cladosporioides* and *Cladosporium herbarum* along with *Penicillium brevicompactum* predominated (46). *Wallemia* was found only in 50–60% of the homes during that time period (46). Another report looking at cultures from bedroom floors and mattresses during October and November (47) found *Alternaria alternata*, *Aspergillus versi-*

color, Aerobasidium pullulans, and *Cladosporium cladosporioides* as the predominant species.

In Belgium homes, Beguin and Noland (48) found *Cladosporium* species, that were predominantly of outdoor origin, in 98% of the homes. Ninety-eight percent of the homes also grew *Penicillium* species, primarily *P. chrysogenum* and *P. brevicompactum* (48). Ninety percent of the homes showed *Aspergillus* species, primarily *Aspergillus versicolor* (48).

Culture samples from dust in German homes revealed a predominance of *Cladosporium, Penicillium, Aspergillus*, and mycelia sterilia (49). In Polish homes, *Penicillium* species, *Aspergillus*, and yeasts predominated (50).

In the desert climate of Saudi Arabia, dust samples in homes also revealed the presence of fungal species including *Aspergillus, Penicillium, Alternaria*, and *Chaetomium* (51).

In the surveys of indoor and fungi recovered in homes in the United States during frost-free periods as well as in Europe, several species appear to predominate. These include *Cladosporium, Alternaria Epicoccum, Fusarium*, and to a lesser degree *Penicillium* and *Aspergillus*. During the cold months, when the outdoor environment is less likely to be contributing to the indoor levels, *Penicillium* and *Aspergillus* predominate.

While the methods employed in the above studies relied on recoverable cultural fungi and in a few cases fungal spores identified by air-sampling devices such as Burkard spore traps, few data are available in terms of fungal allergen recovery from indoor environments as measured by total allergenic activity or specific fungal allergenic protein levels. However, Pacheco et al. (52) conducted limited studies looking for the presence of allergenic activity in the indoor environment and found evidence for the presence of *Penicillium, Alternaria*, and *Cladosporium* allergens in homes in the Kansas City, Missouri, area. Clearly, further studies will need to be done to fully determine the types of fungal exposures occurring in the indoor environment.

Aside from the home environment, individuals are exposed to fungal allergens in their work environment as well. Studies of Canadian office workers indicate that office environments also are potential sources of fungal allergen exposure (53). Culturable fungal samples as well as spore counts collected by volumetric personal samplers indicated that patients with sensitization to fungal allergens such as *Alternaria* experience symptoms of coughing, wheezing, and shortness of breath associated with exposure to these indoor allergens. Most of the symptoms occurred in the skin test positive individuals, as would be expected (53). Clearly, it is important to account for exposure to fungi in the outdoor environment, home environment, and workplace.

VI. Fungal Allergens

Recent advances in molecular biology have led to a better understanding of fungal allergens and their relationships to allergic disease including asthma and allergic bronchopulmonary aspergillosis.

A. *Alternaria alternata* Allergens

A major allergen from *Alternaria*, termed Alt a 1, has been purified, and subunits of it have been molecularly cloned (54,55). The protein is a two-chain dimer with a molecular weight of approximately 30 kDa. Ninety percent of *Alternaria*-allergic individuals have IgE antibodies to this protein. The biological function of this protein has not been elucidated.

Several other minor allergens have been identified, including Alt a 6, which is a P_2 ribosomal protein (56,57). Alt a 7 is homologous with YCP4 yeast protein, and Alt a 10 is an alcohol dehydrogenase (56,57). These appear to be cytoplasmic household proteins that lack glycosylation and are conserved in evolution (56,57).

B. *Cladosporium herbarum* Allergens

The *Cladosporium herbarum* allergens Cla h 1 and Cla h 2 have been purified and found to be major allergens. A third protein known as Cla h 3 has been molecularly cloned (58). Cla h 3 is also a ribosomal P_2 protein that is associated with RNA in the cytosol. In addition, an hsp 70 heat shock protein has also been cloned from *Cladosporium* (59). Approximately 30% of patients allergic to *Cladosporium* have IgE binding to this highly conserved protein.

C. Enolases

Enolases have been obtained from *Cladosporium* and *Alternaria* as well as *Saccharomyces cerevisiae* and *Candida albicans* (60). Approximately 50% of the patients sensitive to *Alternaria* and *Cladosporium* have IgE binding to this protein (60).

D. *Aspergillus* Allergens

Two groups (61,62) molecularly cloned a major allergen from *Aspergillus fumigatus* termed Asp f 1. This protein is a cytotoxin, mitogillin (62). Skin tests were conducted with this protein, and approximately 50% or more of *Aspergillus*-sensitive subjects react to it (63). This protein is excreted into the culture media only during active growth of the organism (62). Asp f 3 is a peroxisomal membrane protein that binds IgE from *Aspergillus*-allergic asthmatic patients at a rate of approximately 72% (64). Asp f 5 is a metalloprotease (65,66). Using a combination of Asp f 1, Asp f 3, and Asp f 5, a diagnostic sensitivity of 97% for *Aspergillus* allergy has been demonstrated (66).

Asp f 2 has been demonstrated to have IgE binding in sera of patients with allergic bronchopulmonary aspergillosis (ABPA) (67). Asp f 4, whose molecular and biological functions are unknown, is an IgE binding protein in many patients with ABPA (66). Asp f 6, which is a manganese superoxide dismutase, is also highly associated with ABPA (66). Using a combination of these specific proteins, a diagnosis of allergic bronchopulmonary aspergillosis may be feasible (66).

Secreted proteins such as Asp f 3 and Asp f 5 are recognized by patients who have a sensitivity to *Aspergillus fumigatus* with or without ABPA, while nonsecreted proteins such as Asp f 4 and Asp f 6 are recognized by patients with allergic bronchopulmonary aspergillosis (66).

E. *Penicillium* Allergens

Several allergens from *Penicillium citrinum* have been identified (68,69). One of these is a 33 kDa major allergen that has been found to be an alkaline serine proteinase (69,70). Approximately 93% of patients with sensitivity to various *Penicillium* species have IgE binding to this protein (69). Further, an hsp 70 heat shock protein has also been identified as an allergen from *Penicillium* (71).

Identification and purification of fungal allergens play a critical role in improving diagnostic capabilities for fungal sensitivity. Further, identification of these allergens provides a basis for the development of immunoassays to quantitate allergenic exposure in the environment.

VII. Fungal Cell Wall Components and Their Relation to Asthma

$(1 \rightarrow 3)$-β-D-Glucans are glucose polymers found in cell walls of fungi, plants, and some bacteria. Methods to measure $(1 \rightarrow 3)$-β-D-glucan have been developed using *Limulus* lysate assays (72). Some evidence has accumulated that $(1 \rightarrow 3)$-β-glucan may produce airway inflammation, although this has not been thoroughly evaluated (29). Indoor exposure to $(1 \rightarrow 3)$-β-glucans has been reported to increase or to cause symptoms of dry cough and wheezing in children exposed to mold growth in school buildings (72). Further studies are required to evaluate the role of this fungal cell wall product in the pathogenesis of asthma.

Extracellular polysaccharides (EPSs) are stable carbohydrates secreted or shed during mold growth. These polysaccharides have antigenic specificity, usually at the genus level. Some extracellular polysaccharides from *Aspergillus* and *Penicillium* have been shown to be cross-reactive. Immunoassays have been developed to measure EPSs (73). They may serve as a marker for fungal exposure; however, no pathogenic role for EPSs in respiratory disease has yet been identified.

VIII. Assessment of Fungal Allergen Exposure

Traditionally, assessment of fungal exposure has relied primarily on spore counts using a volumetric sampler such as the Burkard spore trap. Quantitative assessments of the number of spores per cubic meter of air over a period of time can be obtained. These devices can be used both indoors and outdoors. Identification of fungal spores relies on microscopic characteristics. However, for many spores such as *Penicillium*, *Aspergillus*, and ascospores and basidiomycetes, identification of morphological basis is not entirely possible.

In other instances, viable cultures that can be quantitated as CFU per cubic meter of air sampled have also been utilized as a method of assessing fungal exposure. Usually a device such as an Andersen sampler is used to obtain air samples, which are then grown on appropriate culture media. However, not all fungal material is viable. The culture methodology is also expensive and time-consuming.

Dust samples can also be collected and cultures obtained based on CFU per gram of dust collected. This approach has the same constraints as airborne culture sampling. Since fungal spore and viable culturable levels may vary significantly over a period of time, simple "grab samples" are only reflective of the instantaneous exposures. When obtaining samples it is appropriate to compare both indoor and outdoor levels to assess whether the predominant exposure is coming from indoor or outdoor sources. Sampling is not always necessary if visible fungal growth is occurring in an indoor environment. Sampling may be appropriate under conditions where a source of fungal exposure is not readily apparent and patients are symptomatic.

Since allergic asthma due to fungal exposure is due to allergen exposure, more direct methods are being developed to assess actual allergen levels. An assay for an *Alternaria* allergen, GP70, has been developed that has a detection level limit of 0.2 μg/mL although it has not yet been applied to either dust or airborne samples (74). An Alt a 1 assay has been developed (Chapman MD, personal communication). The development of assays to actually quantitate airborne exposure of levels will be very useful in assessing fungal allergen exposure.

IX. Fungal Allergen Avoidance Measures

Outdoor fungal exposures should be avoided by fungal allergic people with possibly high exposure levels, such as farmers or people working with moldy materials. Wearing a fitted face mask is useful. Since most indoor exposure occurs through outdoor sources, closing windows and running air conditioning can also reduce exposure. Automobiles equipped with air conditioners can also be helpful in reducing exposure (Table 2).

Indoor fungal exposure is, as mentioned, dependent on the outdoor environment; however, when fungal growth occurs indoors it is usually in dark, humid, poorly ventilated areas such as basements. Bathrooms and kitchens or other sites with high humidity are also sources of fungal growth. Humidifier systems with standing water are also subject to fungal growth. If structural leaks occur, these need to be repaired. Water-damaged carpets need to be removed. Kitchens and bathrooms should be ventilated. Materials that cannot be cleaned, e.g., moldy books, clothing, should be discarded. Washable surfaces such as bathroom tiles and other washable surfaces can be treated with 5–10% chlorine bleach with detergent solution or approved fungicidal solution. It is advised that if the person who is cleaning these areas has an allergy, he or she should wear a fitted mask. Air conditioning during periods of high relative humidity to keep humidity levels less than 50% is very helpful in limiting fungal growth (75) (Table 2).

Table 2   Fungal Allergen Control Methods

Indoors
Remove contaminated materials, e.g., carpets, rotted wood, wallpaper.
Treat washable surfaces with 5% chlorine bleach and detergent solution.
Wear mask when cleaning contaminated material.
Reduce relative humidity to ≤50%.
Keep windows and doors closed during periods of high outdoor spore levels.
Seal water leaks.
Outdoors
Wear mask when working with moldy materials, e.g., when gardening.

Use of high efficiency particulate air (HEPA) cleaners or electrostatic air cleaners may decrease fungal spores in the air, but their overall benefits for treating of asthma have not been proven. Other useful methods to reduce indoor airborne fungal concentrations include avoiding indoor clothes drying unless the dryer is vented to the outside, decreasing the number of indoor plants, and having no unheated rooms in the winter or unheated outside wall closets (34).

Although these methods make common sense, they have not been systematically studied to determine their effectiveness.

X. Role of Immunotherapy and Treatment of Fungus-Induced Asthma

Because of problems identifying personal exposure to fungal allergens and the lack of suitable standardized reagents for treatment, there have been limited clinical trials of the use of immunotherapy in the treatment of fungus-induced asthma. Nonetheless, several trials of immunotherapy using *Cladosporium* and *Alternaria* extracts have been reported (76). These studies have shown some benefits in the treatment of fungus-induced asthma. For further discussion, see Chapter 14 by Bousquet.

XI. Summary

Sensitivity to fungi is a major risk factor for the development of asthma. However, the prevalence of fungal sensitivity in asthma is not completely understood, although upward of 80% of asthmatic patients may be sensitized to one or more fungi. Fungal exposure occurs primarily outdoors but can occur in the indoor environment as well. Assessment of fungal exposure requires a multifaceted approach including measurement of airborne spores and culture techniques to identify the relevant organisms. Preventing intrusion of outdoor fungal spores into the indoor environment may be helpful in reducing allergic symptoms. Methods to abate indoor fungal growth include reduction of indoor humidity and removal of water sources. Specifically contaminated areas must be treated with appropriate procedures such as fungicides or dilute bleach–detergent solutions. Fungus-contaminated materials that cannot be cleaned must be removed. Patients with fungal sensitivity should be advised to avoid exposures as much as possible. For patients who have failed to respond to environmental control measures and appropriate medications, it may be reasonable to consider specific immunotherapy.

References

1. Horner E, Lehrer S, Salvaggio JE. Fungi. Immunol Allergy Clin No Amer 1994; 14:551–566.
2. Solomon WR, Platts-Mills TAE. Aerobiology and inhalant allergens. In: Middleton E Jr, Reed CE, Ellis EF, Adkinson NF Jr, Yunginger JW, Busse WW, eds. Allergy Principles and Practice. 5th ed. St. Louis: Mosby, 1998:367–403.
3. Aas K, Leegaard J, Aukrust L. Immediate type hypersensitivity to common moulds. A comparison of different diagnostic materials. Allergy 1980; 35:443–451.
4. Gergen PJ, Turkeltaub PC, Kovar MG. The prevalence of skin test reactivity to eight common aeroallergens in the US population: results from the second National Health and Nutrition Examination Survey. J Allergy Clin Immunol 1987; 80:669–679.
5. Tariq SM, Matthews SM, Stevens M, Hakin EA. Sensitization to Alternaria and Cladosporium by the age of 4 yrs. Clin Exp Allergy 1996; 26:794–798.
6. D'Amato G, Chatzrgeorgiou G, Corsico R, Gioulekas D, Jager L, Jager S, Kontan-Fati K, Kouridakis S, Liccardi G, Meriggi A, Palma-Carlos A, Paliner-Carlos M, Alemar AP, Parmiari S, Puccinelli P, Russo M, Spieksmer FThM, Torrieelli R, Wuthrich B. Evaluation of the prevalence of skin prick test positively to Alternaria and Cladosporium in patients with suspected respiratory allergy. Allergy 1997; 52:711–716.
7. Lehrer SB, Hughes JM, Altnan LC, Bousquet J, Davies RJ, Gell L, Li J, Lopez M, Malling H-J, Mathison DA, Sastre J, Schultze-Weringhaus G, Schwartz HJ. Prevalence of basidiomycete allergy in the USA and Europe and its relationship to allergic respiratory symptoms. Allergy 1994; 49:460–465.
8. Eggleston PA, Rosenstreich D, Lynn H, Gergen P, Baker D, Kattan M, Mortimer KM, Mitchell H, Ownby D, Slavin R, Malveaux F. Relationship of indoor allergen exposure to skin test sensitivity in inner city asthma. J Allergy Clin Immunol 1998; 102:563–570.
9. Lopez M, Salvaggio JE. Mold sensitive asthma. Clin Rev Allergy 1985; 3:183–196.
10. Gergen PJ, Turkeltaub PC. The association of individual allergen reactivity with respiratory disease in a national sample: data from the second National Health and Nutritional Examination Survey, 1976–80 (NHANES 1). J Allergy Clin Immunol 1992; 90:579–588.
11. Peat JK, Tovey E, Mellis CM, Leeder SR, Woolcock AJ. Importance of house dust mite and Alternaria allergens in childhood asthma: an epidemiological study in two climatic regions of Australia. Clin Exp Allergy 1993; 23:812–820.
12. Halonen M, Stern DA, Wright AL, Taussig LM, Martinez FD. Alternaria as a major allergen for asthma in children raised in a desert environment. Am J Respir Crit Care Med 1997; 155:1356–1361.
13. Kauffman HF, Tomee JFC, vanderWerf TS, deMonchy JGR, Koëter GK. Review of fungus-induced asthmatic reactions. Am J Respir Crit Care Med 1995; 151: 2109–2116.
14. Henderson FW, Henry MM, Morris R, Neebe EC, Len S-Y, Stewart DW, Physi-

cians of Raleigh Pediatric Association, PA. Correlates of recurrent wheezing in school-age children. Am J Respir Crit Care Med 1995; 151:1786–1793.

15. Perzanowski MS, Sporik R, Squllace SP, Gelber LE, Call R, Carter M, Platts-Mills TAE. Association of sensitization to Alternaria allergens with asthma among school-age children. J Allergy Clin Immunol 1998; 101:626–632.

16. Bruce CA, Norman PS, Rosenthal PR. The role of ragweed pollen in autumnal asthma. J Allergy Clin Immunol 1977; 59:449–459.

17. Delfino RJ, Coate BD, Zeiger RS, Seltzer JM, Street DH, Koufrakis P. Daily asthma severity in relation to personal ozone exposure and outdoor fungal spores. Am J Respir Crit Care Med 1996; 154:633–641.

18. Rosas I, McCartney HA, Payne RW, Calderon C, Lacey J, Chapela R, Ruiz-Velazco S. Analysis of the relationships between environmental factors (aeroallergens, air pollution, and weather) and asthma emergency admissions to a hospital in Mexico City. Allergy 1998; 53:394–401.

19. Nelson RP Jr, DiNicolo R, Fernandez-Caldas E, Seleznick MJ, Lockey RF, Good RA. Allergic specific IgE levels and mite allergen exposure in children with acute asthma first seen in an emergency department and in non-asthmatic control subjects. J Allergy Clin Immunol 1996; 98:258–263.

20. Salvaggio J, Seabury J, Schoenhardt EA. New Orleans asthma. V. Relationship between Charity Hospital asthma admission rates, semiquantitative pollen and fungal spore counts, and total particulate aerometric sampling data. J Allergy Clin Immunol 1971; 48:96–114.

21. Horner WE, O'Neil C, Lehrer SB. Basidiospore aeroallergens. Clin Rev Allergy 1992; 10:191–211.

22. Frankland AW, Gregory PH. Allergenic and agricultural implication of airborne ascospore concentrations from a fungus, Didymella exitalis. Nature 1973; 245:336–337.

23. Codina R, Lockey RF. Possible role of molds or secondary etiologic agents of the asthma epidemics in Barcelona, Spain. J Allergy Clin Immunol 1998; 102:318–320.

24. O'Hollaren MT, Yunginger JW, Offord KP, Somers MJ, O'Connell EJ, Ballard DJ, Sachs MI. Exposure to an aeroallergen as a possible precipitating factor in respiratory arrest in young patients with asthma. N Engl J Med 1991; 324:359–363.

25. Targonski PV, Persky VW, Ramekrishnan V. Effect of environmental molds on risk of death from asthma during the pollen season. J Allergy Clin Immunol 1995; 95:955–961.

26. Verhoeff AP, Burge HA. Health risk assessment of fungi in home environments. Ann Allergy Asthma Immunol 1997; 78:544–556.

27. Peat JK, Dickerson J, Li J. Effect of damp and mould in the home on respiratory health: a review of the literature. Allergy 1998; 53:120–128.

28. Croft WA, Jarvis BB, Yatawara CS. Airborne outbreak of trichothecene toxicosis. Atmos Environ 1986; 20:549–552.

29. Rylander R. Microbic cell wall constituents in indoor air and their relationship to disease. Indoor Air 1998; 4(suppl):59–65.

30. Beaumont F, Kaufman HF, Sluiter HJ, deVries K. Sequential sampling of fungal air spores inside and outside the homes of mould sensitive, asthmatic patients: a search for a relationship to obstructive reactions. Ann Allergy 1985; 55:740–746.
31. Warburton CJ, Nirven RM, Pickering CAC, Fletcher AM, Hepworth J, Francis HC. Domiciliary air filtration units, symptoms and lung function in atopic asthmatics. Respir Med 1994; 88:771–776.
32. Solomon WR. Assessing fungus prevalence in domestic interiors. J Allergy Clin Immunol 1975; 56:235–242.
33. Hirsh SR, Sosman JA. A one year survey of mold growth inside twelve homes. Ann Allergy 1976; 36:30–38.
34. Prahl P. Reduction of indoor airborne mould spores. Allergy 1992; 47:362–365.
35. Garrett MH, Ratznient PR, Hooper MA, Abramson MJ, Hooper GM. Indoor airborne fungal spores, house dampness and association with environmental factors and respiratory health in children. Clin Exp Allergy 1998; 28:459–467.
36. Rijckaert G. Exposure to fungi in modern homes. Allergy 1981; 36:277–280.
37. Beaumont F, Kaufman HF, Sluiter HJ, deVries K. A volumetric-aerobiologic study of seasonal fungus prevalence inside and outside dwellings of asthmatic patients living in northeast Netherlands. Ann Allergy 1984; 53:486–492.
38. Wood RA, Eggleston PA, Lind P, Ingeman L, Schwartz B, Graveson S, Tervy D, Wheeler B, Adkinson NF Jr. Antigenic analysis of household dust samples. Am Rev Respir Dis 1988; 137:358–363.
39. Hunter CA, Grant C, Flannigan B, Bravery AF. Mould in buildings: the air spora of domestic dwellings. Int Biodeterioration 1988; 24:81–101.
40. Strachan DP, Flannigan B, McCabe EM, McGarry F. Quantification of airborne moulds in the homes of children with and without wheeze. Thorax 1990; 45:382–387.
41. Tarlo SM, Fradkin A, Tobin RS. Skin testing with extracts of fungal species derived from the homes of allergy clinic patients in Toronto, Canada. Clin Allergy 1988; 18:45–52.
42. Wickman M, Gravesen S, Nordvall SL, Pershagen G, Sundell J. Indoor viable dust-bound microfungi in relation to residential characteristics, living habits, and symptoms in atopic and control children. Allergy Clin Immunol 1992; 89:752–759.
43. Li C-S, Hsu L-Y, Chou C-C, Hsieh K-H. Fungal allergens inside and outside the residences of atopic and control children. Arch Environ Health 1995; 50:38–43.
44. Wei D-L, Chen J-H, Jong S-C, Shen H-D. Indoor airborne *Penicillium* species in Taiwan. Curr Microbiol 1993; 26:137–140.
45. Muilenberg M, Burge H, Sweet T, Solomon W. *Penicillium* species in and out of doors in Topeka, KS (abstr). J Allergy Clin Immunol 1990; 85:247.
46. Verhoeff AP, VanWijnen JH, Brunekreef B, Fischer P, VanReenen-Hockstra L-S, Samson RA. Presence of viable mould propagules in indoor air in relation to house damp and outdoor air. Allergy 1992; 47:83–91.
47. Verhoeff AP, VanWijnen JH, VanReenen-Hoestra ES, Sampson RA, VanStrien RT, Brunekreef B. Fungal propagules in house dust II. Relation with residential characteristics and respiratory symptoms. Allergy 1994; 49:540–547.

48. Beguin H, Noland N. Mould biodiversity in homes. I. Air and surface analysis of 130 dwellings. Aerobiologia 1994; 10:157–166.
49. Dill I, Noggemann B. Domestic fungal viable propagules and sensitization in children with IgE mediated allergic disease. Pediatr Allergy Immunol 1996; 7:151–155.
50. Horak B, Dutkiewicz J, Jolarz K. Microflora and acrafauna of bed dust from homes in Upper Silesiu, Poland. Ann Allergy Asthma Immunol 1996; 76:41–50.
51. Bokhary HA, Parvez S. Fungi inhabiting household environments in Riyadh, Saudi Arabia. Mycopathologia 1995; 130:79–87.
52. Pacheco F, Landuyt J, Barnes C, Hu F, Portnoy J. Fungal allergens in house dust (abstr). J Allergy Clin Immunol 1997; 99:584.
53. Merizies D, Comtois P, Pasztor J, Nunes F, Hamleez JA. Aeroallergens and work-related respiratory symptoms among office workers. J Allergy Clin Immunol 1998; 101:38–44.
54. Barnes CS, Pacheco F, Landuyt J, Rosenthal D, Hu F, Portnoy J. Production of a recombinant protein from Alternaria containing the reported N-terminal of the Alt a 1 protein. Adv Exp Med Biol 1996; 409:197–203.
55. DeVonge MW, Thaker AJ, Curran IHA, Zhang L, Muradia G, Rode H, Vijay H. Isolation and expression of a cDNA clone encoding an Alternaria alternata Alt a 1 subunit. Int Arch Allergy Immunol 1996; 111:385–395.
56. Breitenbach M, Achatz G, Oberkofler H, Simon B, Unger A, Lechenauer E, Kandler D, Ebner C, Kraft D. Molecular characterization of allergens of Cladosporium herbarum and Alternaria alternata. Int Arch Allergy Immunol 1995; 107:458–459.
57. Achatz G, Oberkofler H, Lechenauer E, Simon B, Unger A, Kandler D, Ebner C, Prillinger H, Kraft D, Breitenbach M. Molecular cloning of major and minor allergens of Alternaria alternata and Cladosporium herbarum. Mol Immunol 1995; 32:213–227.
58. Zhang L, Muradia G, Curran IHA, Rode H, Vijay HM. A cDNA clone coding for a novel allergen, Cla h III, of Cladosporium herbarum identified as a ribosomal P2 protein. J Immunol 1995; 54:710–717.
59. Zhang L, Muradia G, DeVonge MW, Rode H, Vijay HM. An allergenic polypeptide representing a variable region of hsp 70 cloned from a cDNA library of Cladosporium herbarum. Clin Exp Allergy 1996; 26:88–95.
60. Breitenbach M, Simon B, Probst G, Oberkofler H, Ferreira F, Briza P, Achatz G, Unger A, Ebner C, Kraft D, Hirschwehr R. Enolases are highly conserved fungal allergens. Int Arch Allergy Immunol 1997; 113:114–117.
61. Moser M, Crameri R, Menz G, Schneider T, Dudler T, Virchow C, Gmachi M, Blaser K, Suter M. Cloning and expression of recombinant Aspergillus fumigatus allergen I/a (rAsp f I/a) with IgE binding and type 1 skin test activity. J Immunol 1992; 149:454–460.
62. Arruda LK, Mann BJ, Chapman WD. Selective expression of a major allergen and cytotoxin Asp f 1, in Aspergillus fumigatus. J Immunol 1992; 149:3354–3359.
63. Moser M, Crameri R, Brust E, Suter M, Menz G. Diagnostic value of recombinant

Aspergillus fumigatus allergen I/a for skin testing and serology. J Allergy Clin Immunol 1994; 93:1–11.

64. Hermann S, Blaser K, Crameri R. Allergens of Aspergillus fumigatus and Candida boidinii share IgE-binding epitopes. Am J Respir Crit Care Med 1997; 156:1956–1962.

65. Banerjee B, Kurup VP. Molecular biology of Aspergillus allergens. Immunol Allergy Clin No Amer 1998; 18:601–618.

66. Crameri R. Recombinant Aspergillus fumigatus allergens: from the nucleotide sequences to clinical applications. Int Arch Allergy Immunol 1998; 115:99–114.

67. Banerjee B, Kurup VP, Phadnis S, Greenberger PA, Fink JN. Molecular cloning and expression of a recombinant Aspergillus fumigatus protein Asp f 11 with a significant immunoglobulin E reactivity in allergic bronchopulmonary aspergillosis. J Lab Clin Med 1996; 127:253–256.

68. Shen H-D, Lin W-L, Tsai J-J, Liaw S-F, Han S-H. Allergenic components in three different species of *Penicillium*: cross-reactivity among major allergens. Clin Exp Allergy 1996; 26:444–451.

69. Shen H-D, Lin W-L, Liaw S-F, Tam MF, Han S-H. Characterization of the 33-kilodalton major allergen of *Penicillium* citrinum by using MoAbs and N-terminal amino acid sequencing. Clin Exp Allergy 1997; 27:79–86.

70. Shen H-D, Lin W-L, Wang S-R, Tsai J-J, Chou H, Hans S-H. Alkaline serine proteinase: a major allergen of Aspergillus oryzase and its cross-reactivity with *Penicillium* citrinum. Int Arch Allergy Immunol 1998; 116:29–35.

71. Shen H-D, Au L-C, Lin W-L, Liaw S-F, Tsai J-J, Han S-H. Molecular cloning and expression of a *Penicillium* citrinum allergen with sequence homology and antigenic cross-reactivity to a hsp 70 human heat shock protein. Clin Exp Allergy 1997; 27:682–690.

72. Rylander R, Norrhall M, Engdahl U, Tunsäter A, Holt PG. Airways inflammation, atopy, and $(1{\rightarrow}3)$-β-D-glucan exposures in two schools. Am J Respir Crit Care Med 1998; 158:1685–1687.

73. Kamphuis HJ, deRuiter GA, Veeneman GH, VanBoom JH, Rombouts FM, Notermans SHW. Detection of Aspergillus and *Penicillium* extracellular polysaccharides (EPS) by ELISA: using antibodies raised against acid hydrolyzed EPS. Antonie Van Leeuwenhoek 1992; 61:323–332.

74. Portnoy J, Pacheco F, Upadrashta B, Barnes C. A double monoclonal antibody assay for the Alternaria allergen GP-70. Ann Allergy 1993; 71:401–407.

75. Garrison RA, Robertson LD, Koehn RD, Wynn SR. Effect of heating–ventilation–air conditioning system sanitation on airborne fungal populations in residential environments. Ann Allergy 1993; 71:548–556.

76. Salvaggio JE, Burge HA, Chapman JA. Emerging concepts in mold allergy: what is the role of immunotherapy? J Allergy Clin Immunol 1993; 92:217–222.

77. Solomon WR. From: Bush RK. Fungal extracts in clinical practice. Allergy Proc 1993; 14:383–390, used with permission.

6

Role of Seasonal Pollen Exposure
Assessment and Control

WILLIAM R. SOLOMON

University of Michigan Medical School
Ann Arbor, Michigan

I. Introduction

Periodic asthma that coincides with pollen "seasons" has been described traditionally, in atopic subjects, as a feature of inhalant allergy (1). Affected persons often have allergic rhinitis as a troublesome comorbidity, and many primarily seek relief of nasal symptoms. However, the implication that pollen-induced asthma could impair quality of life, complicate etiological diagnosis, augment bronchial hyperreactivity, facilitate secondary infection, and, potentially, yield to specific immunotherapy continues to justify interest.

In the last quarter-century, the validity of asthma due to natural pollen exposure has been scrutinized and potential mechanisms reevaluated (2). That *per oral* exposure to nebulized pollen extracts can provoke both immediate and late bronchial reactions is well established, challenges often measurably heightening airway reactivity as indicated by PD_{20} values for methacholine and histamine (3). However, such challenges typically deliver extremely high *total* allergen loads at dosing *rates* rarely, if ever, approached in nature. The growing recognition that "acute" laboratory challenge is not a realistic dose–response model seems well founded; however, this view has been expanded to cast doubt on the validity of airway responses with ambient pollen exposure. Several additional concerns reinforce this skepticism; chief among these is the manifest improbability that inhaled pollen grains, sized as inferred from intact reference materials, would reach the subcarinal airways (4). In addition, relatively few subjects are *easily* identified as experiencing pollen-season-associated asthma flares, since additional sensitivities and exposures regularly obscure the identity and relative impact of individual offenders (5). Related studies of the efficacy of specific allergen immunotherapy for pollen-season-associated asthma have been, at best, modestly favorable, reflecting again a paucity of ideally qualified, monosensitive subjects.

Despite these reservations, current clinical evidence supports a role for pollen allergens in many seasonal flares of asthma. Furthermore, recent insight into the nature and dispersion of implicated agents has increasingly implicated pollen as a cause of allergic lower airway response.

II. Nature and Travels of Airborne Pollen

A. Pollen Structure and Function

The reproductive potential of pollen was evident to many early cultures, prompting both ceremonial use to symbolize fertility and hand-pollination of certain crops. However, even today, the complex generative nature of pollen is widely unrecognized. Rather than behaving as a spore, pollen functions as a distinctive *stage* (the "male gametophyte") in the life cycle of most flowering plants. Following transfer to a compatible stigma and germination of the grain, i.e., protrusion of a cellulose-covered pollen tube, (haploid) gametes are formed that, on reaching an ovary, effect fertilization and, ultimately, seed production. Passage of the pollen tube from stigma to ovary requires enzymatic digestion of the intervening tissue (a portion of the usually elongate style). Fusion of other pollen- and ovary-derived nuclei allows development of *endosperm*, a nutritive substance for the prospective plant embryo. These diverse functions mandate a host of constitutive and inducible pollen components—especially subserving grain–stigma compatibility and pollen tube penetration—some of which function as human allergens (6).

Pollen grains form in tetrads, but in most species the individual units or "monads" separate before dispersion occurs. Anther sacs shelter the developing grains, and an inner lining, the *tapetum*, provides both structural substance and nourishment. Of the three principal regions of the grain, the tapetum contributes an outermost layer, the *exine*, composed of sporopollenin, a durable squalene polymer. The exine bears distinctive ornaments and apertures; it thereby contributes most to grain appearance in air samples, and it is exclusively preserved, allowing identification, in lake sediments. A *protoplast* containing genetic material, starch grains, and other organelles occupies the grain's center and secretes an envelope, the *intine*, which underlies the exine. Pollen develops in a liquid medium that facilitates a bidirectional exchange of soluble products. On emergence from the anther (*anthesis*), grains dry and contract, but they can easily expand when rewetted by a receptive style or other moist surface. Pollen can also undergo osmotic lysis in hypotonic media. In rainwater, for example, grain protoplasts swell and often burst, extruding their contents; the exine may rupture (e.g., in *Juniperus* species), but it usually retains its integrity. However, even intact grains release their allergens in a predictable sequence, and some fairly quickly, when moistened (7).

B. Pollen Release and Dispersion

Several studies suggest that anthers ripen and release pollen as a brief, coordinated event orchestrated by temperature, day/night length, and other factors. However, a single plant may mature flowers (florets) during one or more weeks, *possibly* with changing complements of pollen allergens. Similarly, site-to-site differences in pollen allergens have been suggested for single species (e.g., short ragweed), although confirmation is lacking.

Pollen is presented to the environment when mature and may be dispersed in one or more distinctive ways. A majority of flowering plants have coevolved with vectors (e.g., insects, birds, bats) that provide targeted cross-pollination within single species or among closely related species. These types, generically termed "entemophilous," characteristically show attractants (i.e., large colorful flowers, sweet scents, carbohydrate-rich nectaries) for their preferred vectors. [With entemophily, reproductive efficiency is achieved despite relatively low pollen output (i.e., few grains per anther and small numbers of flowers)]. Pollen grains of entemophilous species are often relatively large (i.e., above 30 μm) with a more or less thick lipid coating and prominent surface sculpting. These features should facilitate transport of grains *in groups* by a mobile vector.

By contrast, wind-dispersed grains and their floral sources are modified to maximally exploit dispersion by air currents. These pollen types are often

15–40 μm in size, are relatively smooth ("psilate"), and show thin lipid coatings—features that favor atmospheric dispersion as buoyant, single units. Wind-pollinated (anemophilous) flowers achieve copious pollen outputs, reflecting numerous grains per anther; massed groupings of small, drab, scentless flowers are the norm. These species (e.g., the grasses) are highly successful and are the principal offenders in pollinosis worldwide. In addition, a limited number of *amphiphilous* types enjoy transport by *both* wind *and* flying vectors, often with intermediate floral and pollen features. Actively foraging insects will also, occasionally, produce highly localized "hot spots" of suspended entemophilous grains. A clinical role for resulting exposures has been claimed, but their impact remains speculative (8).

Successful pollination (the transfer of viable grains to a receptive stigma) by wind requires the release of huge numbers of particles under conditions that favor dispersion as viable units. The resulting bioaerosol levels and areas of contamination can be truly astounding, leaving little doubt as to why anemophilous species are such potent pollinosis sources. Access to freely moving air assists dispersion, and anemophilous plants have evolved to favor open areas; those of woodlands are, largely, trees of the canopy and usually flower before leaves emerge. Since low humidity promotes the dispersion of pollen as dry, discrete grains rather than as damp aggregates, a host of adaptations encourage dispersion in dry, breezy periods, usually during daylight hours (9). This pattern also lowers the risk of suspended grains being scavenged by falling raindrops or swelling and falling out more rapidly in humid air. While mulberries (*Morus*), nettles (*Urtica*), and some related species project dry pollen explosively (in visible "puffs"), release by most species is more passive. A multiphase process dependent on falling humidity and rising air motion after sunrise has been shown to direct pollen shedding by short ragweed (10). In this sequence, the protruded anthers desiccate, crack, and spill pollen onto the underlying leaves, where the grains dry and later are refloated by warm air currents. The anthers of several taxa, including some grasses and plantains, have pores that close hygroscopically in damp periods, opening as humidity falls. Related mechanisms to retain mature pollen during damp periods had already evolved in the relatively primitive conifers, and antecedents are known even among nonvascular plants (e.g., mosses) (9).

C. Pollen Exposure: A Complex Function of Prevalence

Several factors in addition to source strength affect risks of human exposure to pollen. These include proximity to discrete or extended ("area") sources, wind speed and direction, degree of air turbulence, and depth of the atmospheric layer in which mixing can occur (described by the *lapse rate*).* Both indoors and out, disturbance of dry surfaces also may refloat previously deposited grains and/or their liberated products. The variable interplay of these factors has frustrated efforts to relate pollen prevalence simply to single environmental variables in prediction models. In rural air, for example, in the Midwest, with wind speeds up to 8–10 mph, ragweed pollen levels rise but then decline as winds grow stronger (often with a deepening mixing layer) (11). Nocturnal data, especially, can vary between urban and rural sites also due to differential effects of surface temperature on vertical air motion (the "urban heat island" phenomenon).†

Particle peaks often vary diurnally when points near and distant from sources are compared, the differences reflecting time required for horizontal transport. Measurable middle- and long-distance carriage of pollen (with prevailing continental flows) is amply documented (9,12); however, most pollinosis probably reflects sources within a few miles. Despite the tonnage of anemophilous pollen produced, much falls out or is intercepted close to its release point.

III. Pollen Allergens and Their Distribution

A. Allergen Designation and Occurrence Patterns

A variety of soluble pollen components sensitize atopic humans and can, with exposure, induce mast-cell-dependent clinical responses. Like most other inhaled IgE-reactive agents, pollen allergens typically are glycoproteins, most sized at 10–80 kDa (13); however, exceptions are recognized. Implicated agents may occur primarily (or exclusively) in pollen, while others are found widely in plant tissues. Among the latter, profilins have attracted attention as

---

*The lapse rate is the rate of fall of air temperature with increasing altitude. As long as greater height offers progressively colder conditions, a parcel of warm air will continue to rise. If warm air lies above cold ("thermal inversion"), air (and aerosols) will rise no higher. Thermal inversions at low altitudes markedly restrict the depth of the mixing layer and serve to concentrate emissions, and so on, near the surface.

†In general, urban areas have higher surface temperatures than surrounding rural land. This prompts the warming, expansion, and consequent rising of air over towns and cities, which opposes the predominant subsidence (descent) of cooling air after sunset.

potential "panallergens," common to many forms (14). Profilins are a family of structural proteins, averaging 14 kDa, that couple metabolic processes with cytoskeletal structures and function importantly to facilitate eukaryotic cell motion (14,15). Enzymes, especially ribonucleases, also include prominent allergens, and their intrinsic activity may contribute to such tissue effects as mucosal penetration and inflammatory cell activation. Sharing of multiply conserved components may explain allergenic similarities among pollens of unrelated taxa (16) as well as conjoint sensitivity to pollens and certain ingested plant products such as nuts and fleshy fruits that may be offenders in an "oral allergy syndrome" (17) described especially in birch pollen reactive subjects.

Techniques allowing the cloning and harvest of gene products, with amplification using expression vectors, have facilitated the characterization and sequencing of several major pollen allergens. Agents studied have typically shown more than one antigenically reactive epitope, often with differential effects on T and B cells of single donors. Multiple isoforms of specific allergens also are found commonly, with differing isoelectric points, reflecting small intermolecular differences in charged amino acids. The biological (especially enzymatic) activity of many pollen components is conspicuous (6) and may affect clinically relevant interactions such as mucosal penetration, processing by antigen-presenting cells, and cytokine responses of T-helper cell subtypes (18).

The increasing usefulness of purified allergens for standardizing diagnostic and treatment reagents has mandated a now widely accepted system for designating defined biogenic sensitizers. This scheme uses the first three letters of the generic epithet and the first letter of the species name to identify allergens of a specific taxon (e.g., a plant species); in this approach, the IgE-reactive agents of short ragweed (*Ambrosia artemisiifolia*) are "Amb a 1" to "Amb a *n*" and those of rye grass (*Lolium perenne*) are identified as "Lol p" (+ number) components. The numerical assignment reflects an allergen's place in the historical sequence of characterized entities from that species. In many instances, the most clinically reactive allergen also has been the first described for its taxon, but this is not invariably true. Reservations may also develop where species (or genera) names begin similarly (e.g., for ragweeds, *Ambrosia artemisiifolia* and *A. acanthicarpa*). Confusion also might result where an allergen shared among species is named for a related but locally minor taxon [e.g., rye grass (Lol p) allergens also present in regional dominants, such as june, orchard, and timothy grass pollens in the Midwest]. Despite such concerns, however, this internationally accepted system remains quite useful, a lingua franca of biogenic sensitizers.

Even by light microscopy, pollen grains show surface debris, including partly organized fragments of exine substance (Übisch bodies), scraps of tapetal tissue, and dried fluid plus a surface lipid layer (pollenkitt) (19). The rapid release of at least some allergens, shown clearly for several pollen types in aqueous media, may, in part, reflect these superficial materials (7,20). Such surface activity and the apparently prompt mobilization of agents from deeper sites in moist pollen have slowed efforts to localize allergens in intact grains. These ultrastructural studies have been especially sensitive to artifacts induced by conditions of fixation and immunochemical staining. However, careful immunogold treatment of electron microscopic (EM) sections has suggested typical sites for several pollen allergens; selective localization to exine, intine, or protoplast has been described (21–24).

B. Pollen Allergens in Diverse Aerosols

Reasons to Pursue Allergen in Small Particle Fractions

The ease of mobilizing allergens from moist pollen and the various particulates that are associated with mature grains (i.e., tapetal tissue and dried fluid, Übisch bodies, etc.) has long suggested that more than one aerosol fraction might provide a vector for pollen allergens. In addition, several groups have described allergens, relatively plentiful in pollen, that occur also in nonfloral plant tissues (25,26). Interest also has been spurred by the improbability that inhaled, *intact* pollen grains should reach subcarinal airways where the primary asthmatic response is expected to occur (27). This theoretical prediction of essentially complete removal of pollen-sized particles by upper airways has been borne out in direct challenge using radiotagged short ragweed grains (4); however, discordant findings also have been reported, suggesting that "nonrespirability" is not absolute (28).

These considerations are especially intriguing when one recalls the difficulty of assessing dose–response relationships for pollinosis. Even for pollen-induced allergic rhinitis, many temporal disparities between parameters of exposure and clinical response are familiar, including the appearance of pollinosis symptoms both before and well after periods of measurable pollen occurrence in air. The paradox of peak pollinosis symptoms occurring at or shortly after sunrise, when numbers of airborne grains reach their diurnal nadir (29), has also prompted a reexamination of response determinants.*

---

*Besides the form of an inhalant allergen, factors meriting attention include direct effects of changing air quality variables and body position, impact of *late* IgE-mediated responses in fostering "priming" phenomena, and dynamics of allergen absorption from the upper airway as well as its subsequent circulation and bioavailability.

Indications of Allergen Transport by Smaller Aerosols

The inferred uncertainties regarding pollen-induced asthma were crystallized by Hoehne and Reed in 1971 (2) and Busse et al. in 1972 (30). These workers challenged various respiratory tract levels of appropriately sensitive subjects extraseasonally with ragweed pollen. Despite previous suggestions of nasal/nasopharyngeal-bronchial reflexes (31), they found no evidence of bronchial response unless allergen physically reached the subglottic airways (3). This result was especially striking, since their methods did not totally preclude the "slippage" (adventitious passage) of some material from the upper to the lower tract (as suspended particles or "allergen-soiled" secretions). The same group went on to search for ragweed allergens in aerosol fractions sized below intact pollen grains, using a sequential sieve impinger (30). They noted allergenic activity in several small micrometric fractions that appeared by light microscopy to have no intact grains. However, since the deposits scanned were quite dense and the possibility of particles rebounding from dry surfaces was real, their findings required confirmation. Collateral evidence of ragweed pollen allergen activity in "paucimicrometric"* aerosol fractions far smaller than single, dry grains was later obtained during periods of active pollination (32). At these times, activity was also demonstrated in submicrometric fractions partitioned by absolute filtration and captured by "freeze-out" in a cold trap (33). More recently, similar findings of allergens in small atmospheric aerosol cuts have been reported for several major pollen sensitizers (34).

Methods used in these studies have emphasized serial (differential) filtration or sequential sieve impingement on special collection surfaces. Both high and low volume air movers have been employed successfully. Where a *comparison* of large and small aerosol-associated activity is the focus, simultaneous collections of both are mandatory, since these fractions tend to vary independently over time. Artifacts due to anisokinetic† sampling is a common risk, but resulting errors probably are small, at least for pollen grains, especially if the sampler is wind-oriented (35). Problems of analysis by ELISA, etc. have included variable rates of allergen elution from particle collections, possible

---

*i.e., with equivalent aerodynamic size of a "few" micrometers.

†Failure of a collector to remain directionally aligned with airflow and/or for the speed of free airflow to equal that in the sampler's entrance orifice results in anisokinetic conditions and collection errors; those due to directional factors are greatest for larger aerosols.

contamination by cross-reactive, allergen-containing aerosols, and the tenacious adherence of allergens to certain filter media. Disparities in which recoveries indicate many pollen grains with little total assayable allergen may indicate refloated particles from which allergen has been thoroughly leached (36); however, direct evidence for this scenario is limited.

Data indicating pollen allergens in outdoor aerosols smaller than intact grains have now been reported for short ragweed, oak, grass, birch, Japanese (Sugi) cypress (*Cryptomeria japonica*) (37), and *Parietaria* (38). Indeed, such polydisperse transport seems to have been shown whenever it was sought and may be a feature of many (perhaps all) common anemophilous types. In most instances, peaks of small-particle-associated allergens have accompanied maximum anthesis, with variably lesser prevalence levels following these periods. In some cases, active small micrometric aerosols have been described *before* pollen shedding (39), although earlier flowering, cross-reactive types might explain certain occurrences (40).

Effects of Weather Conditions on Allergen Transport

Changes in levels of allergenic activity among aerosol fractions have been linked to weather variables (40). However, the interplay of atmospheric factors is sufficiently complex that major determinants and epiphenomena may be indistinguishable. Most studies reflect associations between increases in the larger bioaerosols with high temperature and full solar input, lower relative humidity, and the absence of rainfall—factors that promote pollen shedding and dispersion (9). These particle levels fall sharply during brief convective showers due to scouring by large droplets, and more slowly during sustained (frontal) rain (9). By contrast, during both types of rainfall, particles sized below 5 μm (paucimicrometric), as well as submicrometric units, may rise precipitously; resulting levels of small particles can remain elevated for many hours (40). This effect of rain has been especially marked for grass (34) and birch (40) pollens but is also suggested in our own ragweed-based data (11).

Multiple mechanisms to explain allergen-rich, rainfall-generated paucimicrometric aerosols have been proposed and several supported by aerometric evidence. The best studied example is grass pollen, which undergoes osmotic lysis of its protoplast in rainwater, releasing its content of 1–2 μm starch granules (Fig. 1); approximately 100 such organelles may be liberated per grain, each rich in a principal grass pollen allergen (41). Entire starch granules may be splash-dispersed in the outwash spray from impacting raindrops, especially in thunderstorms. Alternatively, molecular allergens, previously eluted and present in accessible surface films, might be dispersed similarly

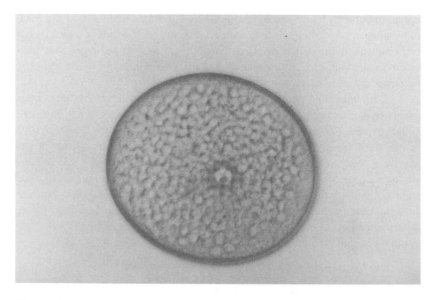

Figure 1 Single timothy grass pollen grain showing the numerous starch granules that it characteristically contains. These granules are allergen associated and can elicit obstructive airway responses when separated and used in bronchial challenge of grass-pollen-sensitive subjects. The single pore with a central dark disk (the operculum) is a feature of grass pollens in general.

(42). The occurrence of (ragweed) pollen allergen associated with submicrometric aerosols collected by freeze-out supports a role for this or related processes (33).

Studies of birch pollen have suggested that allergen-associated, paucimicrometric particles become airborne in a scenario recalling that of grass grains. Specifically, birch grains germinate on natural surfaces when wetted, for example, by dew formed at night. When drying later occurs, these tubes, thinly covered with cellulose, rupture, liberating organelles including as many as 400 starch granules (43). These minute units may be dispersed later by dry or splash-induced disturbance.

Outbreaks of Asthma with Convective Showers

The confirmation of pollen allergens in small respirable aerosols, as described above, has motivated a search for resulting allergic lower airway events; recent interest has focused principally on asthma occurring during and after thunderstorms (41). This association is familiar to many clinicians and may reflect lower atmospheric determinants such as physical properties of air, pollutant levels, barometric or sferic (lightning-associated) effects, and exposure to potential allergens such as ballistospores (e.g., *Didymella*) (44) that require free water for dispersion. While any of these factors might cause asthma flares, exposure to paucimicrometric pollen allergen aerosols has been suggestively associated with several regional epidemics of asthma during thunderstorms (45,46). Recognition of these events has been facilitated by real-time utilization data gathered by national health systems and the focused interest of astute local investigators. Perhaps the most dramatic epidemic event was accompanied by a large convective storm during the night of 24–25 June 1994, close to the local peak of grass pollination in southeastern England (45,46). The storm was mesoscale (i.e., unusually large), with several centers and strong turbulence. A tenfold excess of patients presenting for treatment of asthma (over that expected) was recorded with well above 1000 persons affected regionally; a high percentage of these were grass pollen sensitive. Analyses of this event suggest that it was most notable for its prestorm temperature drop, sferic intensity, and occurrence after several days of peak grass pollen prevalence (46).

Thunderstorms occurring during spring rye grass pollination also have been associated with striking numbers of asthma events requiring emergency room attendance in Melbourne, Australia (47). Here, as in England, there was no suggestion of fossil fuel combustion products as determinants; but, again, grass pollen sensitivity was typical of those affected. Many persons studied had previously experienced only grass pollen induced rhinitis and encountered their first asthma symptoms during the implicated storms.

While sudden, intense exposure to respirable grass pollen aerosols seems critical to these epidemic events, increased emergency room attendance for asthma is often observed in association with storms and the passage of cold fronts (48). At these times, possible effects of gaseous and particulate pollutants (49), humidity, lapse rate, and bioaerosols including ragweed pollen, ascospores, and small basidiospores have all been proposed with variably persuasive supporting data. Any of these factors singly or in concert may determine the impact of an epidemic asthma event. However, recognition of at least some pollen allergens in respirable aerosols provides an additional plausible source for seasonal lower airway symptoms. The dispersion of allergen-rich organelles shown for grass and birch grains remains to be demonstrated for other types of pollen and, if confirmed, does not preclude sources of specific microaerosols, especially at times outside the normal anthesis period.

Additional Sources of Small, Pollen-Specific Allergenic Aerosols

As previously noted, pollen develops in a complex fluid with (friable) tapetal tissue as well as fragments of exine material (Übisch bodies)—all potential allergen vectors and all liberated at anthesis. Furthermore, there is evidence that anemophilous species vary greatly in their outputs of such small particles (50). Takahashi and coworkers (50) studied this question directly using plants undergoing anthesis in the laboratory with particle outputs analyzed by aerosol beam spectrometry. They focused attention on particles sized 20–40 μm (intact grains) and those of 0.4–1.4 μm (approximating the size range of Übisch bodies). Small particles predominated by at least eightfold in emanations of *Cryptomeria japonica* (Sugi cypress), a major pollinosis source in Japan; 99% of these were confirmed as Übisch bodies by electron microscopy. Similar analyses using pollen outputs of *Alnus japonica* (alder), *Quercus serrata* (oak), and *Dactylus glomerata* (orchard grass) found equal numbers of large and small particles as well as many of intermediate (2.5–10 μm) size. However, no particles below 18 μm were described from emanations of *Ambrosia artemisiifolia* (short ragweed) collected from sites in Japan. Whether these findings fully characterize the species studied or vary among clones or with growth conditions remains to be determined (51).

Additional sources of respirable pollen allergen might include physically degraded or naturally shed plant tissues that contain sensitizing factors. Studies of such materials including indument (plant hairs) (52) require comprehensive efforts to avoid incidental contamination by pollen-derived materials. Despite this *caveat*, evidence has been presented for small amounts of "pollen" allergen in somatic tissue of several species (53), at least one report based on tissue culture (54). However, the source of grass allergen microparticulates, apparently dispersed during turf cutting, remains controversial (26).

IV. Evaluation of Exposure

The identification of pollinosis requires, at minimum, demonstration of specific sensitivity and a persuasive association of symptoms with patterns of exposure to suspected (or candidate) allergens. As a consequence, even the earliest studies in this field included aerometric data in attempts to reflect exposure (1). The once elusive goal of describing pollen prevalence as "grains recovered per cubic meter of air sampled" has been achieved using spore traps and rotating arm impactors allowing visual analysis of stained particle deposits. These devices collect intact grains with acceptable (i.e., > 50%) efficiency under most conditions, unbiased by changing wind direction (9). Spore trap performance does vary with wind speed, especially for aerosols below 10 μm and above 40 μm, although for most anemophilous types this effect is small (35). Overloading of both types of samplers, with resulting drops in adhesive efficiency, must be prevented. This risk is greater for impactors and is sharply reduced by limiting total sampling time (55). These resources have favored the establishment of air-sampling networks in several regions, providing detailed synoptical records and forecasting potential (56). However, many areas—especially in Asia and Latin America—remain to be studied systematically.

Recognition of airborne pollen allergens associated with aerosols smaller than intact grains has posed new aerometric challenges in exposure assessment. While a preference for suction collectors is acknowledged, the relative merits of (dry) filtration versus impingement in fluids (e.g., in glass impingers) have not been compared (57). Dry impingement on solid surfaces was employed in the earliest studies (30) but seems to pose unnecessary risks of overloading and particle loss. Both impingers and filters can be designed and sequenced to separate aerosols into fractions of different aerodynamic sizes.

Efforts to assay particle deposits must recognize the ease with which major allergens enter solution as well as their tendency to migrate and bind tenaciously to filter media (as well as glass). The latter risk is not predictably eliminated by addition of unrelated proteins (e.g., human serum albumin) but can be assessed by "spiking" samples with *known* allergen and determining percent recovery. The emergence of defined pollen allergens, their increasing availability as recombinant products, and their use to elicit monoclonal antibodies have greatly aided analysis of paucimicrometric aerosols. Solid-phase immunoassay has been especially useful, although nonspecific binding remains a concern.

While volumetric allergen data (values per unit volume) often are translated directly into respiratory tract dosing (based on defined minute volumes), some reservations are justified. Access to the airways and depth of penetration will depend on the regime of breathing (nasal vs. oral) and the size range of presented aerosols. Total allergen dosing will vary with the speed and direction of ambient air movement relative to the mouth and (more or less) downward-directed human nares.* Impaction on unshielded ocular surfaces also may supply allergen to distant organs following its absorption. Although hematogenous

---

*For the nose, as with (other) suction collectors, nonalignment of intake orifice and flow increases recovery errors, especially for larger (e.g., pollen-sized) units.

dissemination of allergen eluted from mucous surfaces has not been a focus of research in over 50 years (58), evidence suggesting clinically relevant absorption of intact allergens is recognized (59).

Disparities in exposure also can result at sites near and distant from specific sources; barrier-induced flow eddies and stagnation points, local substrate disturbance, or the "shelter" effect of enclosed spaces may all contribute. Exposure in vehicles varies primarily with regimes of ventilation but also with speed of airflow, changing outdoor levels, and residual allergen burdens in cabin interiors (60).

V. The Case for Pollen-Induced Asthma

Recognition of allergen transport by respirable aerosol fractions has removed a significant barrier to acceptance of pollen as a plausible asthma determinant. However, several lines of evidence, besides clinicians' impressions, also lend strong positive support to this view.

Efforts to explain allergic asthma as a reflex response to upper airway inflammation have attracted little supporting evidence, although such pathways may occur in other species (31). In fact, despite risks that aerosol traces might reach lower airways, nasal challenge with pollen extracts only rarely elicits a bronchial response (61). This experience accords well with earlier data in which no airways changes followed whole pollen challenge of nasal and nasopharyngeal sites in specifically sensitive subjects (2). However, inhalation of crushed pollen grains has produced asthma in comparable volunteers (62). These findings imply that a pollen-allergen-specific lower airways response is elicited most readily by bronchial exposure to IgE-reactive *respirable* units; other potent mechanisms may yet be shown to coexist.

This laboratory-based experience is especially intriguing in view of the emerging recognition of allergen transport by an array of particulates smaller than intact pollen grains. Besides directly challenging the airways in their "original" form, these biogenic units can be shown to associate with aerosols such as diesel exhaust particles (63), charge largely determining the binding. The products derived may have greater aerodynamic size than their "parent" units, promoting deposition in more proximal, subcarinal airways (27). Such condensed aerosols also may exceed the size range of 0.1–0.5 µm, which most readily evades pulmonary deposition by gravity *or* diffusion.

Evidence arising from clinical (and basic) research also implicates pollen among the determinants of allergic asthma. Studies of grass pollen sensitive subjects, reporting seasonal deterioration of asthma control, showed this subjective view supported by increased symptom scores and levels of bronchodilator use (64). Furthermore, both sets of parameters rose especially *after* the annual peak of pollen prevalence, suggesting parallels to late-phase IgE-dependent airway responses. Affected asthmatic individuals, on BAL and airway biopsy, have shown evidence of increased mast cell activation (including greater IL-4 release) and loss of metachromatic staining. Increased numbers of mucosal T_H cells were also observed, and those in lavage fluid showed acute activation markers. Methacholine responsiveness rose variably from preseasonal levels during peak pollen exposure, but the differences lacked statistical significance.*

However, other studies have observed the expected rise in bronchial hyperresponsiveness (BHR) during natural exposure of pollen-sensitive asthmatic patients (and its anticipated fall after exposure is ended) (3,66). The effectiveness of corticosteroids (67,68) and of cromones (69) in blunting this exposure-induced rise in airways reactivity also has been amply confirmed. Since the accumulation of activated airway eosinophils is thought critical to BHR, evidence for their *directed* inmigration, in pollen-exposed allergic asthmatic individuals holds special interest. Besides confirming this chemotactic effect, Raq et al. (70) showed that it could be limited by immunotherapy with specific pollen extracts. Not surprisingly, seasonal exposure of pollen-sensitive asthmatic individuals has been found to increase peripheral blood eosinophil activation markers (i.e., surface CD9 and CD11b and granular ECP epitope EG2), although eosinophil numbers did not rise significantly during exposure to local pollen offenders (71). Peripheral blood mononuclear cells of specifically sensitive atopic patients have shown greater T_H cytokine production (IL-2, IL-4, and IL-5) in response to pollen allergens than those of nonatopic controls (72). Among atopic individuals, cells from those with asthma showed high cytokine outputs (especially of IL-5) and greater response during pollen seasons than at other times.

The foregoing findings complement that weight of clinical impression which supports the *tradition* of verifiable pollen-induced asthma. While most providers recognize persons so affected, *formal* indicators of prevalence (i.e.,

---

*Additional reports describe temporal dissociations of bronchial hyperresponsiveness and markers of airway inflammation (65), although a mechanistic relationship is highly probable.

for "asthma as a form of pollinosis") have not been presented; rather, it is in descriptions of study populations, usually assembled incident to interventional trials, that evidence of clinical airways disease *in* pollinosis is manifest. Immunotherapy trials—some classic, some recent (see below)—have recruited appropriate asthmatic populations with great care, documenting specific sensitivity, seasonal morbidity patterns, and (relative) absence of confounding determinants; medication trials of comparable quality also are recorded. In addition, small numbers of pollen-sensitive individuals, with only seasonal cough, who benefit from newer antihistaminic drugs, have been described in Europe (73).

Epidemic seasonal asthma remains the most dramatic, if not typical, expression of pollinosis-induced airways events. Although late summer and autumn episodes in New Orleans involved the largest numbers, their determinants remain incompletely resolved (74). Several asthma outbreaks in pollen-reactive subjects have been reported (see above) in Europe and Australia, associated with thunderstorm activity. A convincing association between clinical asthma and seasonal grass pollen exposure also has been described by Reid et al. (75) during (dry) northern California summers. These workers noted sharp rises in symptoms, emergency room visits, and hospital admissions for asthma that paralleled grass pollen prevalence during a 4 year study period; amelioration of exposure-induced chest symptoms with specific allergen immunotherapy was demonstrated also in a well-blinded trial.

These converging lines of evidence leave little room to doubt the reality of pollen as a determinant of *some* seasonal asthma. Intense symptoms can result, and synergy of pollens with other offending allergens as sources of morbidity (and possibly, mortality) is strongly suggested (76). However, the finite nature of annual pollen exposures serves to limit their potential impact (e.g., in comparison with dust mites, house pets, etc.). Effects of diverse additional allergens and airborne irritants may amplify the health impact of pollen exposure while, paradoxically, obscuring its clinical role (49,62,77,78). It seems clear that the extent of asthma in pollinosis remains to be fully detailed and that its definition will require both innovative study methods and subjects with delimited, specific sensitivities.

VI. Prevention and Mitigation of Pollen-Related Asthma

Because subjects in whom specific pollens, *alone*, determine asthma are uncommon, few controlled trials are available to assist the clinician. However, less formal observations suggest that fundamental approaches (i.e., avoidance, symptom-suppressant drugs, specific immunotherapy), validated in related settings, can be helpful here as well.

A. Limiting Exposure to Pollen Allergens

The impact of pollen allergens usually reflects large area (vs. point) sources. Therefore, effective avoidance generally requires either a major (albeit, often temporary) geographic move or creation, in situ, of a "sanctuary" from exposure. Since the latter option is often the more feasible, it is fortunate that closed (preferably air-conditioned) structures often promote lessening of pollinosis symptoms. Within such enclosures, levels of familiar aeroallergens are greatly decreased (79), although the effect on pauci- and submicrometric units may be less and awaits critical study. Since relative separation of indoor and free air compartments is a critical goal, decreasing the frequency of air exchanges should further reduce exposure intensity.* Especially for the smallest bioaerosols, expected benefits of standard air cleaners are minimal (80) *centrally installed* HEPA filters offering the best hope of reducing total exposure.

Reliance upon indoor "sanctuaries" can fail also due to exposures while in transit between such privileged spaces. Motor vehicle travel can impose especially heavy allergen doses, although they may be substantially decreased by recirculation of air and window closure (60); again the effect of these maneuvers on vehicle penetration by small allergenic particles is unknown. However, it is clear that late IgE-based respiratory reactions may foster recurrent symptoms for days after a single intense exposure (81).

Enclosed spaces also may contain offenders that (paradoxically) nullify any expected benefits of outdoor allergen exclusion. Tobacco smoke in homes or vehicles can be especially troublesome (82), and the avoidance of animal, mite, and insect allergen merits serious consideration in those who are multiply sensitive. Pollens once deposited indoors are easily refloated by human activity; however, *indoor* pollen sources are rarely significant (83).

Although rarely implemented, opportunities to avoid pollen through travel do exist. Periods at sea, for example, often bring relief of pollinosis despite documented bioaerosol transport downwind of continents (9). Periods of tree pollinosis often are relatively short, allowing benefit from brief periods of remote travel (Table 1). However, types such as oaks, ashes, and poplars/aspens are much more widespread, while extended or multiple pollen "sea-

---

*This can be optimized by operating window units with the vent closed.

Table 1 Some Regionally Delimited Allergenic Tree Pollens of North America

Source species	Distribution	Comments
Red alder[a] (*Alnus rubra*)	Pacific Northwest (mid-Feb.–April)	Major allergen 18 kDa, resembles those of birch, hazelnut, etc.
White and paper birch (*Betula alba, B. papyrifera*)	Cold woodlands of northern tier (late Apr.–late May)	Allergens similar to other members of family (Betulaceae).
Australian pine (*Casuarina* species)	Principally S. Florida (Oct.–April)	Not a conifer; fall and spring "seasons."
Box elder[a] (*Acer negundo*)	Upper Midwest (mid Apr.–May)	Weedy, totally wind-pollinated maple.
Sugar maple[b] (*Acer saccharum*)	New England (mid Apr.–May)	Amphiphilous maple.
Hackberry (*Celtis* spp.)	Coastal areas, Texas to N. Florida (Jan.–Apr.)	Birch-like grains; allergens unstudied.
Mountain cedar (*Juniperus ashei* and related species)	Southern Rocky Mtns into northern Mexico (mid-Dec.–mid-Fed.)	Pollinates massively in W. Texas; output reaches S. Great Plains.
Red mulberry[a] (*Morus rubra*)	Upper Midwest (early–mid May)	A formidable weed.
White mulberry[a] (*M. alba*)	Arid Southwest (Feb.–Apr.)	Often escapes from cultivation; introduced.
Olive[b] (*Olea europaea*)	Urban Southwest and S. California (Mar.–May)	Imported; major allergen in Mediterranean basin.
Pecan[b] (*Carya texana, C. pecan*)	S. Atlantic states, lower Midwest (Mar.–early May)	Street and plantation tree.
Sycamore[b] (*Platanus* sp.)	Large Mid-atlantic cities (and river valleys) (mid-Apr.–mid-May)	Prominent in urban air; smallest common tree pollen grains.

[a]Dioecious [i.e., "male" (pollen-producing) and "female" (seed-producing) organs on separate plants].
[b]Popular for urban planting.

sons" are typical of mountain cedar (southern Rocky Mountains) and elms as well as *Casuarina* (Australian pines) of warmer regions.

Grass pollens reflect two major allergen categories: (1) those described from perennial rye grass (*Lolium*) and other cool temperate species and (2) those of Bermuda grass (*Cynodon*) and Johnson grass (*Sorghum*). Bermuda grass predominates in southern and western states as well as in warm temperate and subtropical areas worldwide. Furthermore, its flowering period lengthens as mean annual temperature rises. Effective avoidance of grass pollen is achieved only in forested areas at higher latitudes or at substantial elevations; tropical forests offer effective, but less convenient, havens.

Broad-leafed, nonwoody plants (forbs), often referred to as weeds, are dominant pollinosis factors in many (primarily temperate) areas. Particular concern surrounds the huge impact of ragweeds in North America during their well-known August–September anthesis period. Furthermore, the demonstration of ragweed pollen allergen in small particles adds credence to reports of asthma in late summer pollinosis. Refuges for ragweed sufferers have traditionally been in northern forests; however, for many of these sites, progressive upwind land clearing for agriculture has allowed ragweed growth in profusion. Land cultivation appears to be the principal form of soil disturbance favoring ragweed growth, cultivated fields showing the highest short ragweed densities in midwestern surveys (84). Patients eager to evade ragweed emanations should recognize that several species also flower (May through early June) in the arid southwest. Establishment of short ragweed at Old World sites has created exposure risks in Europe and cooler parts of the Far East; many stations in Balkan countries and around the Black Sea are now appreciated. Both extensive ragweed growth and pollinosis are recognized in Hungary. However, the best established "Old World" site is in the upper Rhône valley of France (near Lyon), where epidemic ragweed pollinosis has been observed for several decades. The extent of this site has expanded progressively since World War II, and its output is known to cause pollinosis also in downwind areas of Switzerland, where *no sources* exist at ground level. Similar examples of meso- or megascale transport are well described (12), although studies of smaller aerosols as allergens in this corridor remain to be pursued.

Additional forbs of the chenopod-amaranth group constitute important pollinosis sources in (western) North America and temperate Eurasia due to diverse "scales," poverty weeds, Russian thistle (*Kochia*), etc. Local cultivation of sugar beets provides a potent related pollen source. Similarly distributed species of *Rumex* (sorrels and docks) are strong sensitizers, forming brief local pollen peaks. Although unstudied, possible dispersion of their prominent starch granules might provide abundant paucimicrometric allergen vectors. A comparable mechanism could explain widespread sensitization to plantain (*Plantago*) pollens despite their usually low prevalence levels in air.

Pollens of *Parietaria* species are not now prominent in North America but are dominantly linked to allergic rhinitis and asthma in the Mediterranean basin (e.g., Italy, Greece, Turkey, Israel) (85). *P. officinalis* and the less cold tolerant *P. judaica* are the principal source species responsible for extended mid- to late-summer symptoms. However, the similar appearing grains of *Urtica* (nettle) species, a related genus, appear to lack the potent *Parietaria* allergens (85). Pollens of *Parietaria* are small and thin-walled and act aerodynamically as even smaller units when dry; in addition, paucimicrometric aerosols with allergen activity have been described (38).

B. Medication Options in Seasonal Asthma

Limited subject pools also have severely restricted the amount of data describing drug trials in exclusively pollen-sensitive asthmatic subjects. However, little current evidence suggests that their responses differ from those with airway disease related to mites, animal allergens, etc. Where nasal blockage is associated, restoration of nasal breathing using alpha agonists and/or corticosteroids can sharply reduce particle dosing to subglottic airways and risks of gravitationally mobile (and potentially infectious) secretions (86,87). Observations in laboratory subjects and patient populations also support the usefulness of beta-adrenergic agonists and ipratropium as "rescue" agents and of salmeterol as a preventive bronchodilator. Effects of anti-inflammatory agents (especially inhaled corticosteroids, antileukotriene drugs, and inhaled cromones) all address fundamental tissue processes of asthma with variable adequacy. While cromolyn sodium and nedocromil seem to display their maximum value in allergen-induced asthma, this may be exceeded (or complemented) by other agents. The cromones are especially adapted to brief prophylactic use before and during predictably potent allergen exposures. More regular use also may blunt airway hyperreactivity due to allergen (including pollen) exposure and the tendency to exercise-induced airway narrowing that often results (69).

C. Specific Immunotherapy for Pollen-Induced Asthma

Pollinosis was the first atopic problem to be treated with injected allergen immunotherapy and the first condition in which this approach was validated using a controlled study design. Remarkably, the initial demonstration of efficacy, using grass pollen extracts, was achieved in a study largely of allergic asthmatic patients, although many also had allergic rhinitis. Frankland and Augustin (88) described significant reduction in (rhinitis and) asthma symptoms in intensively treated adults following just 4 months of *preseasonal* therapy (88). Although blinding was crude by modern standards, many placebo-treated participants believed that they had received *active* extracts. An additional British study, by Hill et al. (89), of young asthmatic individuals with grass pollen-induced symptom flares found no difference in seasonal morbidity between specific pollen extract and placebo-treated volunteers. This latter (single-blinded) report was based on relatively small numbers of subjects who were treated somewhat less intensely (although longer) than those in the prior series. Furthermore, perennial allergen exposures, e.g., dust (mites) and house pets, may have imposed a confounding level of baseline symptoms on Hill's study participants.

As recorded in early controlled studies of immunotherapy, problems of marked placebo "efficacy," low available numbers of suitable subjects, and additional sensitivities that obscure "specific" results have remained formidable. However, several additional studies have confirmed lessening seasonal asthma severity in those receiving grass pollen extracts than in those treated with placebo (90). Similar conclusions resulted from an unblinded study of asthma in birch pollinosis with active extract treatment vs. placebo (70,91). Immunotherapy trials for asthma in ragweed pollinosis have been less than conclusive despite the established value of active treatment in epidemic rhinitis (90). Efficacy in late summer asthma was not observed by the Johns Hopkins group using approaches and materials of demonstrated value in ragweed hay fever (5). More recently, a multicenter study of standardized ragweed pollen extract treatment (vs. placebo) was reported with clinical evaluation spanning at least two pollen seasons (92). Once again, enrollment of suitable subjects was a major hurdle, with some original exclusion criteria (e.g., skin reactivity to fungi) later necessarily compromised. Overall, several criteria reflecting morbidity did significantly favor the actively treated subjects. Differences were especially marked in medication use (versus placebo-treated subjects); however, even here, the superiority of active treatment was not consistent over each study season.

Additional immunotherapy trials have not focused primarily on the lower airway and offer only impressions of effects in asthma. For *Parietaria* pollinosis, as one example, most subjects had both rhinitis *and* asthma (85); significant benefit has been seen overall in trials of injection combined with local nasal immunotherapy (93), but differences in *lower* airway parameters were less convincing. At present, therefore, the question of the efficacy of immunotherapy for pollen-induced asthma admits no single verdict. Evidence of benefit in grass pollinosis seems most persuasive; however, evaluation of other problems will require new initiatives with adequate numbers of selectively sensitive subjects, potent materials, and extended periods of treatment and evaluation.

References

1. Vaughan WT. Practice of Allergy. St. Louis: Mosby, 1939.
2. Hoehne JH, Reed CE. Where is the allergic reaction in ragweed asthma? J Allergy Clin Immunol 1971; 48:36–39.
3. Boulet L-P, Cartier A, Thompson NC, Roberts RS, Dolovich J, Hargreave FE. Asthma and increases in nonallergic bronchial responsiveness from seasonal pollen exposure. J Allergy Clin Immunol 1983; 71:399–406.
4. Wilson AF, Novey HS, Berke RA, Suprenant EL. Deposition of inhaled pollen and pollen extract in human airways. N Engl J Med 1973; 288:1056–1058.
5. Bruce CA, Norman PS, Rosenthal RR, Lichtenstein LM. The role of ragweed pollen in autumnal asthma. J Allergy Clin Immunol 1977; 59:449–459.
6. Kao TH, McGubbin AG. How flowering plants discriminate between self and non-self pollen to prevent inbreeding. Proc Natl Acad Sci USA 1996; 93:12059–12065.
7. Baraniuk JN, Bolick M, Esch R, Buckley CE III. Quantification of pollen solute release using pollen grain column chromatography, 1992; 47:411–417.
8. Lewis HW, Vinay P. North American pollinosis due to insect-pollinated plants. Ann Allergy 1979; 42:309–318.
9. Gregory PH. Microbiology of the Atmosphere. 2nd ed. New York: Wiley, 1973.
10. Bianchi DE, Schwemmen DJ, Wagner WH Jr. Pollen release in common ragweed (Ambrosia artemisiifolia). Bot Gazette 1959; 120:235–243.
11. Solomon WR. Unpublished observations.
12. Frei T. Pollen distribution at high elevation in Switzerland: evidence for medium range transport. Grana 1997; 36:34–38.
13. King TP, Hoffman D, Løwenstein H, Marsh DG, Platts-Mills TAE, Thomas W. Allergen nomenclature. Int Arch Allergy Immunol 1994; 105:224–233.
14. Valenta R, Duchêne M, Pettenburger K, Sillaber C, Valent P, Bettleheim P, Breitenbach M, Rumpold H, Kraft D, Scheiner O. Identification of profilin as a novel pollen allergen; IgE autoreactivity in sensitized individuals. Science 1991; 253:557–560.
15. Baatout S. Profilin: an update. Eur J Clin Chem Clin Biochem 1996; 34:575–577.
16. Pham NH, Baldo BA. Allergenic relationship between taxonomically diverse pollens. Clin Exper Allergy 1995; 25:599–606.
17. Pastorello EA, Ortolani C. Oral allergy syndrome. In: Metcalfe DD, Sampson HA, Simon RA, eds. Food Allergy. 2nd ed. Cambridge, MA: Blackwell Science, 1997.
18. Tomee JFC, van Weissenbruch R, de Monchy JGR, Kauffman HF. Interactions between inhalant allergen extracts and airway epithelial cells: effect on cytokine production and cell detachment. J Allergy Clin Immunol 1998; in press.

19. Davis, GL. The anther tapetum, Übisch granules and hay fever. Aust J Sci 1967; 30(6):235–236.
20. Hussain R, Norman PS, Marsh DG. Rapidly released allergens from short ragweed pollen, II. Identification and partial purification. J Allergy Clin Immunol 1981; 67:217–222.
21. Staff IA, Taylor PE, Smith P, Singh MB, Knox RB. Cellular localization of water soluble allergenic proteins in rye-grass (Lolium perenne) pollen using monoclonal and specific IgE antibodies with immunogold probes. Histochem J 1990; 22:276–290.
22. Miki-Hirosige H, Nakamura S, Yasueda H, Shida T, Takahashi Y. Immunocytochemical localization of the allergenic proteins in the pollen of Cryptomeria japonica. Sex Plant Reprod 1994; 7:95–100.
23. Casas C, Marquez J, Suarez-Cervera M, Seoane-Camba JA. Immunocytochemical localization of allergenic proteins in Parietaria judaica L. (Urticaceae) pollen grains. Eur J Cell Biol 1996; 70:179–188.
24. E;-Gjazaly G, Nakamura S, Takahashi Y, Cresti M, Walles B, Milanesi C. Localization of the major allergen Bet v 1 in *Betula* pollen using monoclonal antibody labelling. Grana 1996; 35:369–374.
25. Fernandez-Caldas E, Bandele E, Dunnette E, Swanson M, Reed C. Rye grass cross-reacting allergens in leaves from seven different grass species. Grana 1992; 31:157–159.
26. Rowe M, Baily J, Ownby DR. Evaluation of the cause of nasal and ocular symptoms associated with lawn mowing. J Allergy Clin Immunol 1986; 77:714–717.
27. Gerrity TR, Lee PS, Hass EJ, Marinelli A, Werner P, Lourenco RV. Calculated deposition of inhaled particles in the airway generations of normal subjects. J Appl Physiol 1979; 47:867–873.
28. Soler, M, LeBouffant L, Charpin J. Retention of pollen grains in human lung. Allergy 1982; 37:373–376.
29. Goodwin JE, McLean JA, Hemphill FM, Sheldon JM. Air pollution by ragweed: medical aspects. Fed Proc 1957; 16:628–631.
30. Busse WW, Reed CE, Hoehne JH. Where is the allergic reaction in ragweed asthma? J Allergy Clin Immunol 1972; 50(5):289–293.
31. Whicker JH, Kern EB. The naso-pulmonary response in the awake animal. Ann Otol 1973; 82:355–358.
32. Solomon WR, Burge HA, Muilenberg ML. Allergen carriage by atmospheric aerosol. I. Ragweed pollen determinants in smaller micronic fractions. J Allergy Clin Immunol 1983; 72:443–447.
33. Habenicht HA, Burge HA, Muilenberg ML, Solomon WR. Allergen carriage by atmospheric aerosol, II. Ragweed-pollen determinants in submicronic atmospheric fractions. J Allergy Clin Immunol 1984; 74:64–67.
34. Emberlin J. Plant allergens on pauci-micronic airborne particles. Clin Exper Allergy 1995; 25:202–205.
35. Watson HH. Errors due to anisokinetic sampling of aerosols. Am Ind Hyg Assoc Quart 1954; 15:21–25.

36. Yli-Panula E, Takahashi Y, Rantio-Lehtimäki A. Comparison of direct immuno-staining and electroimmunoassay for analysis of airborne grass-pollen antigens. Allergy 1997; 52:541–546.

37. Spieksma FTM, Nikkels BH, Dijkman JH. Seasonal appearance of grass pollen allergen in natural, pauci-micronic aerosol of various size fractions. Relationship with airborne grass pollen concentration. Clin Exper Allergy 1994; 25:234–239.

38. D'Amato G, Gentili M, Russo M, Mistrello G, Sagese M, Liccardi G, Falagiani P. Detection of *Parietaria judaica* airborne allergenic activity. Comparison between immunochemical and morphological methods including clinical evaluation. Clin Exper Allergy 1993; 24:566–574.

39. Fernandez-Caldas E, Swanson MC, Pravda J, Welsh P, Yunginger JW, Reed CE. Immunochemical demonstration of red oak pollen aeroallergens outside the oak pollination season. Grana 1989; 28:205–209.

40. Pehkonen E, Rantio-Lehtimäki A. Variations in airborne pollen antigenic particles caused by meteorologic factors. Allergy 1994; 49:472–477.

41. Knox RB. Grass pollen, thunderstorms and asthma. Clin Exper Allergy 1993; 23:354–359.

42. Schlichting HE Jr. Ejections of microalgae into the air via bursting bubbles. J Allergy Clin Immunol 1974; 53:185–188.

43. Schäppi GF, Suphioglu C, Taylor PE, Knox RB. Concentrations of the major birch tree allergen Bet v 1 in pollen and respirable fine particles in the atmosphere. J Allergy Clin Immunol 1997; 100:656–661.

44. Packe GE, Ayres JG. Asthma outbreak during a thunderstorm. Lancet 1985; i:199–204.

45. Venables KM, Allitt U, Collier CG, Emberlin J, Greig JB, Hardaker PJ, Higham JH, Laing-Morton T, Maynard RL, Murray V, Strachan D, Tee RD. Thunderstorm-related asthma: the epidemic of 24/25 June 1994. Clin Exper Allergy 1996; 27: 725–736.

46. Newson R, Strachan D, Archibald E, Emberlin J, Hardaker P, Collier C. Effect of thunderstorms and airborne grass pollen on the incidence of acute asthma in England, 1990–94. Thorax 1997; 52:680–685.

47. Bellomo R, Gigliotti P, Treloar A, Holmes P, Suphioglu C, Singh MB, Knox B. Two consecutive thunderstorm associated epidemics of asthma in the city of Melbourne. Med J Aust 1992; 156:834–837.

48. Celenza A, Fothergill J, Kupek E, Shaw RJ. Thunderstorm-associated asthma: a detailed analysis of environmental factors. Br Med J 1996; 312:604–607.

49. Taggart SCO, Custovic A, Francis HC, Faragher EB, Yates CJ, Higgins BG, Woodcock A. Asthmatic bronchial hyperresponsiveness varies with ambient levels of summertime air pollution. Eur Respir J 1996; 9:1146–1154.

50. Takahashi Y, Sasaki K, Nakamura S, Miki-Hirosige H, Nitta H. Aerodynamic size distribution of the particles emitted from the flowers of allergologically important plants. Grana 1995; 34:45–49.

51. Lee YS, Dickinson DB, Schlager D, Velu J. Antigen E content of pollen from individual plants of short ragweed (*Ambrosia artemisiifolia*). J Allergy Clin Immunol 1979; 63:336–339.

52. Ostrov MR. Oak leaf hairs as aeroallergens. Immunol Allergy Pract 1984; 6:258–262.

53. Rantio-Lehtimäki A, Viander M, Kiovikko A. Airborne birch pollen antigens in different particle sizes. Clin Exper Allergy 1994; 24:23–28.

54. Shafiee A, Staba E. Allergens from short ragweed leaf tissue cultures. In Vitro 1973; 9:23–26.

55. Solomon WR, Cathey J. Collection deficits due to particle loading by rotating arm samplers. J Allergy Clin Immunol 1991; 87:169 (abstract).

56. Emberlin JC. Grass, tree and weed pollens. In: Kay AB, ed. Allergy and Allergic Diseases London: Oxford Univ. Press, 1997.

57. Schäppi GF, Monn C, Wüthrich B, Wanner HU. Direct determination of allergens in ambient aerosols: methodological aspects. Int Arch Allergy Immunol 1996; 110:364–370.

58. Johnson MC, Alexander HL, Alexander JH, Walker JM. Measurement of circulating ragweed antigen. Allergy 1945; 16:261–266.

59. Kontou-Karakitsos K, Salvaggio JE, Mathews KP. Comparative nasal absorption of allergens in atopic and nonatopic subjects. J Allergy Clin Immunol 1975; 55:241–248.

60. Muilenberg ML, Skellinger WS, Burge HA, Solomon WR. Particle penetration into the automotive interior. I. Influence of vehicle speed and ventilatory mode. J Allergy Clin Immunol 1991; 87:581–585.

61. Baur X. Asthmatic reactions after nasal allergen provocation. Respiration 1996; 63:84–87.

62. Rosenberg GL, Rosenthal RR, Norman PS. Inhalation challenge with ragweed pollen in ragweed-sensitive asthmatics. J Allergy Clin Immunol 1983; 71:302–310.

63. Knox RB, Suphioglu C, Taylor P, Desai R, Watson HC, Peng JL, Bursill LA. Major grass pollen allergen Lol p 1 binds to diesel exhaust particles: implications for asthma and air pollution. Clin Exper Allergy 1997; 27:246–251.

64. Djukanovic R, Feather I, Gratziou C, Walls A, Peroni D, Bradding P, Judd M, Howarth PH, Holgate ST. Effect of natural allergen exposure during the grass pollen season on airways inflammatory cells and asthma symptoms. Thorax 1996; 51:575–581.

65. Ferdousi HA, Dreborg S. Asthma, bronchial hyperreactivity and mediator release in children with birch pollinosis. ECP and EPX T levels are not related to bronchial hyperreactivity. Clin Exper Allergy 1997; 27:530–539.

66. Barbato P, Pisetta F, Ragusa A, Marcer G, Zacchello F. Modification of bronchial hyperreactivity during pollen season in children allergic to grass. Ann Allergy 1987; 58:121–124.

67. Sotomayor H, Badier M, Verloet D, Orehek J. Seasonal increase of carbachol airway responsiveness in patients allergic to grass pollen. Eur J Respir Dis 1984; 130:56–58.

68. Prieto, L, Berto JM, Gutierrez V, Tornero C. Effect of inhaled budesonide on seasonal changes in sensitivity and maximal response to methacholine in pollen-sensitive asthmatic subjects. Eur Respir J 1994; 7:1845–1851.

69. Bleecker ER, Mason PL, More WC. Clinical effects of nedocromil sodium. J Allergy Clin Immunol 1996; 98:S118–S123.

70. Rak S, Bjornson A, Håkanson L, Sörenson S, Venge P. The effect of immunotherapy on eosinophil accumulation and production of eosinophil chemotactic activity in the lung of subjects with asthma during natural pollen exposure. J Allergy Clin Immunol 1991; 88:878–888.

71. Fernvik E, Grönneberg R, Lundahl J, Hed J, Andersson O, Johansson SGO, Hallden G. The degree of natural allergen exposure modifies eosinophil activity markers in the circulation of patients with mild asthma. Allergy 1996; 51:697–705.

72. Tang C, Rolland JM, Ward C, Bish R, Thien F, Walters H. Seasonal comparison of cytokine profiles in atopic asthmatics and atopic non-asthmatics. Am J Respir Crit Care Med 1996; 154:1615–1622.

73. Ciprandi G, Tosca M, Ricca V, Passalacqua G, Fergonsese L, Fasce L, Canonica GW. Cetirizine treatment of allergic cough in children with pollen allergy. Allergy 1997; 52:752–754.

74. Salvaggio J, Seabury J, Schoenhardt EA. New Orleans asthma. V. Relationship between Charity Hospital admission rates, semiquantitative pollen and fungal spore counts and total particulate aerometric sampling data. J Allergy Clin Immunol 1971; 48:96–114.

75. Reid MJ, Moss RB, Hsu YP, Kwasnicki JM, Commerford TM, Nelson BL. Seasonal asthma in northern California: allergic causes and efficacy of immunotherapy. J Allergy Clin Immunol 1986; 78:590–600.

76. Targonski PV, Persky VW, Ramekrishnan V. Respiratory pathophysiologic responses: effect of environmental molds on risk of death from asthma during the pollen season. J Allergy Clin Immunol 1995; 95:955–961.

77. Rusznak C, Bayram H, Devalia JL, Davies RJ. Impact of the environment on allergic lung diseases. Clin Exper Allergy 1997; 27(S1):26–35.

78. Seaton A, Soutar A. Oilseed rape and seasonal symptoms. Clin Exper Allergy 1994; 24:1089–1090.

79. Solomon WR, Burge HA, Boise JR. Exclusion of particulate allergens by window air conditioners. J Allergy Clin Immunol 1980; 65:305–308.

80. Fox RW. Air cleaners: a review. J Allergy Clin Immunol 1994; 94:413–416.

81. Newman Taylor AJ, Davies RJ, Hendrick DJ, Pepys J. Recurrent nocturnal asthmatic reactions to bronchial provocation tests. Clin Allergy 1979; 9:213–219.

82. Menon P, Rando RJ, Stankus RP, Salvaggio JE, Lehrer SB. Passive cigarette smoke-challenge studies: increase in bronchial hyperreactivity. J Allergy Clin Immunol 1992; 89:560–566.

83. Burge HA, Solomon WR, Muilenberg ML. Evaluation of indoor plantings as allergen exposure sources. J Allergy Clin Immunol 1982; 70:101–108.

84. Payne WW. Air pollution by ragweed pollen. II. The source of ragweed pollen. J Air Pollut Control Assoc 1967; 17:653–654.

85. Liccardi G, Visone A, Russo M, Saggese M, D'Amato M, D'Amato G. *Parietaria* pollinosis: clinical and epidemiological aspects. Allergy Asthma Proc 1996; 17:23–29.

86. Scadding GK. Could treating asthma help rhinitis? Clin Exper Allergy 1997; 27:1387–1393.

87. Martonen TB, O'Rourke MK. Deposition patterns of ragweed pollen in the human respiratory tract. Grana 1991; 30:82–86.

88. Frankland AW, Augustin R. Prophylaxis of summer hay fever and asthma. A controlled trial comparing crude grass pollen extracts with the isolated main protein component. Lancet 1954; 1:1055–1057.

89. Hill DJ, Hosking CS, Shelton MJ, Turner MW. Failure of hyposensitization in treatment of children with grass-pollen asthma. Br Med J 1982; 284:306–309.

90. Dykewicz MJ. Allergen immunotherapy for the patient with asthma. Immunol Allergy Clin N Am 1992; 12:125–144.

91. Rak S, Löwenhagen O, Vengep. The effect of immunotherapy on bronchial hyperresponsiveness and eosinophil cationic protein in pollen-allergic patients. J Allergy Clin Immunol 1988; 82:470–480.

92. Creticos PS, Reed CE, Norman PS, Khoury J, Adkinson NF, Buncher CR, Busse WW, Bush RK, Gadde J, Li JT, Richerson HB, Rosenthal RR, Solomon WR, Steinberg P, Yunginger JW. Ragweed immunotherapy in adult asthma. N Engl J Med 1996; 334:501–506.

93. D'Amato G, Kordash TR, Liccardi G, Lobefalo G, Cazzola M, Freshwater LL. Immunotherapy with Alpare® in patients with respiratory allergy to *Parietaria* pollen: a two year double-blind placebo controlled study. Clin Exper Allergy 1995; 25:149–158.

7

Air Pollution and Asthma

DAVID B. PEDEN

University of North Carolina School of Medicine
Chapel Hill, North Carolina

I. Introduction

According to recent estimates, up to 5–10% of the U.S. population suffer from asthma. Increases in asthma death and morbidity have been reported in both the United States and Europe in recent years (1,2). Asthma is characterized by reversible airway obstruction and nonspecific bronchial hyperresponsiveness, both of which are associated with increased airway inflammation. This inflammation is characterized as a desquamating eosinophilic bronchitis. For a majority of children with asthma, as well as approximately 50% of adults with this disease, allergic sensitization to allergens (especially indoor allergens) is a driving stimulus for chronic airway inflammation (3,4).

The characteristics of asthma suggest that this segment of the population would be especially susceptible to the effects of air pollutants. Indeed, there is substantial epidemiological evidence demonstrating that exposure to increased levels of ambient air pollutants is associated with increases in asthma morbidity. Among the pollutants of interest are ozone, sulfur dioxide, nitrogen dioxide, and respirable particulate matter (5–12).

There are a number of ways by which air contaminants might influence asthma. One is that these agents might activate bronchial reflexes, analogous to the effects of histamine or methacholine in these individuals. Another is enhancement of underlying airway inflammation, which is associated with both nonspecific airway responses and bronchoconstriction. A third effect is enhancement of either the immediate or late-phase response to inhaled allergens.

Some have suggested that air pollution not only contributes to exacerbation of asthma but also leads to increased asthma incidence. However, this does not appear to be true. This was perhaps best shown in a study that compared respiratory health status of children in western and eastern Germany shortly after reunification (13). In general, air quality in preunification East Germany was thought to be substantially worse than that in West Germany. However, increased atopy, airway reactivity, and asthma episodes were found in children from the West, while increased bronchitis was reported in those from the East. Other lifestyle factors may be equally important in asthma pathogenesis other than air pollution.

This chapter reviews both epidemiological studies of the relationship between exposure to air pollutants and increases in measures of asthma morbidity as well as controlled exposure studies of asthmatic individuals that directly examine the effect of specific pollutants on the airway biology of asthma.

II. Sulfur Dioxide and Acid Aerosols

A. Epidemiology

Total emergency room visits for respiratory problems and increased hospital admission rates have been linked with increased ambient exposure to SO_2 (5). Changes in lung function of children have also been linked to increases in sulfur dioxide levels (14,15). The likelihood of chronic asthma or obstructive lung disease has also been weakly associated with lifetime exposure to SO_2 (16,17). However, in many of these studies, it is difficult to separate effects of sulfur dioxide from that of total suspended particulates. Additionally, ambient SO_2 may contribute to acid aerosol (H_2SO_4) formation. This may be important as some studies suggest that asthma symptoms are increased on days in which increased levels of aerosolized acid is observed (7). Acid (H^+) concentrations of over 100 nmol/m^3 (5 mg/mL H_2SO_4 equivalent) have been observed over 24 hr periods and concentrations over 500 nmol/m^3 (25 mg/mL H_2SO_4 equivalent) over 12 hr. Thus, SO_2 may exert effects either as a gas or by contributing to H_2SO_4 particle formation.

B. Controlled Exposures to SO_2

Sulfur dioxide is a strong inducer of bronchospasm in asthmatics. Bronchoconstriction in asthmatic individuals occurs after exposure to SO_2 at concentrations as low as 0.25 ppm, whereas nonasthmatics experience no effect on pulmonary function following exposure to levels as high as 0.6 ppm (5,8,18–26). In asthmatics, SO_2 has a rapid onset of action with initial bronchoconstrictive responses beginning 2 min into exposure that become maximal in 5–10 min. Spontaneous recovery occurs 30 min after challenge with a refractory period of up to 4 hr. Repeated exposure to low levels of SO_2 induce acute tachyphylaxis. Other reports suggest that repeated exercise during SO_2 exposure is associated with diminished airway responsiveness to SO_2 6 hr after exposure (27–29).

FEV_1 can drop as much as 60% after exposure to SO_2. There is variability in the response of asthmatics to SO_2, with some experiencing bronchoconstriction at levels as low as 0.25 ppm and others having no response at levels as high as 2.0 ppm. However, bronchoconstriction generally occurs in asthmatics exposed to levels of $SO_2 > 0.50$ ppm. Exercise enhances SO_2-induced bronchoconstriction in asthmatics. SO_2-related symptoms in asthmatics include wheezing, chest discomfort, and dyspnea.

The effect of SO_2 on asthmatics can be modified by pharmacological agents, including beta agonists, antimuscarinic agents, cromolyn sodium, and nedocromil. Beta agonists are the most effective at reversing SO_2-induced bronchospasm. However, long-term use of methyl xanthines, inhaled corticosteroids, and short-term administration of antihistamines do not alter the sensitivity of asthmatics to SO_2 (22,30). However, despite the insights provided by these pharmacological observations, the mechanisms by which SO_2 may influence asthma remain incompletely explained.

Nasal breathing largely eliminates the effect of SO_2 on lung function in asthma. This is likely due to absorption of this water-soluble gas by the nasal mucosa. At rest, most airflow occurs through the nasal airway except in those with pathological nasal obstruction. Exercise causes a shift from strictly nasal breathing to oronasal respiration, resulting in a marked decrease in the amount of inspired air that interacts with the nasal mucosa, thus increasing the amount of SO_2 that will reach the lower airway. This may explain how exercise enhances the effect of SO_2. Asthmatics are more likely to have nasal pathology as well (such as allergic rhinitis or sinusitis), which may further decrease nasal airflow during exercise, possibly increasing the percentage of inspired air that is not exposed to nasal tissue (31).

Sulfur dioxide exposure also augments responses to other environmental contaminants. Exposure to ozone prior to exposure to SO_2 increases bronchial sensitivity to SO_2 in asthmatics (32). Exposure to cold dry air also exacerbates the bronchospastic effect of SO_2 in asthmatic patients (28). However, unlike ozone, SO_2 exposure has not been shown to exacerbate allergen-induced bronchospasm. The question of whether there is a relationship between sensitivity to SO_2 and asthma severity has not been resolved, although some observations indicate that SO_2 causes similar effects in those with mild and moderate asthma.

C. Controlled Exposures to Acid Aerosols

Acid aerosols, which result in part from release of SO_2 into the atmosphere, have also been studied for their effect on respiratory function. Repeated studies in nonasthmatic patients demonstrate that acute exposure to H_2SO_4 up to 2000 mg/m^3 for 1 hr does not alter lung function (12,20,33,34). However, similar studies suggest that this population is more susceptible to acid exposure (35,36). This may be particularly true for asthmatic adolescents, in whom lung function decrements were observed at acid levels as low as 100 mg/m^3. In general, it seems that the effect of inhaled aerosolized acid on lung function in asthma roughly correlates with baseline levels of airway hyperresponsiveness. Overall, despite the studies cited above, there is significant debate as to the importance of acid aerosol exposure in asthma exacerbation.

III. Nitrogen Dioxide

A. Epidemiology

Nitrogen dioxide (NO_2), a precursor to photochemical smog, is found in ambient outdoor air in urban and industrial regions and, in conjunction with sunlight and hydrocarbons, results in the production of ozone. Automobile exhaust is the most significant source for outdoor NO_2, although power plants and other industrial sources that burn fossil fuels also release NO_2 into the environment.

However, the most significant exposure to NO_2 occurs indoors in conjunction with the use of gas cooking stoves and kerosene space heaters (5).

The majority of epidemiological studies of the effect of NO_2 on asthma-like symptoms have focused on indoor exposure to NO_2, especially in homes in which natural gas is used for cooking. A number of studies found that increased levels of NO_2 inside dwellings correlate with increased respiratory symptoms in children (37; reviewed in Ref. 5). These studies also link increased reports of cough, wheeze, phlegm, and bronchitis with the annual average household NO_2 concentration (5,38). However, other studies fail to show a relationship between NO_2 concentration and airway symptoms. Thus, the major effect of NO_2 in asthma may lie in its role in production of ozone rather than a direct effect of this gas on the airways.

B. Controlled Exposure Studies with NO_2

As with epidemiological studies, controlled exposure studies of both asthmatic and normal subjects have not consistently demonstrated an effect of NO_2 on airway function. Several investigations of the effect of NO_2 on nonspecific reactivity in asthmatics contradict each other, with some reporting that low levels of NO_2 enhance nonspecific airway reactivity whereas othersl fail to find such an effect (39–41). Higher levels of NO_2 (4.0 ppm) do appear to alter airway function of asthmatics. Also, NO_2 may enhance airway inflammation, a prominent feature of asthma. In nonasthmatics, NO_2 exposure is associated with an influx of airway PMNs (42). NO_2 has been shown to induce proinflammatory cytokine production in epithelial cells following in vitro pollutant exposure (43). Overall, these data suggest that NO_2 could influence airway function of asthmatics by increasing airway inflammation.

Nitrogen dioxide may also enhance the effect of allergen challenge in allergic asthmatics. One hour exposure to 0.4 ppm NO_2 has been reported to enhance bronchospasm associated with challenge to a fixed dose of allergen (44). A combination of 0.2 ppm SO_2 and 0.4 ppm NO_2 for 6 hr was found to enhance immediate bronchial responses of mild asthmatics to inhaled allergen, whereas either gas alone did not have this effect (45). Exposure to NO_2 has also been reported to enhance late-phase responses of asthmatics to inhaled allergen (46). Finally, exposure to 0.4 ppm NO_2 for 6 hr increases allergen-induced ECP, but not mast cell tryptase, in the nasal airways of patients with allergic asthma, suggesting that this gas effects eosinophil responses without having any effect on mast cell degranulation (47). Taken together, these studies demonstrate that NO_2 may alter both allergen-induced and nonspecific airway responses in asthmatic individuals.

IV. Ozone

A. Epidemiology

A number of epidemiological studies indicate that exposure to ambient ozone is related to increased asthma morbidity. Various studies that collectively examined admissions to 79 hospitals in southern Ontario reveal a significant association between O_3 and admissions for respiratory symptoms (5,7). Of note is a 24–48 hr time lag between the ozone exposure and occurrence of hospital admission. White et al. (48) also found an association between ER visits for asthma and ozone levels >0.11 ppm (but not <0.11 ppm) in schoolchildren. Similar observations have been made in Mexico City (49–51). Thus, ozone exposure is strongly associated with increased asthma morbidity.

B. Controlled Exposure Studies to Ozone

Ozone is perhaps the most extensively examined pollutant with regard to its effect on airway function and inflammation in asthmatics. Insight into the likely mechanisms by which ozone alters airway function in asthma has come from controlled exposure studies of both normal subjects and asthmatics.

In normal subjects, ozone has two actions: 1) a reproducible decrease of both FVC and FEV_1 (with increased nonspecific bronchial responsiveness and substernal discomfort when taking a deep breath) (52) and 2) development of neutrophilic inflammation as quickly as 1 hr after exposure (5,53). Interestingly, these two effects are not correlated with each other, suggesting that separate mechanisms mediate these changes.

The effects of ozone on lung mechanics are dependent on the concentration of ozone, duration of exposure, and level of exercise (with corresponding increases in minute ventilation) (52). Exposure to ozone without exercise usually exerts no effect on lung function at levels below 0.50 ppm (52,54–56). With exercise, ozone induces increases in respiratory frequency, and the concentration of ozone required to cause decreases in FEV_1, FVC, airway resistance, and symptoms can be much less (55).

Examination of the action of a variety of pharmacological agents on the effect of ozone on respiratory mechanics has provided some clues as to the mechanisms of this effect. Atropine inhibits ozone-related decreases in airway resistance (though not spirometry), indicating that vagal mechanisms are involved in the respiratory response to ozone (57). Ozone could also directly increase smooth muscle sensitivity to acetylcholine, consistent with the observation that sensitivity to inhaled methacholine is increased after ozone exposure (57,58).

Ozone also effects eicosanoid responses in the airway, which alters airway mechanics. Levels of PGE_2 in BAL recovered from normal subjects after O_3 exposure correlate with observed lung function decrements (53). Additionally, multiple laboratories have shown that cyclooxygenase inhibitors, such as ibuprofen and indomethacin, inhibit ozone-induced decreases in spirometry, although they have little effect on inflammatory responses to ozone (59–62). Airway C fibers can be stimulated by PGE_2, suggesting a mechanism by which ozone-related increases in PGE_2 may also account for changes in lung function due to ozone (63,64). Animal studies in anesthetized dogs also suggest that ozone may act via C fiber-mediated mechanisms in the lung (64). This finding is further supported by recent observations in normal subjects that ozone exposure causes depletion of substance P, but not CGRP, in airway neurons and that levels of substance P and PGE_2 are correlated in BAL fluid after ozone exposure (65).

Pain responses may also play a role in the restrictive pulmonary response to ozone. Lidocaine, when applied to the upper airway, exerts a partial inhibition of ozone-induced decreases in spirometry, suggesting an inhibition of irritant receptors in the upper airway that blunts ozone-induced reflex-mediated decrease in inspiratory effort (20). Also, sufentanyl (a short-acting narcotic) rapidly normalizes lung function in subjects found to have decreases in FVC and FEV_1 after ozone exposure (66). Thus, pain responses that are sensitive to opiates may partially account for the pulmonary response to ozone.

Beta agonists have little effect on the immediate effect of ozone on lung function. While there is a report that they can block some ozone-induced decreases in lung function, most studies indicate that beta agonists have little effect on the impact of ozone on lung function (67). Therefore, it is unlikely that β-adrenergic tone plays a substantial role in the response of humans to ozone exposure.

Initial studies comparing lung function of nonasthmatic subjects to that of subjects with mild asthma demonstrated that the latter were not more sensitive to low level ozone exposure. However, others have demonstrated that, with more robust exposures, asthmatics are more sensitive to the effect of ozone. Kriet and coworkers (68) reported that exposure to 0.4 ppm ozone for 2 hr with rigorous exercise caused asthmatics to have greater increases in both airway resistance and nonspecific airway hyperresponsiveness than normal subjects. Silverman (69) also demonstrated that exposure to 0.25 ppm ozone for 2 hr resulted in decreased pulmonary function in asthmatics. Other studies indicate that ozone not only causes the well-described decrease in FVC but also causes true bronchospasm in asthmatics (23,68,70). Thus, ozone has been demonstrated to directly worsen airflow in asthma.

Recent studies (71,72) revealed that ozone exposure followed by an exercise challenge (without ozone) of persons with exercise-induced bronchospasm (EIB) has no effect on subsequent EIB. Weymer and colleagues (72) found that mild asthmatics with EIB exposed to 0.0, 0.1, 0.25, and 0.40 ppm ozone for 1 hr with mild exercise (VE of 20–30 L/min) followed an hour later with an exercise challenge had no subsequent exercise-induced bronchospasm due to the ozone exposure. Fernandez et al. (71) also examined the effect of 0.12 ppm ozone for 1 hr in asthmatics with EIB and found no exacerbation of EIB attributable to ozone.

In normal subjects, ozone induces neutrophilic influx into the airway as revealed in analysis of BAL fluid and in bronchial mucosal biopsies recovered from subjects following exposures ranging from 0.10 to 0.4 ppm. Neutrophil influx appears to be maximal between 1 and 6 hr after exposure and persists for 18 hr (53,58). Inflammatory mediators such as IL-6, IL-8, PGE_2, LTB_4, TXB_2, fibronectin, plasminogen activator, and elastase are also increased by ozone (reviewed in Ref. 5). Direct comparison of the kinetics of mediator response to ozone shows that changes in IL-6 and PGE_2 peak 1 hr after exposure whereas fibronectin and plasminogen activator are higher 18 hr after exposure (53)

With the exception of PGE_2, none of the above-noted markers of inflammation correlate with immediate changes in lung function of normal subjects. Neither has an association been made between ozone-induced inflammation and airway responsiveness in normal subjects. Thus, the clinical significance of ozone-induced inflammation in normal subjects remains unclear. It has been suggested that this proinflammatory effect of ozone could have a greater significance in asthma, a disorder characterized in part by an eosinophilic inflammation of the lower airways.

Bascom et al. (73) found increased numbers of neutrophils and eosinophils in nasal lavage fluid from patients with allergic rhinitis after 4 hr exposure to 0.5 ppm ozone. Later studies by others found this to be true for mite-sensitive asthmatics as well, following exposure to 0.4 ppm ozone for 2 hr. In the latter study, ozone also caused increases in eosinophil cationic protein, suggesting that eosinophils may have been activated (74). Thus, ozone induces eosinophil as well as PMN influx to the nasal airways of persons with either allergic rhinitis or asthma.

The effect of ozone on bronchial inflammation in asthmatics is not as clear. Some investigators have reported that ozone induces greater numbers of PMNs in asthmatics than normal subjects, without causing any bronchial eosinophilia (75,76). In one of these studies, airway lavage fluid was collected 18 hr after exposure in three different ways. One technique was lavage from an isolated proximal airway, another involved selective analysis of the first 10 mL of traditional BAL (labeled the bronchial fraction), and the final technique was traditional BAL fluid. Asthmatics yielded increased levels of PMNs, LDH, total protein, MPO, fibronectin, and IL-8 with each of the sampling techniques following ozone exposure. In BAL fluid, asthmatics also had a greater PMN response than nonasthmatics, with a trend for increased IL-8 levels as well.

On the other hand, other investigators have reported that ozone induces eosinophils into the bronchial airways, as it does into the nasal airways. An investigation of the effect of exposure to 0.16 ppm ozone for 8 hr in eight mite-sensitive asthmatics revealed a notable increase in both PMNs and eosinophils in BAL fluid. Bronchial samplings included traditional BAL fluid as well as separate examination of the first 20 mL recovered (the bronchial fraction), with the bronchial fraction yielding more striking differences between air and ozone exposure (77). Consistent with this are preliminary data reported by Framptom and colleagues (78) in which a twofold increase in eosinophils was observed in asthmatics following ozone exposure. In these asthmatics, ozone caused both neutrophil and eosinophil influx to the airway. Despite their differences, each of the four studies cited above suggest that asthmatics have stronger inflammatory responses to ozone than normal subjects (78).

Exposure to ozone has also been reported to enhance both immediate and late-phase responses to inhaled allergen. This was first suggested by Molfino et al. (79), who observed decreased PD_{20} values to inhaled allergen from seven grass-sensitive subjects challenged immediately after exposure to 0.12 ppm ozone for 1 hr at rest. A study of 12 subjects employing this same exposure regimen failed to find a significant effect of ozone on bronchial reactivity to allergen (80). However, 0.25 ppm ozone exposure over 3 hr with moderate exercise does enhance the bronchial reactivity of persons with both allergic asthma and allergic rhinitis to inhaled allergen (81). Preliminary data from our group also indicate that exposure to 0.16 ppm ozone for 8 hr with moderate exercise increases sensitivity of mite-sensitive asthmatics to bronchial challenge with mite allergen 18 hr after the exposure.

Late-phase response to allergen is also influenced by ozone. In nasal studies of allergic asthmatics, 0.4 ppm ozone was found to enhance allergen-induced eosinophil influx, ECP levels, and IL-8 levels (74). A study in which exposure to 0.2 ppm ozone for 3 hr was followed by inhaled allergen challenge did not show any effect of allergen-associated levels of eosinophils, neutrophils, ECP, or IL-8 recovered in nasal fluid. Taken together, these studies suggest that the effect of ozone on inhaled allergen challenge is dose-related. Also, all of these studies were performed in mild asthmatics. It is possible that persons with more severe disease may be more sensitive to the effect of ozone on both immediate and late-phase responses to allergen.

V. Particulate Matter

Respirable particulate matter (that less than 10 μm) is also associated with episodes of increased asthma exacerbation. Increased requirement for asthma medication in a cohort of asthmatics in Utah was correlated with increased particulate levels. A study in the Seattle area demonstrates that hospitalization for increased asthma severity occurs in conjunction with increases in airborne particulate matter. Similar observations have been made in Mexico City (11,50,82–87). These data demonstrate the important role that particulates could play in asthma morbidity.

However, identification of specific agents that may mediate asthma exacerbation is difficult, as there is a vast array of particles that have been identified and shown to have biological effects in animal and in vitro studies. Active agents in particulate matter include silica, metal ions (such as iron, vanadium, nickel, and copper), organic residues (polyaromatic hydrocarbons found on diesel exhaust particles), acid aerosols, and biological contaminants such as endotoxin (5). To date, few human exposure data are available for controlled exposures to metal-containing particles. However, there are some human exposure studies that examine the effect of diesel exhaust particles and endotoxin on the airway.

A. Controlled Exposure to Diesel Exhaust Particles

Numerous animal and in vitro studies have demonstrated that diesel exhaust particles (DEPs) enhance both inflammation and airway hyperresponsiveness following allergen exposure (88–92). This includes increasing IgE production and enhancing cytokines involved in eosinophilic or allergic inflammation, especially IL-4, IL-5, and GM-CSF. DEPs also induce B- lymphocyte immunoglobulin isotype switching to IgE (93). Polyaromatic hydrocarbon residues on DEPs may be responsible for this effect on allergic inflammation (94).

Nasal challenge studies in humans have been used to examine the effect of DEPs on allergic inflammation. Diaz-Sanchez et al. (93) found that exposure of volunteers (four atopic and seven nonatopic) to DEP increased nasal IgE production 4 days after DEP challenge without any effect on IgG, IgA, or IgM. There were also shifts in the ratio of the five isoforms of IgE noted with the challenge. This effect was very dose-specific, as only a dose of 0.3 mg DEP caused this result.

This same group also found that DEP challenge of the nasal mucosa causes increased cytokine production by cells recovered in lavage fluid. Subjects underwent lavage before and after challenge with 0.3 mg of DEP, with the recovered cells being analyzed for mRNA levels of certain cytokines. Cells recovered before challenge had detectable mRNA levels for γ-interferon, IL-2, and IL-13, whereas DEP challenge was associated with detectable levels of IL-2, IL-4, IL-5, IL-6, IL-10, IL-13, and γ-interferon in recovered cells. IL-4 protein was also measured in postchallenge lavage (95). While it is unclear which types of cells were present in lavage fluid before or after challenge, it was not thought to be due to an increase in the number of lymphocytes. The general conclusion is that DEPs do appear to enhance Th2 type inflammation. Also examined was the effect of combined challenge of DEP with ragweed allergen vs. challenge with ragweed alone on allergen-specific IgE and IgG in ragweed-sensitive subjects. DEP plus allergen resulted in significant increases in allergen-specific IgE and IgG_4 without an increase in total IgE and IgG. DEP plus allergen, compared to DEP alone, was also associated with increased expression of IL-4, IL-5, IL-6, IL-10, and IL-13 and decreased expression of γ-interferon and IL-2.

Compared to other pollutants, such as ozone, DEP appears to be unique in its effect on IgE production. The in vivo effect of DEP on IgE isotype switch can be replicated in vitro with extracts from DEP containing the polyaromatic hydrocarbon (PAH) fraction from these particles, as well as specific PAH compounds phenanthrene and 2,3,7,8-tetrachlorodibenzo-*p*-dioxin (93–96). Thus, polyaromatic hydrocarbons, by their action on B cells, appear to play a central role in the effect of diesel exhaust on allergic inflammation.

B. Controlled Exposure to Endotoxin

While endotoxin has not been shown to affect atopic subjects without asthma (97), it may be an important contributor to asthma morbidity (98). This is most strongly suggested by an observation that for house dust mite sensitive asthmatics, disease severity correlates better with LPS levels in house dust than with mite allergen levels in these same samples (99). Previous to that study, Michel and colleagues performed a series of challenge studies examining the response of asthmatics to inhaled endotoxin challenge (98,100,101). In one study, a 7% decrease in FEV_1 was observed 30 min after inhalation of 22,222 ng of the lipid moiety of endotoxin. Five hours after the challenge, the FEV_1 was only partially recovered with an increase in nonspecific bronchial reactivity (NSBR) to histamine. A study of 16 asthmatics (eight of whom were atopic) confirmed that endotoxin challenge resulted in bronchospasm and increased

NSBR to histamine in a fashion that correlated with baseline histamine NSBR but not state of atopy or history of tobaco use. A third study, which entailed inhalation of 20,000 ng of LPS, resulted in a decrease in the FEV_1 45 min after challenge (which persisted for 5 hr), and increases in peripheral blood TNFga after 60 min, in histamine NSBR after 5 hr, and in peripheral blood neutrophils at 6 hr post LPS challenge. These results all suggest that respiratory responses to LPS involve an inflammatory process.

Inhaled LPS is clearly able to cause neutrophilic inflammation in both atopic and nonatopic subjects and is a key feature of many occupational lung diseases (102,103). The apparent interaction between LPS and allergen exposure reported by Michel et al. (99) indicates that endotoxin can modulate allergen related airway inflammation. However, it is unclear that LPS has an effect on the eosinophilic inflammation characteristic of asthma.

Endotoxin-contaminated allergen solutions, when instilled into a segment of the lower airway, caused a marked neutrophilic inflammatory response that was observed on follow-up bronchoscopy 18 hr later (104). This contrasts with the more typical allergen-induced inflammation, characterized by influx of both neutrophils (PMNs) and eosinophils, that was observed when endotoxin-free allergen was used. These data would suggest that LPS dominates, rather than enhances, allergen-induced inflammation in the airway. However, there are animal studies that suggest that LPS can influence eosinophilic inflammation.

Macari and colleagues (105) reported that 30 ng of LPS injected into the skin of guinea pigs has no direct effect on eosinophil influx, yet it does cause a threefold increase in eosinophil responses to dermally applied allergen without an enhancement of PMN influx. LPS at doses of 50–1000 ng of LPS cause a dose-dependent eosinophil influx in guinea pig skin (106). This activity may be mediated by de novo generation of TNFα. This is supported by studies that show that both actinomycin D (which inhibits protein synthesis) and soluble TNFα fusion protein (which binds TNFα) blunt LPS-induced eosinophil influx (107). In studies employing a murine pleurisy model, LPS was found to induce a significant influx of PMNs in 4 hr and eosinophils in 24 hr.

Peripheral human blood monocytes stimulated with LPS also yield a supernatant that enhances eosinophil degranulation and survival in vitro (108). Comparison of LPS-induced cytokine responses of peripheral blood monocytes and alveolar macrophages recovered from asthmatic and normal subjects demonstrate increased cytokine responses in cells from asthmatics (109). Likewise, depletion of lymphocytes with appropriate monoclonal antibody also blunts LPS-induced pleural eosinophilia in a rat model (110,111). Thus, LPS appears to have a proinflammatory effect on the airway, mediated by monocytes or lymphocytes, which may be greater in asthmatics than nonasthmatics.

Also, asthmatics acutely exposed to allergen may have enhanced responses to endotoxin because of increased levels of soluble CD14 and LPS-binding protein in bronchoalveolar lavage fluid after allergen challenge (112). Taken together, these results demonstrate that LPS is an important air contaminant for asthmatics.

VI. Summary

Both epidemiological and controlled exposure studies indicate that air pollutants can induce asthma exacerbations. This may be due to direct effects on the airway or to priming of the airway such that responses to inhaled allergen are enhanced. In either case, it is likely that individuals with more significant asthma (such as those with moderate or severe disease) will be affected more than those with mild disease, due to increased levels of inflammation in the airway.

While it does not appear that asthma prevalence is altered by air pollution, it is unknown how the severity of chronic asthma in those who already have asthma may be a affected by poor air quality. Occupational exposures, especially with diisocyanates, have profound long-term effects on airway morbidity. It seems reasonable that measures to decrease airway inflammation, including avoidance of either allergens or pollutants and anti-inflammatory therapy, may be useful. However, decreased release of pollutants into the air is a key component in a public health strategy designed to decrease asthma exacerbations. Rational intervention strategies depend on improved understanding of both the biological effects of pollutants in asthma and the atmospheric chemistry that may result in production of the ultimately important pollutants from precursor molecules.

References

1. Crain EF, Weiss KB, Bijur PE, Hersh M, Westbrook L, Stein RE. An estimate of the prevalence of asthma and wheezing among inner-city children. Pediatrics 1994; 94(3):356–362.
2. Weiss KB, Gergen PJ, Wagener DK. Breathing better or wheezing worse? The changing epidemiology of asthma morbidity and mortality. Annu Rev Publ Health 1993; 14:491–513.
3. Henderson FW, Henry MM, Ivins SS, Morris R, Neebe EC, Leu SY, Stewart PW. Correlates of recurrent wheezing in school-age children. The Physicians of Raleigh Pediatric Associates. Am J Respir Crit Care Med 1995; 151(6):1786–1793.

4. Rosenstreich DL, Eggleston P, Kattan M, Baker D, Slavin RG, Gergen P, Mitchell H, McNiff-Mortimer K, Lynn H, Ownby D, Malveaux F. The role of cockroach allergy and exposure to cockroach allergen in causing morbidity among inner-city children with asthma. N Engl J Med 1997; 336(19):1356–1363.

5. Anonymous. Health effects of outdoor air pollution. Committee of the Environmental and Occupational Health Assembly of the American Thoracic Society. Am J Respir Crit Care Med 1996; 153(1):3–50.

6. Balmes JR. The role of ozone exposure in the epidemiology of asthma. Environ Health Perspect 1993; 101:219–224.

7. Bates DV, Sizto R. Relationship between air pollutant levels and hospital admissions in southern Ontario. Can J Publ Health 1983; 74:117–122.

8. Gong H Jr. Health effects of air pollution. A review of clinical studies. Clin Chest Med 1992; 13:201–214.

9. Koren HS, Bromberg PA. Respiratory responses of asthmatics to ozone. Int Arch Allergy Immunol 1995; 107(1-3):236–238.

10. Peden DB. Mechanisms of pollution-induced airway disease: in vivo studies. Allergy 1997; 52(38 suppl):37–44.

11. Schwartz J, Slater D, Larson TV, et al. Particulate air pollution and hospital emergency room visits for asthma in Seattle. Am Rev Respir Dis 1993; 147: 826–831.

12. Utell MJ, Morrow PE, Speers DM, et al. Airway responses to sulfate and sulfuric acid aerosols in asthmatics. Am Rev Respir Dis 1983; 128:444–450.

13. von Mutius E, Martinez FD, Fritzsch C, Nicolai T, Roell G, Thiemann HH. Prevalence of asthma and atopy in two areas of West and East Germany. Am J Respir Crit Care Med 1994; 149:358–364.

14. Dassen W, Brunekreef B, Hoek P, et al. Decline in children's pulmonary function during an air pollution episode. J Air Pollut Control Assoc 1986; 32:937–942.

15. Dockery DW, Ware JH, Ferris BG, et al. Change in pulmonary function associated with air pollution episodes. Am J Publ Health 1982; 81:90–97.

16. Schenker MB, Samet JM, Speizer FE, et al. Health effects of air pollution due to coal combustion in the Chestnut Ridge region of Pennsylvania: results of cross-sectional analysis. Arch Environ Health 1983; 38:325–330.

17. Van De Lende R, Kok TJ, Reig RP, et al. Decreases in VC and FEV1 with time: indicators for the effects of smoking and air pollution. Bull Eur Physiopathol Respir 1981; 17:775–792.

18. Boushey HA. Bronchial hyperreactivity to sulfur dioxide: physiologic and political implications. J Allergy Clin Immunol 1982; 69(4):335–338.

19. Folinsbee LJ, Bedi JF, Horvath SM. Pulmonary response to threshold levels of sulfur dioxide (1.0 ppm) and ozone (0.3 ppm). J Appl Physiol: Respir Environ Exercise Physiol 1985; 58:1783–1787.

20. Folinsbee LJ. Human health effects of air pollution. Environ Health Perspect 1993; 100:45–56.

21. Hackney JD, Linn WS, Bailey RM, et al. Time course of exercise-induced bronchoconstriction in asthmatics exposed to sulfur dioxide. Environ Res 1984; 34: 321–327.

22. Heath SK, Koenig JQ, Morgan MS, et al. Effects of sulfur dioxide exposure on African-American and Caucasian asthmatics. Environ Res 1994; 66:1–11.

23. Horstman D, Roger LJ, McDonnell W, et al. Increased specific airway resistance (SR_{aw}) in asthmatics exercising while exposed to 0.18 ppm ozone (O_3). Physiologist 1984; 27:212.

24. Horstman D, Roger LJ, Kehrl H, et al. Airway sensitivity of asthmatics to sulfur dioxide. Toxicol Ind Health 1986; 2(3):289–298.

25. Kehrl HR, Roger LJ, Hazucha MJ, et al. Differing response of asthmatics to sulfur dioxide exposure with continuous and intermittent exercise. Am Rev Respir Dis 1987; 135:350–355.

26. Witek TJ, Schachter EN. Airway responses to sulfur dioxide and methacholine in asthmatics. J Occup Med 1985; 27(4):265–268.

27. Horstman DH, Seal E Jr, Folinsbee LJ, et al. The relationship between exposure duration and sulfur dioxide-induced bronchoconstriction in asthmatic subjects. Am Ind Hyg Assoc J 1988; 49(1):38–47.

28. Pierson WE, Koenig JQ. Respiratory effects of air pollution on allergic disease. J Allergy Clin Immunol 1992; 90:557–566.

29. Roger LJ, Kehrl HR, Hazucha MJ, et al. Bronchoconstriction in asthmatics exposed to sulfur dioxide during repeated exercise. J Appl Physiol: Respir Environ Exercise Physiol 1985; 59(3):784–791.

30. Bigby B, Boushey H. Effects of nedocromil sodium on the bronchomotor response to sulfur dioxide in asthmatic patients. J Allergy Clin Immunol 1993; 92:195–197.

31. Linn WS, Shamoo DA, Spier CE, et al. Respiratory effects of 0.75 ppm sulfur dioxide in exercising asthmatics: influence of upper-respiratory defenses. Environ Res 1983; 30:340–348.

32. Koenig JQ, Covert DS, Hanley QS, et al. Prior exposure to ozone potentiates subsequent response to sulfur dioxide in adolescent asthmatic subjects. Am Rev Respir Dis 1990; 141:377–380.

33. Koenig JQ, Pierson WE. Air pollutants and the respiratory system: toxicity and pharmacologic interventions. Clin Toxicol 1991; 29(3):401–411.

34. Aris R, Christian D, Sheppard D, et al. Lack of bronchoconstrictor response to sulfuric acid aerosols and fogs. Am Rev Respir Dis 1991; 143:744–750.

35. Koenig JQ, Pierson WE, Korike M. The effects of inhaled sulfuric acid on pulmonary function in adolescent asthmatics. Am Rev Respir Dis 1983; 128:221–225.

36. Koenig JQ, Covert DS, Pierson WE. Effects of inhalation of acidic compounds on pulmonary function in allergic adolescent subjects. Environ Health Perspect 1989; 79:173–178.

37. Dijkstra L, Houthuijs D, Brunekreef B, et al. Respiratory health effects of the indoor environment in a population of Dutch children. Am Rev Respir Dis 1990; 145:1172–1178.

38. Neas LM, Dockery DW, Ware JH, et al. Association of indoor nitrogen dioxide with respiratory symptoms and pulmonary function in children. Am J Epidemiol 1991; 134:204–209.

39. Bauer MA, Utell MJ, Morrow PE, et al. Inhalation of 0.30 ppm nitrogen dioxide potentiates exercise-induced bronchospasm in asthmatics. Am Rev Respir Dis 1986; 134:1203–1208.

40. Linn WS, Shamoo DA, Spier CE, et al. Controlled exposure of volunteers with chronic obstructive pulmonary disease to nitrogen dioxide. Arch Environ Health 1985; 40(6):313–317.

41. Anto JM, Sunyer J. Nitrogen dioxide and allergic asthma: starting to clarify an obscure association. Lancet 1995; 345:402–403.

42. Sandstrom T, Stjernberg N, Eklund A, et al. Inflammatory cell response in bronchoalveolar lavage fluid after nitrogen dioxide exposure of healthy subjects: a dose-response study. Eur Respir J 1991; 4:332–333.

43. Devalia JL, Campbell AM, Sapsford RJ, et al. Effect of nitrogen dioxide on synthesis of inflammatory cytokines expressed by human bronchial epithelial cells in vitro. Am J Respir Cell Mol Biol 1993; 9:271–278.

44. Tunnicliffe WS, Burge PS, Ayres JG. Effect of domestic concentrations of nitrogen dioxide on airway responses to inhaled allergen in asthmatic patients. Lancet 1994; 344(8939–8940):1733–1736.

45. Rusznak C, Devalia JL, Davies RJ. Airway response of asthmatic subjects to inhaled allergen after exposure to pollutants. Thorax 1996; 51(11):1105–1108.

46. Strand V, Rak S, Svartengren M, Bylin G. Nitrogen dioxide exposure enhances asthmatic reaction to inhaled allergen in subjects with asthma. Am J Respir Crit Care Med 1997; 155(3):881–887.

47. Wang JH, Devalia JL, Duddle JM, Hamilton SA, Davies RJ. Effect of six-hour exposure to nitrogen dioxide on early-phase nasal response to allergen challenge in patients with a history of seasonal allergic rhinitis. J Allergy Clin Immunol 1995; 96(5 Pt 1):669–676.

48. White MC, Etzel RA, Wilcox WD, Lloyd C. Exacerbations of childhood asthma and ozone pollution in Atlanta. Environ Res 1994; 65(1):56–68.

49. Romieu I, Meneses F, Sienra-Monge JJ, Huerta J, Ruiz Velasco S, White MC, Etzel RA, Hernandez-Avila M. Effects of urban air pollutants on emergency visits for childhood asthma in Mexico City. Am J Epidemiol 1995; 141(6):546–553.

50. Romieu I, Meneses F, Ruiz S, Sienra JJ, Huerta J, White MC, Etzel RA. Effects of air pollution on the respiratory health of asthmatic children living in Mexico City. Am J Respir Crit Care Med 1996; 154(2 Pt 1):300–307.

51. Romieu I, Meneses F, Ruiz S, Huerta J, Sienra JJ, White M, Etzel R, Hernandez M. Effects of intermittent ozone exposure on peak expiratory flow and respira-

tory symptoms among asthmatic children in Mexico City. Arch Environ Health 1997; 52(5):368–376 (abstract).

52. McDonnell WF, Horstman DH, Hazucha MJ, et al. Pulmonary effects of ozone exposure during exercise: dose–response characteristics. J Appl Physiol: Respir Environ Exercise Physiol 1983; 54(5):1345–1352.

53. Koren HS, Devlin RB, Becker S, et al. Time-dependent changes of markers associated with inflammation in the lungs of humans exposed to ambient levels of ozone. Toxicol Pathol 1991; 19(4):406–411.

54. Bates DV, Hazucha MJ. The Short-Term Effects of Ozone on the Human Lung. Washington, DC: US Govt Printing Office 93-15 1973; 507–540.

55. McDonnell WF, Kehrl HR, Abdul Salaam S, et al. Respiratory response of humans exposed to low levels of ozone for 6.6 hours. Arch Environ Health 1991; 46:145–150.

56. Folinsbee LJ, Horstman DH, Kehrl HR, et al. Respiratory responses to repeated prolonged exposure to 0.12 ppm ozone. Am J Respir Crit Care Med 1994; 149:98–105.

57. Beckett WS, McDonnell WF, Horstman DH, et al. Role of the parasympathetic nervous system in acute lung response to ozone. J Appl Physiol: Respir Environ Exercise Physiol 1985; 59:1879–1885.

58. Holtzman MJ, Fabbri LM, O'Byrne PM, et al. Importance of airway inflammation for hyperresponsiveness induced by ozone. Am Rev Respir Dis 1983; 127:686–690.

59. Ying RL, Gross KB, Terzo TS, et al. Indomethacin does not inhibit the ozone-induced increase in bronchial responsiveness in human subjects. Am Rev Respir Dis 1990; 142:817–821.

60. Schelegle ES, Adams WC, Siefkin AD. Indomethacin pretreatment reduces ozone-induced pulmonary function decrements in human subjects. Am Rev Respir Dis 1987; 136:1350–1354.

61. Eschenbacher WL, Ying RL, Kreit JW, et al. Ozone-induced lung function changes in normal and asthmatic subjects and the effect of indomethacin. Atmos Ozone Res Policy Implic 1989; 493–499.

62. Hazucha MJ, Madden M, Pape G, Becker S, Devlin R, Koren HS, Kehrl H, Bromberg PA. Effects of cyclo-oxygenase inhibition on ozone-induced respiratory inflammation and lung function changes. Eur J Appl Physiol Occup Physiol 1996; 73.

63. Coleridge HM, Coleridge JCG, Ginzel KH, et al. Stimulation of "irritant" receptors and afferent C-fibers in the lungs by prostaglandins. Nature (Lond) 1976; 264:451–453.

64. Coleridge JCG, Coleridge HM, Schelegle ES, et al. Acute inhalation of ozone stimulates bronchial C-fibers and rapidly adapting receptors in dogs. J Appl Physiol 1993; 74:2345–2352.

65. Krishna MT, Springall D, Meng QH, Withers N, Macleod D, Biscione G, Frew

A, Polak J, Holgate S. Effects of ozone on epithelium and sensory nerves in the bronchial mucosa of healthy humans. Am J Respir Crit Care Med 1997; 156(3 Pt 1):943–950.

66. Passannante A, Hazucha MJ, Seal E, et al. Nociceptive mechanisms modulate ozone-induced human lung function decrements. Anesth Analg 1995; 80:S371 (abstract).

67. Gong H Jr, Bedi JF, Horvath SM. Inhaled albuterol does not protect against ozone toxicity in nonasthmatic athletes. Arch Environ Health 1988; 43(1):46–53.

68. Kreit JW, Gross KB, Moore TB, et al. Ozone-induced changes in pulmonary function and bronchial responsiveness in asthmatics. J Appl Physiol: Respir Environ Exercise Physiol 1989; 66:217–222.

69. Silverman F. Asthma and respiratory irritants (ozone). Environ Health Perspect 1979; 29:131–136.

70. Horstman DH, Ball BA, Brown J, Gerrity T, Folinsbee LJ. Comparison of pulmonary responses of asthmatic and nonasthmatic subjects performing light exercise while exposed to a low level of ozone. Toxicol Ind Health 1995; 11(4): 369–385.

71. Fernandes ALG, Molfino NA, Mcclean PA, et al. The effect of pre-exposure to 0.12 ppm of ozone on exercise-induced asthma. Chest 1994; 106:1077–1082.

72. Weymer AR, Gong H, Lyness A, et al. Pre-exposure to ozone does not enhance or produce exercise-induced asthma. Am J Respir Crit Care Med 1994; 149:1413–1419.

73. Bascom R, Naclerio RM, Fitzgerald TK, et al. Effect of ozone inhalation on the response to nasal challenge with antigen of allergic subjects. Am Rev Respir Dis 1990; 142:594–601.

74. Peden DB, Setzer RW Jr, Devlin RB. Ozone exposure has both a priming effect on allergen-induced responses and an intrinsic inflammatory action in the airways of perennially allergic asthmatics. Am J Respir Crit Care Med 1995; 151:1336–1345.

75. Basha MA, Gross KB, Gwizdala CJ, et al. Bronchoalveolar lavage neutrophilia in asthmatic and healthy volunteers after controlled exposure to ozone and filtered purified air. Chest 1994; 106:1757–1765.

76. Scannell CH, Chen LL, Aris R, et al. Greater ozone-induced inflammatory responses in subjects with asthma. Am J Respir Crit Care Med 1996; 154:24–29.

77. Peden DB, Boehlecke B, Horstman D, Devlin RB. Prolonged acute exposure to 0.16 ppm ozone induces eosinophilic airway inflammation in asthmatic subjects with allergies. J Allergy Clin Immunol 1997; 100:802–808.

78. Frampton MW, Balmes JR, Cox C, Krein PM, Speers DM, Tsai Y, Utell MJ. Mediators of inflammation in bronchoalveolar lavage fluid from nonsmokers, smokers and asthmatic subjects exposed to ozone: a collaborative study. Health Effects Inst Res Rep 1997; 78:73–79.

79. Molfino NA, Wright SC, Katz I, et al. Effect of low concentrations of ozone on inhaled allergen responses in asthmatic subjects. Lancet 1991; 338:199–203.

80. Ball BA, Folinsbee LJ, Peden DB, Kehrl HR. Allergen bronchoprovocation of patients with mild allergic asthma after ozone exposure. J Allergy Clin Immunol 1996; 98(3):563–572.

81. Jorres R, Nowak D, Magnussen H. The effect of ozone exposure on allergen responsiveness in subjects with asthma or rhinitis. Am J Respir Crit Care Med 1996; 153(1):56–64.

82. Schwartz J, Dockery D. Particulate air pollution and daily mortality in Stubenville, Ohio. Am J Epidemiol 1992; 135:12–19.

83. Schwartz J, Dockery DW. Increased mortality in Philadelphia associated with daily air pollution concentrations. Am Rev Respir Dis 1992; 145:600–604.

84. Peters A, Dockery DW, Heinrich J, Wichmann HE. Short-term effects of particulate air pollution on respiratory morbidity in asthmatic children. Eur Respir J 1997; 10(4):872–879.

85. Pope CAI. Respiratory illness associated with community air pollution in Utah, Salt Lake and Cache Valleys. Arch Environ Health 1991; 46:90–97.

86. Pope CA, Dockery DW, Schwartz J. Review of epidemiological evidence of health effects of particulate air pollution. Inhal Toxicol 1995; 7:1–18.

87. Timonen KL, Pekkanen J. Air pollution and respiratory health among children with asthmatic or cough symptoms. Am J Respir Crit Care Med 1997; 156(2 Pt 1): 546–552.

88. Takafuji S, Suzuki S, Koizumi K, Tadakoro K, Miyamoto T, Ikemori R, Muranaka M. Diesel-exhaust particulates inoculated by the intranasal route have an adjuvant activity for IgE production in mice. J Allergy Clin Immunol 1987; 79:639–645.

89. Takafuji S, Suzuki S, Muranaka M, Miyamoto T. Influence of environmental factors on IgE production, IgE, mast cells and the allergic response. Ciba Found Symp 1989; 147:188–204.

90. Takafuji S, Suzuki S, Koizumi K, Tadakoro K, Ohashi H, Muranaka M, Miyamoto T. Enhancing effect of suspended particulate matter on the IgE antibody production in mice. Int Arch Allergy Appl Immunol 1989; 90:1–7.

91. Takano H, Yoshikawa T, Ichinose T, Miyabara Y, Imaoka K, Sagai M. Diesel exhaust particles enhance antigen-induced airway inflammation and local cytokine expression in mice. Am J Respir Crit Care Med 1997; 156(1):36–42.

92. Muranaka M, Suzuki S, Koizumi K, Takafuji S, Miyamoto R, Ikemori R, Tokiwa H. Adjuvant activity of diesel exhaust particulates for the production of IgE antibody in mice. J Allergy Clin Immunol 1986; 77:616–623.

93. Diaz-Sanchez D, Dotson AR, Takenaka H, Saxon A. Diesel exhaust particles induce local IgE production in vivo and alter the pattern of IgE messenger RNA isoforms. J Clin Invest 1994; 94:1417–1425.

94. Takenaka H, Zhang K, Diaz-Sanchez D, Tsien A, Saxon A. Enhanced human IgE production results from exposure to the aromatic hydrocarbons from diesel exhaust particles: direct effects on B-cell IgE production. J Allergy Clin Immunol 1995; 95:103–115.a

95. Diaz-Sanchez D, Tsien A, Fleming J, Saxon A. Combined diesel exhaust partic-
     ulate and ragweed allergen challenge markedly enhances human in vivo nasal
     ragweed-specific IgE and skews cytokine production to a T helper cell 2-type
     pattern. J Immunol 1997; 158(5):2406–2413.
96. Peterson B, Saxon A. Global increases in allergic respiratory disease: the possi-
     ble role of diesel exhaust particles. Ann Allergy, Asthma, Immunol 1996;
     77(4):263– 268.
97. Blaski CA, Clapp WD, Thorne PS, Quinn TJ, Watt JL, Fress KL, Yagla SJ,
     Schwartz DA. The role of atopy in grain dust-induced airway disease. Am J
     Respir Crit Care Med 1996; 154(2 Pt1):334–340.
98. Michel O, Duchateau J, Sergysels R. Are endotoxins an etiopathogenic factor in
     asthma? Am J Ind Med 1994; 25:129–130.
99. Michel O, Kips J, Duchateau J, Vertongen F, Robert L, Collet H, Pauwels R, Ser-
     gysels R. Severity of asthma is related to endotoxin in house dust. Am J Respir
     Crit Care Med 1996; 154(6 Pt1):1641–1646.
100. Michel O, Ginanni R, Le Bon B, Content J, Duchateau J, Sergysels R. Inflam-
     matory response to acute inhalation of endotoxin in asthmatic patients. Am Rev
     Respir Dis 1992; 146(2):352–357.
101. Michel O, Ginanni R, Sergysels R. Relation between the bronchial obstructive
     response to inhaled lipopolysaccharide and bronchial responsiveness to hista-
     mine. Thorax 1992; 47(4):288–291.
102. Sandstrom T, Bjermer L, Rylander R. Lipopolysaccharide (LPS) inhalation in
     healthy subjects causes bronchoalveolar neutrophilia, lymphocytosis, and fibro-
     nectin increase. Am J Ind Med 1994; 25(1):103–104.
103. Schwartz DA, Thorne PS, Yagla SJ, Burmeister LF, Olenchock SA, Watt JL,
     Quinn TJ. The role of endotoxin in grain dust-induced lung disease. Am J Respir
     Crit Care Med 1995; 152(2):603–608.
104. Hunt LW, Gleich GJ, Ohnishi T, Weiler DA, Mansfield ES, Kita H, Sur S. Endo-
     toxin contamination causes neutrophilia following pulmonary allergen chal-
     lenge. Am J Respir Crit Care Med 1994; 149(6):1471–1475.
105. Macari, DM, Teixeria MM, Hellewell PG. Priming of eosinophil recruitment in
     vivo by LPS pretreatment. J Immunol 1996; 157:1684–1692.
106. Weg VB, Walsh DT, Faccioli LH, Williams TJ, Feldman, M, Nourhargh S. LPS-
     induced 111In-eosinophil accumulation in guinea pig skin: evidence for a role
     for TNF-alpha. Immunology 1995; 84:36–40.
107. Henriques GM, Miotla JM, Cordeiro SB, Wolitsky BA, Woolley ST, Hellewell
     PG. Selectins mediate eosinophil recruitment in vivo: a comparison with their
     role in neutrophil influx. Blood 1996; 87:5297–5304.
108. Kita H, Mayeno AN, Weyand CM, Goronzy JJ, Weiler DA, Lundy SK, Abrams
     JS, Gleich GJ. Eosinophil-active cytokine from mononuclear cells cultured with
     L-tryptophan products:an unexpected consequence of endotoxin contamination.
     J Allergy Clin Immunol 1995; 95:1261–1267.

109. Hallsworth MP, Soh CP, Lane SJ, Arm JP, Lee TH. Selective enhancement of GM-CSF, TNF-alpha, IL-1 beta and IL-8 production by monocytes and macrophages of asthmatic subjects. Eur Respir J 1994; 7(6):1096–1102.
110. Bozza PT, Castro-Faria-Neto HC, Penido C, Larangeria AP, das Gracas M, Henriques MO, Silva PM, Martins MA, dos Santos RR, Cordeiro RS. Requirement for lymphocytes and resident macrophages in LPS-induced pleural eosinophil accumulation. J Leukocyte Biol 1994; 56:151–158.
111. Bozza PT, Castro-Faria-Neto HC, Penido C, Larangeira AP, Silva PM, Martins MA, Cordeiro RS. IL-5 accounts for the mouse pleural eosinophil accumulation triggered by antigen but not by LPS. Immunopharmacology 1994; 27(2):131–136.
112. Dubin W, Martin TR, Swoveland P, Leturcq DJ, Moriarty AM, Tobias PS, Bleecker ER, Goldblum SE, Hasday JD. Asthma and endotoxin: lipopolysaccharide-binding protein and soluble CD14 in bronchoalveolar compartment. Am J Physiol 1996; 270(5 Pt 1):L736–L744.

8

Indoor Environment and Asthma

REBECCA BASCOM

Penn State College of Medicine
Hershey, Pennsylvania

JOHN J. OUELLETTE

University of Wisconsin Medical School
Madison, Wisconsin

I. Introduction

The purpose of this chapter is to summarize recent information about the non-industrial indoor environment and asthma, with particular attention to nonallergenic factors. Chapter 1 presents the evidence that allergens in the indoor environment contribute to asthma. This chapter addresses the topic of allergens only in the context of interactions with nonallergenic pollutants. Excellent compilations exist for readers interested in specific topics (1–3).

On average, people spend over 90% of their time indoors and at least 50% of that time in the home (4). More than half the adult workforce in North America and western Europe works in an office or nonindustrial environment (5,6). The newly developed controlled indoor environment typically exists within the sealed exterior shell of modern office buildings. Highly automated heating, ventilation, and air-conditioning systems are controlled by one or two

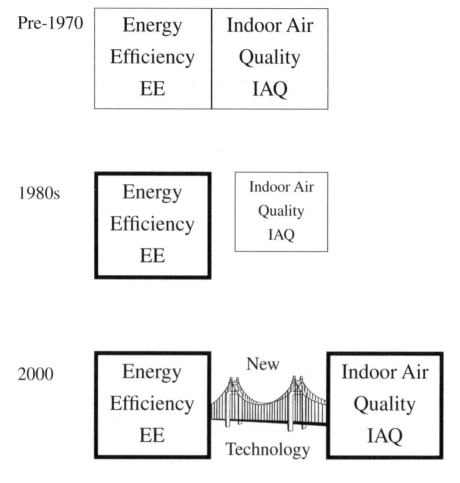

Figure 1   Prior to 1970, the relationship between energy efficiency (EE) and indoor air quality (IAQ) was not a consideration. The supply of energy was thought to be infinite and indoor air quality was not thought to be a problem. In the 1980s, energy efficiency over-ran indoor air quality. After the energy embargo of 1973, new home construction had no regard for indoor air quality. At the present time, new technologies have bridged the gap and allowed us to combine energy efficiency and indoor air quality for health and comfort.

technicians who have no ability to sample indoor air pollutants and little direct contact with occupants (6).

The 1970s gasoline crisis shifted the fundamental assumptions that determined how buildings and homes were constructed and heated (Fig. 1). Builders, engineers, and building maintenance crews struggled to adapt to the urgent need to cut energy consumption in the face of skyrocketing oil costs. The primary design requirement given to them by the health and human performance and industrial hygiene scientists was to maintain "thermal comfort." The chill of the medieval castle had taught humans that drafts and cold were undesirable, an observation quantified in chamber studies in the 1960s. The advent of air conditioning after World War II taught manufacturers that productivity improved when workers were cooler.

The building and engineering communities achieved their goal admirably; energy efficiency soared in the 1980s. The health community began to hear complaints of mucosal irritation, fatigue, and cognitive dysfunction. Human performance experts guessed, but could not readily show, that productivity was altered. The industrial hygiene community could not determine a physical, chemical, or biological explanation for the complaints. Absent an explanation or an easy fix, a complex series of psychosocial dynamics developed in workplaces. Requests for health hazard evaluations flooded the National Institute for Occupational Safety and Health from around the country (7). Frustrated investigators returned empty-handed from what became known as the "hunt a smell" request. Fifteen years later, we understand better how to describe the indoor environment. The pendulum has shifted from an "air-sampling" approach that focused on identifying specific toxicants to a comprehensive approach that identifies and integrates the multiple determinants of the air in indoor environments.

II. Determinants of the Air in Indoor Environments

Table 1 shows the determinants of air in indoor environments. Climate and geology establish the background physical factors that must be modified to achieve thermal comfort. These factors vary widely, from hot, humid climates to cold, dry climates. Pollutants such as radon vary according to geology. Radon does not alter asthma, but the need to reduce the quantity of radon in the air may affect the ventilation requirements of a building.

Regional factors influencing indoor air include the motor vehicle traffic (mobile source pollutants) and power generation facilities (stationary source pollutants). Factories or even small businesses create point source pollution that may influence domestic air quality. The siting of a structure is key, since

Table 1 Determinants of the Indoor Environment

Factor	Examples
Climate	Temperature, humidity, sunlight
Geology	Radon
Region, neighborhood	Rural, industrial, motor vehicular traffic
Siting	High water table, shady area
Structure	Steel, brick, wood, stucco, mud
Surfaces	Concrete, wood, rugs and carpets, mud
Heating and ventilation	Passive, window units, radiator, forced air, electric, gas, oil, coal or wood, kerosene
Occupants	People, cats, dogs
Activities	Cooking, smoking, hobbies

placement in a shady area or in an area of poor drainage may increase moisture problems.

The structural materials may influence indoor air quality either by emitting vapors, such as occurred with ureaformaldehyde foam insulation, or by forming improper moisture barriers or leaky roofs. Within the structure, the surfaces can emit vapors or can serve as reservoirs, collecting then reemitting pollutants. The thermal gradients that occur within surface materials vary widely, and dew points often occur within surface materials.

The heating, ventilation, and air-conditioning system determines the mix of outside and inside air, the temperature and humidity of the inside space, and the water flux in the building. Materials used to clean or disinfect the system can in turn become source pollutants. Improper drainage of pans can provide reservoirs for bioaerosols.

Furnishings and equipment within spaces serve as pollutant sources and also contribute to the thermal load. The occupants contribute their own pollutants, including carbon dioxide, human source bacteria, and allergens. Copiers may emit ozone, which can reach high concentrations when local ventilation is poor. Finally, the activities that occur within the space also serve as source pollutants.

III. Terminology

We support the use of the term "building-related illness" for illnesses that arise in nonindustrial, nonresidential buildings (6). The term "specific building-related illness" refers to a group of illnesses with a homogeneous clinical picture, objective clinical abnormalities, and identifiable sources and pathogens for the allergic, infectious, or immunological disease (6). The term "nonspecific building-related illness" refers to a heterogeneous group of work-related symptoms including irritation of the skin and mucous membranes of the eyes, nose, and throat; headache; fatigue; and difficulty concentrating (6). The term "indoor air quality complaints" (IAQ complaints) refers to a similar symptom cluster but does not label it as an illness. We also support avoiding the terms "sick building" or "healthy building," since they oversimplify a complex environment in which many people, but not all, may be healthy.

IV. The Modern Indoor Environment and Asthma

Does the modern indoor environment adversely affect people with asthma? Surveys often show higher rates of IAQ complaints in patients with asthma (see Table 2).

A survey of 225 female hospital workers in a southern county in Sweden examined the relationship between personal and environmental factors and an overall symptom score (0–26 scale) (11). Symptoms that were enumerated because they are typical of indoor air quality (IAQ) complaints were fatigue, feeling heavy-headed, headache, nausea or dizziness, difficulty concentrating, itching, burning or irritated eyes, irritated or runny nose, hoarseness, dry throat, throat pain, cough, dry facial skin, flushed facial skin, and an itchy, stinging, tight, or burning sensation in facial skin. Multiple linear regression with the overall symptom score indicated that asthma or hay fever had a coefficient of 3.3 (95% CI 1.9–4.7), psychosocial dissatisfaction index had a coefficient of 12.8 (95% CI 7.4–18.2), exhaust ventilation flow had a coefficient of 0.1 (95% CI 0.01–0.9), and perception of static electricity had a coefficient of 1.6 (95% CI 0.2–3.0).

This study illustrates a typical dilemma. We know that mucosal and constitutional symptoms are characteristic of asthma, and so the increase in symptoms among people with asthma is expected. But are these symptoms present in excess? Are people with asthma less able to tolerate environmental variation without adverse health effects? Certainly, a mite-allergic person cannot tolerate the same level of mite allergen that a nonallergic person can. But what about variation in temperature, humidity, ventilation flow, static electricity, and volatile organic compounds?

Table 2 Studies Showing an Association Between Atopy, Allergy, and Asthma, and Symptoms of Nonspecific Building-Related Illnesses Among Office Workers[a]

Author, year	Country	Number of workers	Factors associated with increased symptoms	Ref.
Skov, 1989	Denmark	3507/4369	Females, job category (clerks had more mucous membrane irritation), high surface area)	8
Stenberg, 1993		4943	Females, asthma/rhinitis, high psychosocial load, videodisplay terminals	9
Sundell, 1994			—	10
Nordstrom, 1995	Sweden	225	Asthma or hay fever, psychosocial dissatisfaction index, exhaust ventilation flow, perception of static electricity	11
Bourbeau, 1996	Canada	1371	Females, chronic pulm. disease or asthma, smoking, high job stress, low social support, >4 hrs of computer use per day, working within 5m of a photocopier	12
Wallace, 1993	United States		—	13
Zweers, 1992	Netherlands		—	14
Stenberg, 1994		464	Atopy, photosensitive skin, outdoor air flow, photocopiers	15
Menzies, 1993	Canada	1546	Females, atopic illness, >4 hrs of computer use per day, working in an open area, younger age	16

[a]No studies finding no association were identified.
Source: Ref. 6.

V. Why There Are Problems with Indoor Air Quality

There are many possible ways to link indoor air quality and respiratory health or disease. Broad societal characteristics or trends have been examined, including outdoor air, urbanization, and westernization as well as site-specific factors such as dampness and the presence of combustion products. Another approach has been to perform detailed studies of homes with particular characteristics such as leaky construction or formaldehyde insulation. Other investigators focus on the role of specific toxicants such as steam additives or plasticizers. Each of these areas is discussed now in turn.

A. Outdoor Air

Three common outdoor air pollutants have been linked to exacerbations of asthma: ambient ozone, particulate matter, and sulfur dioxide. This topic has recently been reviewed in detail (17) and is further discussed in Chapter 7. The association with nitrogen dioxide is less well established. Outdoor air pollutants influence indoor air pollution to varying degrees. Ozone is typically an outdoor source pollutant, with reductions of 30–90% occurring as air moves indoors. Ozone is a regional pollutant, increasing during the day over the spring and summer months in many areas of the United States. Ozone is adsorbed to surfaces, and lower rates of removal occur when there is free movement of air through windows unimpeded by curtains.

B. Urbanization

In Africa, urbanization has been linked to the increased prevalence of asthma (18–20). Urbanization has also been associated with increased rates of skin test reactivity in the U.S. National Health and Nutrition Evaluation Survey.

C. Westernization

The importance of environmental factors in relation to asthma was demonstrated in population studies conducted in the former East and West Germany at the time of the reunification (21). Population studies of 9–11-year-old children (5030 in West Germany, 2623 in East Germany) consisted of a parental questionnaire, cold air challenges, and allergy skin prick tests. Atopic sensitization was more frequent in West Germany than in East Germany (37% vs. 18%, odds ratio 2.6, $p < 0001$); the prevalence of current asthma was also more frequent (5.9% vs. 3.9%, odds ratio 1.5, $p < 0.0001$). Bronchitis, however, was more prevalent in East Germany (8.3% vs. 5.5%, odds ratio 1.6, $p < 0.0001$). Once sensitization was taken into account, residence in West Germany was no longer an independent predictor of asthma. Since reunification, rates from East Germany have approached those of West Germany.

One explanation for this finding could be that allergen exposure was greater in West Germany and thus this difference is due to allergic mechanisms. Alternatively, nonallergenic factors may influence the likelihood of sensitization. Subsequent studies by this group support the latter alternative and point to wood or coal stoves as a factor that reduces the risk of sensitization and bronchial hyperreactivity (22).

D. Ventilation Rate

The ventilation rate is defined as the amount of outdoor air supplied to the indoor environment. As summarized by Menzies and Mendell (23), the prevalence of symptoms is higher in buildings with an outdoor air supply of less than 10 L/sec, and typically symptoms were reduced by increasing the ventilation rate if ventilation was previously below this level but not if ventilation was already above the recommended level.

Carbon dioxide is exhaled by humans, and the concentration of carbon dioxide is commonly used as an index of the adequacy of ventilation. In Sweden, for example, a comfort value of 1000 ppm has been adopted (24). Norback et al. (24) found a significant relationship between the concentration of carbon dioxide and nocturnal asthma symptoms.

E. Relative Humidity

Relative humidity is defined as the amount of moisture in the air compared to the maximum possible at that temperature. The capacity of air to hold water varies tremendously with temperature, and condensation occurs at sites of temperature gradients. Diverse factors cause homes to be damp. Placement of the house with siting on a water table with inadequate drainage is a major cause. Vegetation and trees may be dense. Leakage through the basement, roof, or walls may also contribute. An increasing cause of damp homes is the increase in insulation and the changing dynamics of heating, ventilation, and air-conditioning systems.

People contribute humidity to indoor air, both through exhaled air and through common activities such as cooking and bathing. Opening and closing of doors and windows can also change local temperature and humidity gradients. Indirect effects of humidity on indoor air quality relate primarily to whether or not conditions support the growth of molds or fungi or whether condensation occurs at sites of thermal gradients such as windows and other cold surfaces. The biological burden resulting from high humidity is diverse. Infectious bacteria may propagate or may produce biologically active bacterial products such as endotoxin. Molds can exert effects as allergens, as nonallergenic mycotoxins, or by rotting other materials. Arthropods, such as dust and domestic mites, grow more readily.

F. Dampness

Large epidemiological studies in the 1980s concluded that dampness in the home is common in many areas of the United States and that home dampness is a strong predictor of symptoms of respiratory and other illness symptoms, particularly among children (25,26).

In 1986, a random sample of 1000 seven-year-old children in Edinburgh received a postal survey designed to investigate the relationship between damp housing and childhood asthma (27). Of those living in homes reported as damp, 22% were affected by wheeze, while only 11% of those living in homes reported as dry were affected by wheeze. Measurement of ambient temperature and humidity in a stratified sample of 317 bedrooms showed no association with the same respiratory symptoms. The authors acknowledge that their findings run counter to popular wisdom and acknowledge that their findings do not directly exclude effects due to mites or molds, which grow in damp microenvironments.

In 1988, a questionnaire-based study of 17,962 Canadian schoolchildren examined associations between indoor environmental factors and childhood asthma. The children lived in 30 communities across Canada with varying amounts of sulfate outdoor air pollution. None of the communities had local industrial point source pollution. The questionnaire was developed from the 1978 American Thoracic Society—Division of Lung Disease questionnaire, the questionnaire used in the Harvard Six Cities study, the questionnaire used in the Canadian Community Child Health study, and the Environmental Inventory Questionnaire. Children were excluded if they were under 5 or over 8 years old, if they had cystic fibrosis, or if they lived in a mobile home, tent, van, trailer, or boat. Children were also excluded if they reported wheezing only with colds, previous but not current asthma, or persistent cough. The final analysis group consisted of 10,819 children divided into three groups: 978 children who did not report physician-diagnosed asthma but did report wheezing most days or nights, or wheezing apart from colds, or attacks of shortness of breath with wheezing ("Wheezing without a diagnosis of asthma"); 634 children with current asthma and physician-diagnosed asthma; and 9207 children without persistent cough, wheezing, or persistent phlegm and who had reported no chest illness, pneumonia, or bronchitis within the past year. Wheezing without a diagnosis of asthma was associated with ETS [odds ratio (OR) 1.4], home dampness (OR 1.6), and humidifier use (OR 1.4) but not with gas cooking. Increased reports of physician-diagnosed asthma were significantly associated with exposure to environmental tobacco smoke (OR 1.4), living in a damp home (OR 1.5), the use of gas for cooking (OR 2.0), and the use of a humidifier (OR 1.7) (28).

The Canadian investigators also administered questionnaires to 14,799 adults aged 21 or over. Thirty-eight percent of the respondents reported the presence of home dampness and/or mold, as indicated by damp spots, visible mold or mildew, water damage, or flooding. Results were analyzed separately for current smokers, ex-smokers, and lifetime nonsmokers. In all three groups, those with home dampness or mold had a higher prevalence of lower respiratory symptoms defined as any cough, phlegm, wheeze, or wheeze with dyspnea. The adjusted odds ratio was 1.62 and persisted despite stratification by the presence of allergies or asthma (29).

A case control study of 77 schoolchildren with asthma and age-and gender-matched controls examined associations between asthma and home environment factors. Asthma was defined as a history of wheeze, a doctor diagnosis of asthma, or a positive response to an exercise challenge. The investigator was blinded as to the status of the children in the home and performed a visual inspection during a home visit, recording on a checklist the type of building materials, ventilation characteristics (number of windows and presence or absence of a chimney), the type of bedding material, floor coverings, type of cooking fuel, and visible air pollution within the house. The crowding index, vaccination coverage, and parental status were not significantly different between cases and controls. The socioeconomic status of the children varied and influenced the building material of the home: Of the 30 children living in the slums, 88% lived in a mud or semicompleted house while 96% used a pit latrine. In contrast, 89% of the 58 middle class and upper-middle class children lived in brick houses, none had mud homes, and 83% had flush toilets. In multivariate analysis, factors associated with asthma included dampness in the child's sleeping area (adjusted odds ratio 4.9; 95% CI 2–11.7), air pollution in the home (OR 2.5; 95% CI 2–6.4), and the presence of rugs or carpets in the child's bedroom (OR 3.6; 95% CI 1.5–8.5) (30). The survey showed an expected strong association between mud walls and mud floors with damage caused by dampness. An unexpected finding was that children living in homes with mud floors but not mud walls were significantly less likely to have asthma. The factors of dampness and rugs were independently associated risk factors. The authors speculated that differences in allergen or fungal reservoirs could account for these findings.

Investigators in Uppsala, Sweden, investigated possible relationships between symptoms of asthma and building characteristics (24). Their study comprised 88 subjects, aged 20–45 years, selected by stratified random sampling. Subjects underwent a structured interview, spirometry, peak expiratory flow maneuvers, methacholine challenge, and skin prick tests. Environmental factors were measured at a home inspection. Symptoms related to asthma were more common in dwellings with visible signs of dampness or microbial growth in the building, as observed at a home inspection (crude OR 3.9; 95% CI 1.1–14.1). Twenty-three percent of homes of people with symptomatic asthma had visible signs of dampness, while only 7% of those of people without symptoms had visible signs of dampness. None of the other characteristics of the dwellings differed significantly, including the dwelling age, type of house, presence of tobacco smoking indoors, type of ventilation system, or proximity to heavy traffic.

Case Study: Inadequate Moisture Control

The following case study illustrates some of the typical dimensions of asthma and other respiratory illnesses that may occur in damp indoor environments. A damp indoor environment resulted from improper vapor barriers used in home construction. There was a high frequency of respiratory illness and objective evidence of disease. The pattern was not the classic pale, boggy mucosa of allergic rhinitis, however, and skin tests did not demonstrate a single responsible allergen. There was ample evidence of moisture damage and "bioaerosol" reservoirs. Common activities disrupted reservoirs and briefly caused huge increases in exposure levels. Remediation of the obvious problems resulted in measurable reduction of recognized hazards and reduced illness.

In the 1970s, wall construction of the Tri-State Homes consisted of hardboard lap siding, followed by heavy asphalt-coated building paper, followed by plywood sheathing, 3.5 in. of insulation between studs, and interior gypsum board. During 1970–1974 and 1975–1976, the inside and outside facings were Kraft paper. From 1974 to 1976, the inside facing was polyethylene, and from 1977 on it was aluminum. Placement of vapor barriers with new home construction is essential for adequate moisture control.

A questionnaire administered to 268 of the occupants of the Tri-State Homes compared with 181 occupants of comparison homes showed significantly higher levels of chronic cough (29% vs. 17%), shortness of breath (30%

vs. 20%), and nighttime wheezing (16% vs. 8%). Mucosal symptoms were also increased, including burning eyes (11% vs. 3%), burning throat (4% vs. 1%), stuffy nose at home (32% vs. 9%), and frequent colds (11% vs. 1%).

Physical examination of these individuals showed increased rates of pharyngeal redness (27% vs. 17%), nasal redness (24% vs. 11%), sinus drainage (9% vs. 4%), and lung rhonchi (15% vs. 8%). Allergy skin test results showed similar rates of skin test reactivity to molds including *Alternaria* (5% vs. 4%), *Cladosporium* (1% in both groups), *Aspergillus* (0.4% and 1.6%), and *Penicillium* (0.8% and 2.1%). Rates of skin test reactivity to house dust mite were also similar in the two groups (21% and 19%). RAST tests to extracts of the rotten plywood were negative. Occupants with respiratory symptoms had a high frequency of positive skin tests to mite allergens, but the amount of mite allergen in carpet dust was similar in homes of asthmatic and non asthmatic individuals.

The Tri-State Homes had 4.7 air changes per hour, while comparison homes had 9.3 air changes per hour. Twenty percent of the occupants reported current mold or mildew on their walls or ceilings; 43% reported heavy condensation on their windows; 26% reported warping, streaking, or staining of the siding; 14% reported bowing or crumbling of the walls or roof; 40% reported a wet or damp basement; and 30% reported ice buildup on the roof.

Environmental testing results showed increased relative humidity (42% vs. 39%) and higher concentrations of carbon dioxide (1121 vs. 847 ppm), formaldehyde (0.017 vs. 0.011 ppm), and total airborne particles (156 $\mu g/m^3$ vs. 85 $\mu g/m^3$). Airborne fungal spores averaged 315 CFU/m^3 in Tri-State Homes, and 238 CFU/m^3 in the comparison homes.

Carpet dust from the Tri-State Homes contained heavy mite contamination with abundant *D. pteronyssinus* and *D. farinae. Glycophagus* and *Tarsonemus* mites were also present. Occupants with respiratory symptoms had a high frequency of positive skin tests and RAST to mite allergens. The *Dematophagoides* allergens were present in the unrepaired homes at a concentration of 22 μg allergen per gram of dust. Control homes had a concentration of 12 μg/gram of dust. Mite allergy was a major cause of respiratory disease in this environment, but the amount of mite allergen in carpet dust was similar in homes of asthmatics and nonasthmatics. Vacuuming resulted in a 10–100-fold increase over background exposure to mite allergens. Bed-making and going to bed entailed a 100-fold increase in mite allergen exposure.

Repair of the moisture damage required removing the improperly placed vapor barrier, replacing rotten sheathing, and replacing damaged insulation. These repairs resulted in a reduced indoor humidity and a reduction in dust mite allergen to 7.6 $\mu g/g$ dust.

Dust mites and dust mite antigen will vary with the percent relative humidity. While typically the outdoor humidity serves as a surrogate for indoor humidity (and thus high, dry cities have few dust mite problems), local factors that increase indoor humidity can create a microenvironment in which dust mites will proliferate.

G. Ventilation System Additives or Contaminants

New onset asthma occurred in 14 of 2500 office workers after a leak in the steam heating system of a large office building resulted in the release of 2-diethylaminoethanol into the ambient air. The asthma developed within 3 months of the release, and most of the 2500 employees experienced symptoms of irritation at the time of the exposure. Investigators used the National Institute for Occupational Safety and Health surveillance case definition of occupational asthma and reviewed medical records and environmental exposure monitoring data. Of the 14 cases, seven met criteria for "confirmed" and seven met criteria for "suspect" occupational asthma. Investigators concluded that acute exposure to this agent contributed to the development of occupational asthma in this population (31).

H. Indoor Combustion Sources

Combustion occurs in indoor environments in order to generate ambient heat, to prepare meals, or to enable personal activities such as cigarette smoking.

Fuel Combustion

Wood smoke contains carbon monoxide, nitrogen oxides, sulfur oxides, aldehydes, polycyclic aromatic hydrocarbons, and fine respirable particulate matter. The vessel in which a wood fire burns determines the impact of the wood smoke on the indoor environment (32), Wood burned in traditional fireplaces has a fuel efficiency of only 10%, exhausting combustion products, indoor moisture, and 90% of the generated heat up the chimney. In contrast, wood stoves approach 60% fuel efficiency by controlling the air supply and the rate of combustion. Although typically vented to the outside, wood stoves leak smoke into the home through cracks or leaks in the stovepipe or negative pressure indoors.

About half the world's households use biofuels such as wood, crop residues, or animal dung for cooking daily (30). Poor ventilation and the absence of chimneys lead to high levels of smoke indoors (33). In Kenya, visible indoor air pollution was five times more likely if kerosene was used as a primary cooking fuel and three times more likely if charcoal was used than in homes using neither (30). In Britain and North America, domestic air pollution is not consistently associated with asthma (34,35).

Wood Smoke and Incident Respiratory Disease

Infants and young preschool children exposed to wood-burning stoves in the home have an increased risk of pneumonia, bronchiolitis, and wheezing bronchitis and increased incidence of more severe respiratory illness (36). These exposures may increase the risk of upper and lower respiratory tract infections in early childhood.

A study of fourth grade children in rural Bavaria examined the relationship between wood and coal smoke exposure and the development of atopy, atopic disease, and bronchial hyperreactivity (22). "Rural" was defined as fewer than 10,000 cars passing through town each day, and no industry. After controlling for possible confounders, the risk of developing hay fever (OR 0.57; 95% CI 0.34–0.98), atopy defined as at least one positive reaction to a panel of common aeroallergens (OR 0.67; 95% CI 0.49–0.93), sensitization to pollen (OR 0.60; 95% CI 0.41–0.87), and bronchial hyperresponsiveness (OR 0.55; 95% CI 0.34–0.90) was significantly lower in children living in homes where coal or wood was used for heating than in children living in homes with other heating systems.

Bronchial hyperresponsiveness was 11.3% in homes with central heating (57/506), 5.7% in homes heated with coal or wood (31/545), and 8.4% with other gas or oil stoves as the heat source. This protective effect was not simply due to cold bedrooms and lower mite concentrations, since mite sensitization was comparable (6.4% vs. 5.1% vs. 7.9%) in the three groups. Cat allergy was 3.6% vs. 2.0% vs. 4.7%. Pollen sensitization was twofold greater with central oil or gas heat compared to wood or coal stoves (18.8% vs. 10.5% vs. 21.4%). Prevalence of pneumonia in the first year of life was 1.3% vs. 2.4% vs. 1.7%. In the discussion of this paper, the authors speculate that factors directly related to home wood or coal combustion could explain these findings. Alternatively, the use of wood or coal stoves could be an indicator of a protective factor that is part of the more traditional lifestyle of these homes. A third possibility would be that a genetic selection bias occurred over time, resulting in outmigration from the farming community of people with allergic disease.

A study of 4–5-year-old children in Australia had a similar finding of reduced prevalence of asthma, current wheeze, and hay fever but not of eczema in preschool children whose homes were heated with wood or coal (37).

An earlier study of schoolchildren living in East and West Germany showed decreased prevalence of atopic sensitization to a panel of common aeroallergens and of asthma, hay fever, and bronchial hyperresponsiveness in the East German children. One of the differences between children in these two areas of Germany was that coal was used for heating in most households in East Germany or as the energy source for power stations (38).

Wood Smoke Exposure in Patients with Asthma

A panel of 164 nonsmoking asthmatic patients in the Denver, Colorado metropolitan area in 1987–1988 recorded in a daily diary the occurrence of several respiratory symptoms, nocturnal asthma, medication use, and restrictions in activity (39). Patients also reported the use of gas stoves, wood stoves, or fireplaces and environmental tobacco smoke. The mean age was 45 years; 32% were male, 97% were white, 63% college-educated, and 70% employed outside the home. The subjective asthma rating was mild (43%), moderate (36%), or severe (21%). Of the group, 58% took daily theophylline and 19% took daily oral steroids. Multiple logistic regression estimated coefficients for four indoor sources and outdoor hydrogen ion. Of the indoor sources, gas stove use was most strongly associated with moderate or severe cough (OR 2.08; 95% CI 1.77–2.44) and moderate or severe shortness of breath (OR 1.89; 95% CI 1.61–2.21). Gas stove use was also associated with nocturnal asthma (OR 1.3; 95% CI 1.07–1.58). The use of a gas stove was also associated with physician or emergency room visits (OR 2.52; 95% CI 1.45–4.37) and less strongly with an absence from work (OR 2.01; 95% CI 0.92–4.40). The use of a wood stove or fireplace was associated with cough (OR 1.44; 95% CI 1.05–1.99), shortness of breath (OR 1.70; 95% CI 1.24–2.31), and nocturnal asthma (OR 1.59; 95% CI 1.28–1.97).

Investigators in Seattle, Washington, examined the relationship between fine particulate matter and pulmonary function in 326 elementary schoolchildren, 24 of whom were asthmatic (40). The high particulate concentrations derived primarily from wood smoke, since 60% of Washington households burn wood, at a cumulative rate of 2.2 million cords yearly (32). FEV_1 and FVC were measured before, during, and after the 1988–1989 and 1989–1990 winter heating seasons. A light-scattering instrument quantified fine particulate matter. An increase in particulate matter was associated with a decline in asthmatic children's pulmonary function. The FEV_1 and FVC in the asthmatic children dropped an average of 34 and 37 mL for increases in $PM_{2.5}$ of 20 $\mu g/m^3$.

Environmental Tobacco Smoke

Environmental tobacco smoke (ETS) is defined as the products of tobacco combustion inhaled by nonsmokers. The largest source of ETS is the smoke issued from the burning tip of the cigarette, but exhaled mainstream smoke also contributes. In the prenatal period, placental transport of tobacco combustion products occurs when exposure is through active maternal smoking or when the mother is exposed to environmental tobacco smoke. Assessment of ETS occurs by self-report, by parental report, by air sampling for ETS indicators such as carbon monoxide or nicotine, or by analysis of body fluids for the nicotine metabolite cotinine.

ETS can affect asthma risk in several ways. Smoking alters the quantity or characteristics of other asthma risk factors in the home environment. In Sweden, investigators showed higher mite allergen concentrations in the dust from homes with smokers. The quantity of allergen per gram of dust in smokers' homes averaged 200 ng (bedroom) to 157 ng (living room), while the dust in nonsmokers' homes averaged 120 ng (bedroom) to 79 ng (living room) ($p < 0.05$) (41).

ETS can act as an adjuvant, increasing the rate of IgE sensitization in people passively exposed to tobacco smoke. Active smokers have increased levels of IgE and higher rates of sensitization to antigens encountered for the first time in an occupational setting. Rugtveit (42) showed that ETS exposure in the first months of life was related to the development of hypersensitivity.

Epidemiological studies have examined the association between ETS exposure and the prevalence of asthma. Studies have shown an association of parental smoking with persistent wheeze and cough among children (34,43). In the Kenya study, cigarette smoking by any family member was somewhat associated with asthma (OR 1.6; 95% CI 0.8–3.2). Smoking in the home was not associated with visible indoor air pollution as determined by the home inspector.

Cuijpers et al. (44) studied 470 Dutch schoolchildren and defined asthma as a report in the past 12 months of chronic cough, shortness of breath, wheeze, or attacks of shortness of breath with wheeze. Twenty-three percent of the children had one or more of these symptoms. Multiple logistic regression analysis showed an association of maternal smoking of one-half to one pack of cigarettes daily with the presence, in boys only, of chronic cough, shortness of breath, or attacks of shortness of breath and wheezing. Passive smoking was also associated with lower lung function in both girls and boys (44).

Some data point to gender differences in the risk of environmental tobacco smoke for childhood asthma. Passive smoking had a greater effect on asthmatic boys than on asthmatic girls (45). A two-year longitudinal study followed 1812 children (initially 6.7–8.1 years old) in urban areas of southwestern Germany. Parents completed questionnaires, while children performed serial peak flow measurements and provided urine specimens for quantification of urinary cotinine excretion. Cotinine excretion was higher in children of parents who smoked than in these with nonsmoking parents (3.2 ng/mg vs. 0

ng/mg). In boys ($p = 0.00001$), but not girls (0.31), there was a strong association between urinary cotinine excretion and peak flow variability (46).

Other epidemiological studies have examined the association between ETS exposure and asthma severity. In a prospective cohort study of 451 nonsmoking adults with asthma, Eisner et al. (47) evaluated the impact of ETS exposure on asthma severity, health status, and health care utilization over 18 months. There were 129 subjects (29%) who reported regular ETS exposure falling into three categories: exposure at baseline but none at follow-up ($n = 43$, 10%), no baseline exposure and new exposure on follow-up ($n = 56$, 12%), and exposure at both baseline and follow-up ($n = 30$, 7%). In cross-sectional analyses, subjects with baseline ETS exposure had greater severity-of-asthma scores (score difference 1.7, 95% CI 0.2–3.1), worse asthma-specific quality of life scores (score difference 3.5, 95% CI 0.03–7), and worse scores on the Medical Outcomes Study SF-36 physical component summary (score difference 3.0; 95% CI, 0–6.0) than unexposed subjects. They also had greater odds of emergency department visits (OR 2.1; 95% CI 1.2–3.5), urgent physician visits (OR 1.9; 95% CI, 1.1-3.3), and hospitalizations (OR = 0.2; 95% CI, 0.04–0.97) after adjustment for covariates. Environmental tobacco smoke initiation was associated with greater asthma severity, worse health status, and increased health care utilization in adults with asthma.

The panel study of 164 asthmatic patients in Denver also assessed the effects of exposure to environmental tobacco smoke on self-reported symptoms (39). Reporting the presence of smokers in the home was associated with an 8.9% increase in the probability of experiencing daily moderate or severe shortness of breath (OR 1.85; 95% CI 1.57–2.18, $p < 0.0001$) and a 2.8% increase in the probability of experiencing moderate or severe cough (OR 1.21; 95% CI 1.01–1.46, $p = 0.04$). Nocturnal asthma (OR 1.24; 95% CI 1.00–1.53) and restricted activity (OR 2.08; 95% CI 1.63–2.64) also increased.

I. Volatile Organic Compounds

Volatile organic compounds (VOCs) are numerous and diverse in indoor spaces. The TEAM studies by the U.S. Environmental Protection Agency demonstrated that indoor sources were typically more important than outdoor sources in determining indoor space concentrations. The use of cleaning agents, introduction of newly dry-cleaned clothes, personal hygiene products, gas heat, or cigarette smoking may all introduce VOCs into a space. Dampness also results in an increase in VOCs either by emission of VOCs by the proliferating microbes (e.g., 1-octen-3-ol) or by degradation of building materials (e.g., 2-ethylhexanol from hydrolysis of phthalates in floor material) (24).

Table 3 Adjusted Odds Ratios (95% Confidence Interval) for Nocturnal Breathlessness in Relation to Carbon Dioxide, Formaldehyde, and Significant Types of Volatile Organic Compounds[a]

Type of compound	Adjusted OR (95% CI)
Carbon dioxide	20 (2.7–146)
Formaldehyde	12.5 (2.0–77.9)
Toluene	4.9 (1.1–22.8)
C_8-aromatics	6.7 (1.0–45.1)
Terpenes	4.0 (1.2–13.4)
Low retention volatile organic compounds	4.4 (1.3–15.0)
Total volatile organic compounds	9.9 (1.7–58.8)

[a]Logarithmic values were used in the regression models, and odds ratios calculated for a 10-fold increase of the indoor concentrations (except a 1000 ppm increase for carbon dioxide) adjusted for age, sex, current smoking, presence of wall-to-wall carpets, and presence of house dust mites. The C_8-aromatics were ethylbenzene, *m*-xylene, *p*-xylene, and *o*-xylene. The terpens were α-pinene, δ-carene, and limonene. Low retention volatile organic compounds had a retention time below that of benzene.
Source: Ref. 24.

Investigators in Uppsala, Sweden, measured indoor concentrations of selected VOCs in dwellings of subjects with and without nocturnal attacks of breathlessness (Table 3). This analysis was possible because there was no gas cooking or gas heating in the region, sources that would have confounded the analysis. Air sampling was performed during the day without any subjects in the bedroom. This was done to isolate the contribution of the building and its interior to the level of VOCs in the air. In the initial analysis, there was a significant relationship between any type of symptom related to asthma and the concentration of total VOCs ($p < 0.01$) (24). Significant relationships between nocturnal breathlessness and various subclasses of VOCs were detected. The average concentration of toluene was sixfold higher in homes of subjects reporting nocturnal dyspnea; C_8-aromatics, *n*-alkanes, terpenes, and butanols each were twofold higher. Unidentified compounds with a boiling point below benzene were three -to fourfold higher in homes of symptomatic subjects. The total VOCs, meaning the sum or all identified and unidentified compounds, was 780–790 $\mu g/m^3$ in symptomatic subjects compared to 300–310 $\mu g/m^3$ in the bedroom and living room of asymptomatic subjects (24).

Bronchial hyperresponsiveness was related to the indoor concentration of limonene, the most prevalent terpene, while variability in peak expiratory flow was related to two other terpenes, α-pinene and δ-carene.

Controlled human exposure studies have examined the effects of VOC exposures on symptoms, airway inflammation, and lung function. The "Molhave mixture," a representative mixture of VOCs, has been used in chamber studies at concentrations of 25 mg/m³ and shown to cause respiratory symptoms and to induce a neutrophil inflammation at the mucosal surface (48,49).

J. Soft Fiber Wall Materials

The use of textile and other soft fiber wall materials is yet another change in indoor environments over the past several decades. Investigators in Finland studied the relationship between these materials and an asthma reaction score (wheezing, breathlessness, and cough) in 400 workers who occupied two mechanically ventilated eight-story office buildings (50). Exposure was defined as the surface area of textile or other soft wall material, and the outcomes were 7 day prevalences of symptoms. Logistic regression accounted for demographic characteristics including age, gender, and allergic disease history, smoking status, work stress, type of work (photocopying and video display unit work), and the presence of passive smoking, open shelves, and carpeting. While the aggregate asthma symptom score was not associated with exposure, the symptom score of wheezing showed point estimates of greater than unity with a dose–response pattern (OR 1.45 for the low exposure group and 1.78 for the high exposure group). Only 6% of the occupants reported asthma, so the statistical power was limited. Allergic symptoms of rhinorrhea and sneezing were significantly associated with soft wall materials, with a low exposure odds ratio of 1.82 (95% CI 1.14–2.9) and a high exposure odds ratio of 3.16 (95% CI 1.41–7.09). Mucosal irritation symptoms were significantly associated with soft wall materials [OR 1.82 (95% CI 1.14–2.9) for the low exposure vs. 2.46 (95% CI 1.15–5.28) for the high exposure group]. Symptoms included in the mucosal irritation score included eye dryness, itch, or irritation; nasal dryness or congestion; and pharyngeal irritation. The authors speculate that pollutants emitted from the source material could be responsible for the symptoms. Alternatively, the soft wall material could serve as a reservoir or sink for pollutants from other sources.

VI. Environmental Hygienics: Efficiency, Comfort, and Health

An adequate indoor air quality system provides suitable air for both comfort and health. "Environmental hygienics" describes the aggregate effort to address indoor air quality issues for both comfort and health. "Comfort" refers to the physical characteristics of indoor spaces that most humans prefer. Although intersubject variability is acknowledged, human "thermal comfort" was considered achievable. Temperature and humidity are the most important factors, with airflow, temperature gradients, and light also important. Odor control is desirable, but the human nose can perceive very small concentrations of a pollutant, even below levels thought to affect health.

A.   Energy Efficiency and Indoor Air Quality

Energy efficiency influences the cost of heating and cooling an indoor space. The higher the energy efficiency, the lower the yearly energy cost. Air pollutants are anthropogenic (human source) airborne materials that, at low concentrations, may be harmful to plants, animals, or humans. "Mass balance" is the method to estimate the quantity of a pollutant in a particular environment. Mass balance is the net sum of the factors that introduce the pollutant to the environment and factors that remove the pollutant from the environment. Factors that introduce a pollutant to the environment include the size and strength of the pollutant source and its rate of initial entry into the environment and of reentry after deposition into reservoirs or sinks within the environment. Factors that remove the pollutant include the intrinsic rate of inactivation of the pollutant, its inactivation as the result of contact with surfaces or substances in the environment, and the mixing with air that is then exhausted outside the space. When a heating and cooling system becomes more energy-efficient, the ventilation in the space typically decreases, which in turn reduces the amount of dilution of source pollutants. Source strength may need to be reduced in turn to maintain an acceptable mass balance. Typically, however, building operators perform alterations in ventilation independent of an assessment of indoor point sources.

Industrial hygienists identify a generic hierarchy of control strategies. The primary control strategy is source control, accomplished by product substitution, source enclosure or encasement, or source removal. A second control strategy is to dilute the source, such as with ventilation. Filtration can both remove and dilute a source. A third strategy is to protect the individual from the source, such as with respirators or other personal protective equipment.

B.   Ventilation

Some researchers advocate maintaining indoor humidity levels between 40% and 60%, even claiming that this measure would minimize the majority of adverse health effects (51). "This would require humidification during winter in areas with cold winter climates. Humidification should preferably use evaporative or steam humidifiers, as cool mist humidifiers can disseminate aerosols contaminated with allergens."

VII. Conclusion

Asthma is a common chronic disease, so even weak associations between environmental factors and asthma may translate into a large public health burden. People with asthma have mucosal disease and thus may sense environmental factors as adverse, even when no substantial change to their disease state is occurring. Susceptible populations, including children, the elderly, and people with chronic diseases, spend even more time in their home. The concentration of some pollutants is higher indoors than outdoors, and the presence of chronic point sources results in chronic exposures. The strength of the association varies, and the fraction of asthma attributable to that factor can only be estimated. The worldwide increase in the rates of allergic sensitization and asthma spurs the search for contributing factors (indoor allergens).

Two decades after the energy crisis shifted the energy–ventilation trade-off, we can better describe the simple effects of this change than we can understand the health consequences. The technology probably exists to restore indoor air quality without sacrificing energy efficiency. But clinicians and scientists still struggle to understand and define "good" versus "bad" indoor air quality. The multidisciplinary science of indoor air quality offers complex solutions, while a burgeoning consumer product market offers quick fixes, at least some of which are of dubious value.

Clinicians are asked to guide patients, and several practical points emerge from this review. First, damp houses are associated with increased symptoms, and attention must be paid to the fundamentals of moisture control and water balance. Second, the factors in the "modern" house that encourage asthma deserve continued intensive study. Third, accumulating data point to passive smoking as a factor that increases asthma severity for adults as well as children.

References

1. Samet J, Marbury M, Spengler J. Health effects and sources of indoor pollution. Part 1. Am Rev Respir Dis 1987; 136:1486–1508.
2. Samet JM, Marbury MC, Spengler JD. Health effects and sources of indoor air pollution. Part II. Am Rev Respir Dis 1988; 137:221–242.

3. Bardana EJ Jr, Montanaro A, eds. Indoor Air Pollution and Health. Clinical Allergy and Immunology, Vol. 9. New York: Marcel Dekker, 1997:1–520.

4. Spengler J, Sexton K. Indoor air pollution: a public health perspective. Science 1992; 221:9–17.

5. Christie B, ed. Human Factors of Information Technology in the Office. Chichester, England: Wiley, 1985.

6. Menzies D, Bourbeau J. Building-related illness. N Engl J Med 1997; 337(21): 1524–1531.

7. Melius J, Wallingford K, Kennlyside R, Carpenter J. Evaluating office environmental problems. Ann Am Conf Gov Ind Hyg 1984; 10:3–8.

8. Skov P, Valbjorn O, Pedersen B. Influence of personal characteristics, job-related factors and psychosocial factors on the sick building syndrome. Scand J Work Environ Health 1989; 15:286–295.

9. Stenberg B, Hansson MK, Sandstrom M, Sundell J, Wall S. A prevalence study of the sick building syndrome (SBS) and facial skin symptoms in office workers. Indoor Air 1993; 3:71–81.

10. Sundell, J, Stenberg B, Lindvall T. Associations between type of ventilation and air flow rates in office buildings and the risk of SBS-symptoms among occupants. Environ Int 1994; 20:239–251.

11. Nordstrom K, Norback D, Akselsson R. Influence of indoor air quality and personal factors on the sick building syndrome (SBS) in Swedish geriatric hospitals. Occup Environ Med 1995; 52:170–176.

12. Bourbeau J, Brisson C, Allaire S. Prevalence of the sick building syndrome symptoms in office workers before and after exposure to a building with an improved ventilation system. Occup Environ Med 1996; 58:204–210.

13. Wallace L, Nelson CJ, Highsmith R, Dunteman G. Association of personal and workplace characteristics with health, comfort and odor: a survey of 3948 office workers in three buildings. Indoor Air 1993; 3:193–205.

14. Zweers T, Preller L, Brunekreef B, Boleij, JSM. Health and indoor climate complaints of 7043 office workers in 61 buildings in the Netherlands. Indoor Air 1992; 2:127–136.

15. Stenberg B, Eriksson N, Hoog J, Sundell J, Wal S. The sick building syndrome (SBS) in office workers: a case referent study of personal, psychosocial and building related risk indicators. Int J Epidemiol 1994; 23:1190–1197.

16. Menzies R, Tamblyn R, Farant J-P, Hanley J, Nunes F, Tamblyn R. The effect of varying levels of outdoor air supply on the symptoms of sick building syndrome. N Engl J Med 1993; 328:821–827.

17. Bascom R, Bromberg P, Costa D, Devlin R, Dockery D, Frampton M, Lambert W, Samet J, Speizer F, Utell M. Health effects of outdoor air pollution. State of the art review. Am J Respir Crit Care Med 1996; 153:3–50.

18. Godfrey RC. IgE levels in rural and urban communities of Gambia. Clin Allergy 1975; 5:201–207.

19. Van Niekerk CH, Weinberg EG, Shore SC, Heese HdeV, Van Schalkwyk DJ.

Prevalence of asthma: a comparative study of urban and rural Xhosa children. Clin Allergy 1979; 9:319–324.

20. Warrell DA, Fawcett IW, Harrison BDW, Agamah AJ, Ibu JO, Pope HM. Bronchial asthma in the Nigerian savannah region. Q J Med 1975; 44:325–347.

21. von Mutius E, Martinez FD, Fritzsch C, Nicolai T, Roell G, Thiemann H-H. Prevalence of asthma and atopy in two areas of West and East Germany. Am J Respir Crit Care Med 1994; 149:358–364.

22. von Mutius E, Illi S, Nicolai T, Martinez FD. Relation of indoor heating with asthma, allergic sensitization and bronchial responsiveness: survey of children in South Bavaria. Br Med J 1996; 312:1448–1450.

23. Mendell M. Non-specific symptoms in office workers: a review and summary of the literature. Indoor Air 1993; 3:227–236.

24. Norback D, Bjornsson E, Janson C, Widstrom J, Boman G. Asthmatic symptoms and volatile organic compounds, formaldehyde, and carbon dioxide in dwellings. Occup Environ Med 1995; 52:388–395.

25. Brunekreef B, et al., Am Rev Respir Dis 1989; 140:1363–1367.

26. Platt SD. Damp housing, mould growth and symptomatic health state. Br Med J 1989; 298:1673–1678.

27. Strachan DP, Sanders CH. Damp housing and childhood asthma; respiratory effects of indoor air temperature and relative humidity. J Epidemiol Community Health 1989; 43:7–14.

28. Dekker C, Dales R, Bartlet S, Brunekreef B, Zwaneburg H. Childhood asthma and the indoor environment. Chest 1991; 100:922–926.

29. Dales RE, Burnett R, Zwanenburg H. Adverse health effects among adults exposed to home dampness and molds. Am Rev Respir Dis 1991; 143:505.

30. Mohamed N, et al., Home environment and asthma in Kenyan schoolchildren: a case-control study. Thorax 1995; 50(1):74–78.

31. Gadon M, Melius JM, McDonald GJ, Orgel D. New-onset asthma after exposure to the steam additive 2-diethylaminoethanol. A descriptive study. J Occup Med 1994; 36(6):623–626.

32. Pierson WE, Koenig JQ, Bardana EJ. Potential adverse health effects of wood smoke. West J Med 1989; 151:339–342.

33. Smith KR. Biofuels, Air Pollution and Health—A Global Review. New York: Plenum Press, 1987.

34. Dijkstra L, Houthuijs D, Brunekreef B, Akkerman I, Bojeij J. Respiratory health effects of the indoor environment in a population of Dutch children. Am Rev Respir Dis 1990; 142:1172–1178.

35. Speizer FE, Ferris Jr. B, Bishop YMM, Spengler J. Respiratory disease rates and pulmonary function in children associated with nitrogen dioxide exposure. Am Rev Respir Dis 1980; 121:3–10.

36. Morris K, Morganlander M, Coulehan JL, Gahagen S. Wood-burning stoves and lower respiratory tract infections in Indian children. Am J Dis Child 1990; 144:105–108.

37. Volkmer R, Ruffin RE, Wigg NR, Davies N. The prevalence of respiratory symptoms in South Australian preschool children. II. Factors associated with indoor air quality. J Paediatr Child Health 1995; 31:112–115.

38. von Mutius E, Fritzsch C, Weiland SK, Roell G, Magnussen H. Prevalence of asthma and allergic disorders among children in united Germany: a descriptive comparison. Br Med J 1992; 305:1395–1399.

39. Ostro BD, Lipsett MJ, Mann JK, Wiener MB, Selner J. Indoor air pollution and asthma. Results from a panel study. Am J Respir Crit Care Med 1994; 149:1400–1406.

40. Koenig JQ, Larson TV, Hanley QS, Rebolledo V, Damler K, Checkoway H, Wang SZ, Lin D, Pierson W. Pulmonary function changes in children associated with fine particulate matter. Environ Res 1993; 63:26–38.

41. Munir A, Bjorksten B, Einarsson R, Ekstrand-Tobin A, Moller C, Warner A, Kjellman NIM. Mite allergens in relation to home conditions and sensitization of asthmatic children from three climatic regions. Allergy 1995; 50:55–64.

42. Rugtveit J. Environmental factors in the first months of life and the possible relationship to later development of hypersensitivity. Allergy 1990; 45:154–156.

43. Burchfiel CM, Higgins MW, Keller JB, Howatt WF, Butler WJ, Higgins ITT. Passive smoking in childhood. Respiratory conditions and pulmonary functions in Tecumseh, Michigan. Am Rev Respir Dis 1986; 133:966–973.

44. Cuijpers C, Swaen GMH, Wesseling G, Sturmans F, Wouters EFM. Adverse effects of the indoor environment on respiratory health in primary school children. Environ Res 1995; 68:11–23.

45. O'Connor GT, Weiss ST, Tager IB, Speizer FE. The effect of passive smoking on pulmonary function and nonspecific bronchial responsiveness in a population-based sample of children and young adults. Am Rev Respir Dis 1987; 135:800–804.

46. Kuehg J, Frischer T, Karmaus W, Meinert R, Pracht T, Lehnert W. Cotinine excretion as a predictor of peak flow variability. Am J Respir Crit Care Med 1998; 158:60–64.

47. Eisner MD, Yelin EH, Henke J, Shiboski SC, Blanc PD. Environmental tobacco smoke and adult asthma. The impact of changing exposure status on health outcomes. Am J Respir Crit Care Med 1998; 158:170–175.

48. Harving H, Dahl R, Molhave L. Lung function and bronchial reactivity in asthmatics during exposure to volatile organic compounds. Am Rev Respir Dis 1991; 14:751–754.

49. Koren H, Graham D, Devlin R. Exposure of humans to volatile organic mixture. III. Inflammatory response. Arch Environ Health 1992; 47:39–44.

50. Jaakkola JJ, Tuomaala P, Seppanen O. Textile wall materials and sick building syndrome. Arch Environ Health 1994; 49(3):175–181.

51. Arundel AV, et al., Environ Health Perspect 1986; 65:351–361.

9

Environmental Aspects of Asthma

Special Problems in Urban Populations

JEAN G. FORD, JAVED IQBAL, and JOANNE K. FAGAN

School of Public Health
The Harlem Lung Center
Harlem Hospital Center
Columbia University College of Physicians and Surgeons
New York, New York

I. Introduction

Asthma, a chronic inflammatory disorder of the airways, affects approximately 15 million persons in the United States, including 4.8 million children (1). In the United States, asthma-related morbidity and mortality have increased significantly since the late 1970s, with disproportionate impact in urban underserved populations. During this period, the greatest increase in asthma-related morbidity has been observed in African Americans and Hispanics (especially Puerto Ricans), two U.S. minority groups whose members are most likely to live in an urban setting (2,3). Within these groups, children and young adults have been most severely impacted (4–7).

Despite increasing knowledge about the pathophysiology and therapy of asthma, significant gaps persist in understanding the etiological factors that might explain the epidemic rise in morbidity. Consequently, efforts to reduce the impact of asthma on the nation's health have focused principally on strategies to reduce exacerbations in individuals with asthma. Asthma morbidity has been linked to a variety of factors, including environmental factors, lack of access and/or poor adherence to medical care, exposure to psychosocial stressors, exposure to multiple caretakers, lack of non-emergency care, impaired self-efficacy, and deficient problem-solving skills (8–10). However, our increased knowledge about these risk factors and asthma morbidity has not translated into effective community-wide interventions.

Perhaps reflecting the lack of understanding of etiological factors that drive asthma morbidity within urban populations, the term "inner city asthma" has gained widespread acceptance. Considering the complexity of urban populations, strictly speaking, the term "inner city" could describe the residential area for communities rich or poor and of diverse ethnic/racial backgrounds. Contributing causes of asthma-related morbidity in impacted communities are often ascertainable, and appropriate research and intervention strategies must be targeted to these communities to address the public health dimensions of asthma in the United States.

In this chapter, we review potential risk factors for excess morbidity in disadvantaged urban communities, speculate on reasons for possible differential susceptibility to exposure, and summarize the implications for health care policy and research. We examine the differentials in potential exposure to airborne allergens and indoor and outdoor air pollutants. We cite examples from our experience in Harlem and suggest potential directions for future research and intervention to reduce asthma morbidity in economically disadvantaged urban populations.

II. Estimating Exposures Relevant to Asthma

A. Approaches for Estimating Exposure

Environmental exposures are important in the development and maintenance of the abnormal pattern of airway responsiveness that is characteristic of asthma. The risk caused by an environmental exposure depends on the route, magnitude, frequency, and duration of the exposure. The exposures that are relevant to asthma are usually airborne. To effectively assess and manage the risk of asthma in urban populations, it is important to understand the distribution of individual exposures in different populations, the causes of high exposure, and the relationship between exposure and dose (11,12). Because it is often impractical and nearly impossible to measure urban air pollution and allergen exposures, surrogate and mathematical models are commonly used to measure exposures in urban populations (e.g., emission estimates, ambient air quality, skin reactivity to indoor allergens).

B. Role of Time–Activity Patterns in Exposure Estimation

It is often assumed that differences in asthma morbidity are due exclusively to differences in the magnitude of exposures in both indoor and outdoor settings. Little is known, however, about the contribution of time–activity patterns to apparent differences among socioeconomic and ethnic/racial subgroups in exposure to air pollutants, including those in urban communities. Data are lacking on differences in daily activity by age, gender, and work status (12,13). In the aggregate, all, especially children, spend most of their time (~90%) indoors (14). Two recent studies on the relationship between time–activity patterns and short-term exposure to air pollutants with measures of asthma morbidity found a significant correlation among these variables. Analyses also revealed that the children spent more time outdoors and were more physically active in the spring than during other seasons. Girls spent less time outdoors and were less physically active than boys (15,16).

The exposure that occurs in the home "microenvironment" is very important in relation to asthma. Compared to suburban middle class communities, the homes of urban low income minority groups are more likely to harbor increased levels of air pollutants because of greater use of unvented combustion appliances (wood-burning stoves or fireplaces) and exposure to indoor pollutants such as tobacco smoke and chemical sprays. These homes, on average, also exhibit higher levels of dust mite and cockroach allergens, both of which can cause airway sensitization and asthma exacerbations (17,18). Thus, the amount of time spent in different microenvironments is critical to an understanding of the level of exposure to potential triggers of asthma symptoms.

III. Risk Factors for Asthma in Urban Populations

It is widely believed that the onset of asthma follows exposure to significant concentrations of airborne allergens for a duration sufficient to cause sensitization of the airways of susceptible individuals (19–21). In asthmatic individuals, such sensitization usually leads to a complex immunological response in the airways that is characterized by inflammation, nonspecific bronchial hyperresponsiveness, and airway narrowing that is reversible, at least to some degree (22). Thus, any discussion of risk factors for asthma would focus on exposures that have the potential to sensitize the airways and thus cause this abnormal immune response and its physiological consequences. However, most asthma begins early in life (23), and currently only a few of the myriad of environmental exposures that have the potential of sensitizing the airways have been identified (8). Moreover, our understanding of the contribution of these exposures to the incidence of asthma remains limited. Consequently, most studies of risk factors for asthma have focused on factors that maintain the physiological characteristics of asthma (e.g., airway hyperresponsiveness) or cause exacerbation.

We hypothesize that the disproportionate burden of asthma morbidity in urban populations can be explained, in part, by relatively greater levels of exposures with potential to (1) cause airway sensitization and (2) contribute to the maintenance of airway inflammation and its physiological consequences.

A. Risk Factors for (the Onset of) Asthma

Cohort studies on the relationship between early life exposures and asthma (24,25) have found that most cases of asthma begin during infancy and early childhood, with 80% of children who develop asthma having their first episode of wheeze before the age of 3 years (23). Early-life wheezing presents, however, as separate phenotypes at different ages, with each phenotype having distinct characteristics, risk factors, and prognoses for the development of asthma (24,26,27). A number of early-life exposures have been shown to be critical to the development of asthma later in childhood, including allergen exposure and viral infections (19,28–30). There is evidence of prenatal sensitization to airborne allergens such as dust mites that are known to cause airway sensitization and asthma (31). These exposures occur at high levels in urban homes and are associated with increased asthma morbidity (17). Therefore, we hypothesize that the excessive burden of early-life exposure in urban communities contributes to the incidence of asthma and thus to asthma morbidity in general.

It is widely believed that the risk for the onset of asthma represents an interaction between genetic susceptibility, particularly atopic predisposition (29), and relevant environmental exposures. The clustering of asthma morbidity and mortality within specific racial/ethnic groups has raised important questions about the contribution of genetic factors to the rise in asthma morbidity. Current evidence suggests a major hereditary contribution to the etiology of asthma and allergic diseases. However, the inheritance pattern of asthma demonstrates that it is a "complex genetic disorder" (32), polygenic in origin. Asthma cannot be classified simply as having an autosomal dominant, recessive, or sex-linked mode of inheritance. In addition, little is known about the interaction between genetic predisposition and environmental exposures in causing asthma.

In several epidemiological studies it has been shown that asthma is more common in first-degree relatives of asthmatics. The prevalence of asthma is 4–5% in the U.S. population at large, for example, but 20–25% among those who have a sibling or parent with asthma (33,34). Children born to a family with one asthmatic parent have a risk of developing the disease several times that of a child born to nonasthmatic parents. The risk is greater still if both parents have asthma (35). Studies of asthma in sets of identical (monozygotic) twins also show a higher correlation (concordance) with respect to asthma than those of dizygotic twins (36). Genetic factors have been shown to play a significant role in initiating specific immune responses to aeroallergens, in the production of IgE, in the release of cytokine mediators, and in the development of bronchial hyperresponsiveness. Several recent developments present important opportunities for identification and characterization of possible candidate genes for asthma. These include the linkage of the high affinity IgE receptor, the cytokine gene cluster and bronchial hyperresponsiveness to chromosome 5q; the linkage of asthma to chromosome 11q13 (37); and the linkage of the T-cell antigen receptor to chromosome 14q (38).

Although little is known about the genetic control of many elements involved in the development of asthma, genetic factors appear to play an important role at the individual level. The significant rise in asthma morbidity in urban populations during the past two decades cannot be explained, however, solely or primarily on the basis of genetic factors. It can be plausibly explained by a significant change in environmental exposures that interact with genetic determinants of the heterogeneous condition commonly known as "asthma." This is fertile ground for future research with the still elusive goal of primary prevention.

B. Environmental Risk Factors for Asthma Morbidity

Indoor Allergens and Asthma

Indoor allergens (e.g., cockroach, dust mite, and rodent) are ubiquitous, especially in urban communities, and present a significant exposure, based on estimates that Americans spend most of their time indoors (14). Allergy to common indoor aeroallergens can be shown in up to 90% of asthma patients (39). In the National Cooperative Inner City Asthma Study (NCICAS), cockroach allergen exposure was shown to play a role in childhood asthma morbidity in an urban population (17). Cockroach exposure is highly prevalent and is associated with sensitization in asthmatic patients in urban environments, including New York City (17,40–43). This relationship appears to be dose-dependent, with some risk for sensitization at low doses of allergen, 2 μg or less with the risk for sensitization reaching a plateau at levels above 4 μg (44). A correlation has also been demonstrated between cockroach sensitization and the amount of cockroach allergen in bedroom dust samples (45). The NCICAS found an association between the level of cockroach allergen in house dust and both the prevalence of cockroach protein sensitization and asthma severity among children sensitized to cockroach allergen (17).

Dust mite species *Dermatophagoides pteronyssiunus* and *Dermatophagoides farinae* have long been known to play an important etiological role in the development of asthma, atopic dermatitis, and allergic rhinitis (46). Sporik et al. (47) found that exposure to house dust mite allergens at an early age is an important determinant of subsequent development of asthma. In a birth cohort of New Zealand children, Sears et al. (19) noted that sensitivity to dust mite allergen was significantly associated with the development of asthma. Bjornsson et al. (48) reported odds ratios of 7.9 for asthma-related symptoms and 6.2 for nocturnal breathlessness independently related to exposure to dust mites. Chan-Yeung et al. (49) explored the relationships between dust mite levels in the home, skin test reactivity, and severity of asthma in 120 asthmatic subjects (children and adults). In children with positive skin tests to either mite allergen, total mite (sum of Der p 1 and Der f 1) allergen level was positively related to the mean daily symptom score and negatively related to the daily mean peak expiration flow (PEF) (percent of predicted). A dose–response relationship has been demonstrated in adults between the level of dust mite exposure and disease severity and clinical activity (50).

The poor housing conditions that are commonly found in urban neighborhoods have been associated with increased asthma exacerbations in adults and children. Water damage, a common occurrence in urban homes, contributes to household dampness, which promotes the growth of and exposure to cockroaches, mites, molds, and fungi (51,52).

Indoor Air Pollutants

Many air pollutants (e.g., benzene, NO_2, carbon monoxide, ETS, radon.) are found in higher concentrations indoors than outdoors. Levels of carbon monoxide and nitrogen dioxide in Harlem and Washington Heights, two low income communities in northern Manhattan in New York City, are higher than outdoor concentrations and EPA standards (53). Unvented gas-fired cooking stoves, used frequently for space heating, constitute additional possible causes of indoor air pollution.

The effects of environmental tobacco smoke (ETS) on the development of asthma have been inconclusive (54–56). However, some investigators have found that environmental tobacco smoke caused increased risk for asthma (57), bronchial reactivity (58), and emergency visits for asthma (59). Sharing a bedroom with a smoker increased the risk of respiratory symptoms in a case control study of children admitted to the hospital for asthma for the first time (60). Data from the Third National Health and Nutrition Examination survey (1988–1994) (NHANES III) demonstrated that ETS exposure is very common in children in the United States and that the odds of asthma and wheezing increase for children living in households where >20 cigarettes are smoked per day (61). These findings are supported by a 1996 critical review of available data on the health effects of ETS in children (62).

The effect of environmental tobacco smoke (ETS) exposure on adults with asthma has not been well characterized. In a prospective cohort study of 451 nonsmoking adults with asthma, ETS exposure was associated with a greater asthma severity score, worse health status, and increased health care utilization for asthma; and a reduction in ETS exposure resulted in an improvement in health status and a reduction in health care utilization (63).

The burden of asthma-related morbidity attributed to ETS and other indoor air pollutants is likely to be most significant in communities where smoking is highly prevalent. While African Americans, on average, take up smoking at a later age than Caucasians, they are less likely to quit (64,65). This contributes to a relatively higher prevalence of smoking among African Americans and a higher prevalence of exposure to ETS in African American communities. Between 1992 and 1994, the Harlem Health Survey found a high prevalence of self-reported current smoking among both men (48%) and women (41%), including highly educated men (38%) (66). These statistics demonstrate an increased level of exposure to ETS in minority, low income communities, supporting the need for targeted intervention strategies.

Outdoor Air Pollution

Because of the variety of potential sources, both outdoors (e.g., industrial factories, motor vehicles, residential wood burning) and indoors (e.g., combustion appliances, consumer products, tobacco smoke), people living in urban areas are exposed to air pollutants at higher than average levels.

Consequently, in evaluating an asthmatic patient, it is important to consider the air quality in the patient's various personal "microenvironments" at home, work, and elsewhere as well as overall air quality in the community (67). Many outdoor air pollutants readily penetrate indoors. Indoor air quality can deteriorate quickly when persistent and uncontrolled emissions occur and the ventilation/air exchange rate is reduced. Children are highly susceptible to certain environmental toxicants. Those who live in urban underserved communities may be particularly at risk because environmental pollution has been found to be disproportionately distributed among communities (68). The National Ambient Air Quality Standards (NAAQS) criteria air pollutants include ozone, CO, NO_2, SO_2, and PM10. Gelobter (68) noted that high concentrations of these pollutants are most likely to be found in areas with low income, poor housing, and African American and Hispanic populations. Air pollution exposures have also been shown to be the highest for young people who work in low-paying jobs and live in low-rent districts, particularly Blacks and Hispanics. It is also clear that many urban areas are out of compliance with NAAQS guidelines (69), and these urban areas are disproportionately populated by people of color (68).

Studies have demonstrated significant associations between urban air pollutants—NO_2, SO_2, and particulate matter—and asthma-related morbidity and mortality (70–72).

Other investigators have shown that diesel exhaust particles (DEPs) coupled with outdoor and indoor pollutants increase the risk of exacerbations (73). Evidence also points to the role of DEPs in increasing the likelihood of an IgE-mediated immune response and induction of allergic inflammation. A close review of experimental studies in animals and human beings shows that DEPs enhance IgE production by a variety of mechanisms, including effects on cytokine and chemokine production as well as activation of macrophages and other mucosal cell types (74). In New York City, six out of seven diesel bus terminals are located in low income communities in northern Manhattan, including Harlem. These potentially contribute to the burden of exposure and probably disease in these communities (75).

Although ambient air quality has generally improved, these improvements have not reached U.S. minority and low income communities in equal proportions (68). The environmental justice movement has clearly identified urban asthma as a marker condition for environmental inequity. For example, in Hunt's Point, South Bronx, New York, the community began to organize against the continued operation of a medical waste incinerator based on suspicions that pollutants emitted from the incinerator increased asthma prevalence in the area (76). However, it has not been possible, in this community, to narrowly define the independent contribution of specific outdoor air pollutants to asthma morbidity, because other relevant exposures, including cockroach allergens, are also significant. The recent closure of the medical waste incinerator in the South Bronx as a result of community activism is an example of what communities can do, in partnership with academic institutions, to address an identified problem—in this case, asthma. Whether this will result in reduced asthma morbidity in the South Bronx remains an open question.

C. Psychosocial Factors

Race/Ethnicity

The age-adjusted asthma mortality rate in white males increased from 1.0 to 1.4 per 100,000 between 1979 and 1994, an increase of 40%. During the same period, the mortality rate in white females increased from 1.2 to 2.4 per 100,000, an increase of almost 100%. The age-adjusted mortality rate increased by 100% in black males and 111% in black females over this time span.

In 1994, the age-adjusted death rate for asthma in the black population was 3.7 per 100,000. This was almost three times the rate in the white population (1.2 per 100,000) (77).

Racial/ethnic differences have also been noted in asthma prevalence and asthma hospitalization rates. Weitzman et al. (78), using data from the Child Health Supplement of the National Health Interview Survey from 1981 to 1988, noted that black children have higher rates of asthma than white children. In a previous study using data from the 1981 survey (79), Weitzman et al. demonstrated that when social and environmental characteristics were controlled the increased risk of asthma in black children lost significance. Schwartz et al. (80) and Gold et al. (81), however, continued to find asthma significantly associated with race (black vs. white) after adjusting for socioeconomic factors, environmental exposures, and other confounding factors. Nearly 80% of asthma deaths occur in urban areas, with data from New York City and Cook County Chicago showing a serious upward trend (2,82). Hospitalization rates among blacks and Hispanics were 3–5.5 times those for whites (6). The rates of asthma among Puerto Rican children living in the New York City area are among the highest in the United States (83,84). Interestingly, among U.S. soldiers morbidity and mortality related to asthma do not differ significantly between blacks and whites, suggesting that apparent ethnic differences in asthma morbidity disappear under standardized living conditions, environmental exposures, and access to medical care (85).

Socioeconomic Status and Poverty

Asthma morbidity and mortality are more common among the poor than among the more affluent. In Philadelphia, asthma death rates were significantly higher in census tracts with higher percentages of blacks, Hispanic women, and a population with incomes in the poverty range (86). Similar results were found in New York City (6) and Chicago (82). Indeed, socioeconomic status is a strong predictor of death or near death from asthma (87,88). New York City's large population of African Americans and Puerto Rican Hispanics has a high prevalence of poverty and a high rate of health care utilization for asthma (6,89). In 1991, the poverty rate for African Americans was 28.4%, 3 times as high as the poverty rate for white Americans. Hispanic persons had the highest poverty rate (29.4%) of all ethnic groups in 1996 (90). It is unclear the extent to which being poor increases the likelihood of exposure to ubiquitous precipitants of asthma, or whether poverty makes asthma worse because it is associated with less access to medical care.

D. Access to Medical Care

A number of studies have assessed health care access and utilization by U.S. minority populations (91,92). Compared to Caucasian asthmatics, urban minority asthmatic patients are less likely to have primary care visits and more likely to use the emergency department for asthma management. Emergency department use is highest among African American males, and adolescent black males have the highest rate of hospitalizations (93). In New York City, communities such as Harlem and the South Bronx, with high asthma prevalence, have ongoing shortages of primary care resources (94). Such shortages are manifest in part-time, unstable practices, "Medicaid mills," lack of after-hours access to a provider, and a myriad of other problems that translate into a lack of continuity of care. Many asthmatic patients are uninsured, but the provision of emergency care for asthma is mandatory during acute exacerbations. In addition, due to lack of patient education on the preventive management of asthma, patients commonly perceive that the medical care offered in the emergency department is superior, because relief is obtained for acute symptoms in a very short period of time, in contrast to long waiting periods in clinics. Under these circumstances, the emergency department becomes the provider of choice. It is not surprising that several surveys have failed to find a protective effect of access to a provider against asthma-related emergency visits; under prevailing conditions, primary care—an established, continuous relationship with a provider—may be functionally inaccessible. Similarly, language and cultural issues may act as barriers to health care utilization for certain minority populations (92,95).

Recently, Zorratti et al. (96) examined health service use by African Americans and Caucasians with asthma in a managed care setting. Compared with Caucasians, African Americans had fewer visits to an asthma specialist (0.32 vs. 0.50 visit per year) and filled fewer prescriptions for inhaled medications. Several other studies suggest that ethnic differences in patterns of asthma-related health care persist within a managed care setting and are only partially due to financial barriers. In addition, participation in a given managed care plan is often short-lived, with many transitions from plan to plan requiring a change of medical care provider (96).

IV. Conclusions

The observed disparities in asthma morbidity among urban communities are most likely due, at least in part, to exposure differentials between urban populations. While genetic predisposition contributes to asthma morbidity, it probably does not play a predominant role in the recent epidemic rise in asthma morbidity. Socioeconomic status and access to medical care, on the other hand, appear to be important correlates of asthma. Indeed the term "inner city asthma" offers a convenient cliché that fails to capture the complexity of culture, socioeconomic status, and, ultimately, exposure, as determinants of asthma in urban populations of color.

Clearly, a great deal more needs to be learned about etiological factors and potential interventions to reduce the burden of asthma-related morbidity in urban populations. Indoor and outdoor exposures need to be further characterized, including the contribution of time–activity patterns. More research is needed on the effects of age, gender, and genetic factors on the observed differentials in morbidity.

Finally, because much of the relevant exposures occur in the intimacy of the home environment, research strategies must rely on the development of trust and true partnerships with the impacted communities. This is the context in which communities and collaborating academic institutions will succeed in understanding etiological factors and prevention strategies for asthma.

References

1. CDC. Surveillance of asthma. MMWR Surveill Summ 1998; 47 (SS-1):1–28.
2. Weiss KB, Wagener DK. Changing patterns of asthma mortality. Identifying target populations at high risk. JAMA 1990; 264:1683–1687.
3. Sexton K, Gong H Jr, Bailar JC III, Ford JG, Lambert WE, Utell M. Air pollution health risks: do class and race matter? Toxicol Indl Health 1993; 9:843–877.

4. Weiss KB, Gergen PJ, Crain EF. Inner-city asthma. The epidemiology of an emerging US public health concern. Chest 1992; 101(6 suppl):362S–367S.
5. Gergen PJ, Mullaly DI, Evan R III. National survey of prevalence of asthma among children in the United States, 1976 to 1980. Natl Acad Pediatr 1988; 81:1–7.
6. Carr W, Zeitel L, Weiss K. Variations in asthma hospitalizations and deaths in New York City. Am J Public Health 1992; 82(1):59–65.
7. CDC. Asthma mortality and hospitalization among children and young adults— United States, 1980–1993. MMWR Weekly 1996; 45(17):350–353.
8. Peat JK. Prevention of asthma. Eur Respir J 1996; 9(7):1545–1555.
9. Malveaux FJ, Fletcher-Vincent SA. Environmental risk factors of childhood asthma in urban centers. Environ Health Perspect 1995; 103(suppl 6):59–62.
10. Eggleston PA, Buckley TJ, et al. The environment and asthma in US inner cities. Environ Health Perspec 1999; 107(suppl 3):439–450.
11. Sexton K, Ryan PB. In: Watson AY, Bates, eds. Assessment of Human Exposure to Air Pollution: Methods, Measurements and Model. Washington, DC: National Academy Press, 1988.
12. Shwab M. The influence of daily activity patterns and differential exposure to carbon monoxide among social groups. In: Clark TH, ed. Proceedings of the Research Planning Conference on Human Activity Patterns. EPA/600/4-89/004. Washington, DC: EPA, 1991.
13. Avol EL, Navidi WC, Rappaport EB, Peters JM. Acute effects of ambient ozone on asthmatic, wheezy, and healthy children. Res Rep Health Effects Inst 1998; (82):iii, 1–18; discussion pp 19–30.
14. Pope AM, Patterson R, Burge H. Indoor Allergens: Assessing and Controlling Health Effects. Washington, DC: National Institutes of Medicine, National Academy Press, 1993.
15. Linn WS, Shamoo DA, Anderson KR, Peng RC, Avol EL, Hackney JD, Gong H Jr. Short-term air pollution exposures and responses in Los Angeles area schoolchildren. J Expo Anal Environ Epidemiol 1996; 6(4):449–472.
16. Shamoo DA, Linn WS, Peng RC, Solomon JC, Webb TL, Hackney JD, Gong H Jr. Time–activity patterns and diurnal variation of respiratory status in a panel of asthmatics: implications for short-term air pollution effects. Expo Anal Environ Epidemiol 1994; 4(2):133–48.
17. Rosenstreich DL, Eggleston P, Kattan M, Baker D, Slavin RG, Gergen P, Mitchell H, McNiff-Mortimer K, Lynn H, Ownby D, Malveaux F. The role of cockroach allergy and exposure to cockroach allergen in causing morbidity among inner-city children with asthma. N Engl J Med 1997; 336(19):1356–1363.
18. Goldstein IF, Hartel D, Andrews LR, Weinstein AL. Indoor air pollution exposures of low-income inner-city residents. Environ Int 1986; 12:211–219.
19. Sears MR, Herbison GP, Holdaway MD, Hewitt CJ, Flannery EM, Silva PA. The relative risk of sensitivity to grass pollen, house dust mite and cat dander in the development of childhood asthma. Clin Exp Allergy 1989; 19:419–424.

20. Peat JK, Woolcock AJ. Sensitivity to common allergens: relation to respiratory symptoms and bronchial hyperresponsiveness in children from three different climatic areas of Australia. Clin Exp Allergy 1991; 21:573–581.
21. Gergen PJ, Turkeltaub PC. The association of individual allergen reactivity with respiratory disease in a national sample: data from the second National Health and Nutrition Examination Survey, 1976–1980 (NHANES II). J Allergy Clin Immunol 1992; 90:579–588.
22. O'Byrne PM. Airway inflammation and asthma. Aliment Pharmacol Ther 1996; 10(suppl 2):18–24.
23. Yunginger JW, Reed CE, O'Connell EJ, Melton LJ 3d, O'Fallon WM, Silverstein MD. A community-based study of the epidemiology of asthma. Incidence rates, 1964–1983. Am Rev Respir Dis 1992; 146(4):888–894.
24. Wright AL, Taussig LM. Lessons from long-term cohort studies. Childhood asthma. Eur Respir J Suppl 1998; 27:17s–22s.
25. Martinez FD. Maternal risk factors in asthma. Ciba Found Symp 1997; 206: 233–239; discussion, pp 239–243.
26. Martinez FD, Wright AL, Taussig LM, Holberg CJ, Halonen M, Morgan WJ. Asthma and wheezing in the first six years of life. The Group Health Medical Associates. N Engl J Med 1995; 332(3):133–138.
27. Stein RT, Holberg CJ, Morgan WJ, Wright AL, Lombardi E, Taussig L, Martinez FD. Peak flow variability, methacholine responsiveness and atopy as markers for detecting different wheezing phenotypes in childhood. Thorax 1997; 52(11): 946–952.
28. Kuehr J, Frischer T, Meinert R, Barth R, Schraub S, Urbanek R, Karmaus W, Forster J. Clinical aspects of allergic disease: sensitization to mite allergens is a risk factor for early and late onset of asthma and for persistence of asthmatic signs in children. J Allergy Clin Immunol 1995; 95:655–662.
29. Weiss ST. Environmental risk factors in childhood asthma. Clin Exp Allergy 1998; 28(suppl 5):29–34; discussion, pp 50–51.
30. Martinez FD. Viral infections and the development of asthma. Am J Respir Crit Care Med 1995; 151(5):1644–1647; discussion 1647–1648.
31. Warner JA, Jones AC, Miles EA, Colwell BM, Warner JO. Prenatal origins of asthma and allergy. Ciba Found Symp 1997;206:220–228; discussion 228–232.
32. Lander ES, Schork NJ. Genetic dissection of complex traits. Science 1994; 265(5181):2037–2048.
33. Abdulrazzaq YM, Bener A, DeBuse P. Association of allergic symptoms in children with those in their parents. Allergy 1994; 49:737–743.
34. Dold S, Wjst M, von Mutieu E, Reitmeir P, Stiepel E. Genetic risk of asthma, allergic rhinitis, and atopic dermatitis. Arch Dis Child 1992; 67:1018–1022.
35. Litonjua AA, Carey VJ, Burge HA, Weiss ST, Gold DR. Parental history and the risk for childhood asthma. Does mother confer more risk than father? Am J Respir Crit Care Med 1998; 158(1):176–181.

36. Duffy DL, Mitchell CA, Martin NG. Genetic and environmental risk factors for asthma: a cotwin-control study. Am J Respir Crit Care Med 1998; 157(3, Pt 1): 840–845.

37. Hizawa N, Freidhoff LR, Ehrlich E, Chiu YF, Duffy DL, Schou C, Dunston GM, Beaty TH, Marsh DG, Barnes KC, Huang SK. Genetic influences of chromosomes 5q31-q33 and 11q13 on specific IgE responsiveness to common inhaled allergens among African American families. Collaborative Study on the Genetics of Asthma (CSGA). J Allergy Clin Immunol 1998; 102(3):449–453.

38. Hall IP. Genetics and pulmonary medicine 8: asthma. Thorax 1999; 54(1):65–69.

39. Platt-Mills TA, Sporik RB, Chapman MD, Heymann PW. The role of indoor allergens in asthma. Allergy 1995; 50(22 suppl):5–12.

40. Kang BC, Johnson J, Veres-Thorner C. Atopic profile of inner-city asthma with a comparative analysis on the cockroach-sensitive and ragweed-sensitive subgroups. J Allergy Clin Immunol 1993; 92(6):802–811.

41. Kang BC, Wilson M, Price KH, Kambara T. Cockroach-allergen study: allergen patterns of three common cockroach species probed by allergic sera collected in two cities. J Allergy Clin Immunol 1991; 87(6):1073–1080.

42. Pollart SM, Chapman MD, Fiocco GP, Rose G, Platts-Mills TA. Epidemiology of acute asthma: IgE antibodies to common inhalant allergens as a risk factor for emergency room visits. J Allergy Clin Immunol 1989; 83(5):875–882.

43. Menon P, Menon V, Hilman B, Stankus R, Lehrer SB. Skin test reactivity to whole body and fecal extracts of American (*Periplaneta americana*) and German (*Blatella germanica*) cockroaches in atopic asthmatics. Ann Allergy 1991; 67(6): 573–577.

44. Eggleston PA, Rosenstreich D, Lynn H, Gergen P, Baker D, Kattan M, Mortimer KM, Mitchell H, Ownby D, Slavin R, Malveaux F. Relationship of indoor allergen exposure to skin test sensitivity in inner-city children with asthma. J Allergy Clin Immunol 1998; 102:563–570.

45. Sarpong SB, Hamilton RG, Eggleston PA, Adkinson NF Jr. Socioeconomic status and race as risk factors for cockroach allergen exposure and sensitization in children with asthma. J Allergy Clin Immunol 1996; 97(6):1393–1401.

46. Voorhorst R. To what extent are house-dust mites (Dermatophagoides) responsible for complaints in asthma patients? Allerg Immunol (Leipz) 1972; 18(1):9–18.

47. Sporik R, Holgate S, Platts-Mills TAE, Cogswell JJ. Exposure to house-dust mite allergen (Der p I) and the development of asthma in childhood: a prospective study. N Engl J Med 1990; 323:502–507.

48. Bjornsson E, Norback D, Janson C, Widstrom J, Palmgren U, Strom G, Boman G. Asthmatic symptoms and indoor levels of micro-organisms and house dust mites. Clin Exp Allergy 1995; 25(5):423–431.

49. Chan-Yeung M, Manfreda J, Dimich-Ward H, Lam J, Ferguson A, Warren P, Simons E, Broder I, Chapman M, Platts-Mills T, et al. Mite and cat allergen levels

in homes and severity of asthma. Am J Respir Crit Care Med 1995; 152(6, pt 1): 1805–1811.

50. Custovic A, Green R, Taggart SC, Smith A, Pickering CA, Chapman MD, Woodcock A. Domestic allergens in public places. II: Dog (Can f 1) and cockroach (Bla g 2) allergens in dust and mite, cat, dog and cockroach allergens in the air in public buildings. Clin Exp Allergy 1996; 26(11):1246–1252.

51. Gold DR. Indoor air pollution. In: Epler GR, ed. Clinics in Chest Medicine vol. 13, Occupational Lung Diseases. 1992:215–229.

52. Dales RE, Burnett R, Zwanenburg H. Adverse health effects among adults exposed to dampness and molds. Am Rev Respir Dis. 1991; 143:505–509.

53. Goldstein IF, Hartel D. Critical assessment of epidemiological studies of environmental factors and asthma. In: Goldsmith J, ed. Environmental Epidemiology: Community Studies. Boca Raton, FL: CRC Press, 1986:101–114.

54. Gelber LE, Seltzer LH, Bouzoukis JK, Pollart SM, Chapman MD, Platts-Mills TA. Sensitization and exposure to indoor allergens as risk factors for asthma among patients presenting to hospital. Am Rev Respir Dis 1993; 147(3):573–578.

55. Infante-Rivard C. Childhood asthma and indoor environmental risk factors. Am J Epidemiol 1993; 137(8):834–844.

56. Samet JM. Asthma and the environment: do environmental factors affect the incidence and prognosis of asthma? Toxicol Lett 1995; 82–83:33–38.

57. Gortmaker SL, Walker DK, Jacobs FH, Ruch-Ross H. Parental smoking and the risk of childhood asthma. Am J Public Health 1982; 72(6):574–579.

58. Knight A, Breslin AB. Passive cigarette smoking and patients with asthma. Med J Aust 1985; 142(3):194–195.

59. Evans D, Levison MJ, Feldman CH, Clark NM, Wasilewski Y, Levin B, Mellins RB. The impact of passive smoking on emergency room visits of urban children with asthma. Am Rev Respir Dis 1987; 135(3):567–572.

60. Azizi BH, Zulkifli HI, Kasim S. Indoor air pollution and asthma in hospitalized children in a tropical environment. J Asthma 1995; 32(6):413–418.

61. Gergen PJ, Fowler JA, Maurer KR, Davis WW, Overpeck MD. The burden of environmental tobacco smoke exposure on the respiratory health of children 2 months through 5 years of age in the United States: Third National Health and Nutrition Examination Survey, 1988 to 1994. Pediatrics 1998; 101:1–6.

62. DiFranza JR, Lew RA. Morbidity and mortality in children associated with tobacco products by other people. Pediatrics 1996; 97:560–568.

63. Eisner MD, Yelin EH, Henke J, Shiboski SC, Blanc PD. Environmental tobacco smoke and adult asthma. The impact of changing exposure status on health outcomes. Am J Respir Crit Care Med 1998; 158(1):170–175.

64. Headen SW, Bauman KE, Deane GD, Koch GG. Are the correlates of cigarette smoking initiation different for black and white adolescents? Am J Public Health 1991; 81(7):854–858.

65. Siegel D, Faigeless B. Smoking and socioeconomic status in a population-based inner city sample of African Americans, Latinos and whites. J Cardiovasc Risk 1996; 3(3):295–300.

66. Northridge ME, Morabia A, Ganz ML, Bassett MT, Gemson D, Andrews H, McCord C. Contribution of smoking to excess mortality in Harlem. Am J Epidemiol 1998; 147(3):250–258.

67. Hackney JD, Linn WS. Environmental factors: air pollution, weather and noxious gases. In: Weiss EB. Textbook of Bronchial Asthma. 3rd ed. New York Little Brown, 1993:577–578.

68. Gelobter M. The distribution of outdoor air pollution by income and race. Master's Thesis, University of California at Berkeley, 1986.

69. Chow JC. Measurement methods to determine compliance with ambient air quality standards for suspended particles. J Air Waste Manag Assoc 1995; 45:320–382.

70. Ackermann-Liebrich U. Lung functions and long-term exposure to air pollutants in Switzerland. Am J Respir Crit Care Med 1997; 155:122–129.

71. Delfino RJ, Moulton-Murphy AM, Burnett RT, Brook JR. Effect of air pollution on emergency room visits for respiratory illnesses in Montreal, Quebec. Am J Respir Crit Care Med 1997; 155:568–576.

72. Sunyer J, et al. Urban air pollution and Emergency admissions for asthma in four European cities: the APHEA project. Thorax 1997; 52:760–765.

73. Platts-Mills TA, Sporik RB, Chapman MD, Heymann PW. The role of domestic allergens. Ciba Found Symp 1997; 206:173–185; discussion, pp 185–189.

74. Nel AE, et al. Enhancement of allergic inflammation by the interaction between diesel exhaust particles and the immune system. J Allergy Clin Immunol. 1998; 102(4, pt 1):539–554.

75. Northridge ME, Yankura J, Kinney PL, Santella RM, Shepard P, Riojas Y, Aggarwal M, Strickland P. Diesel exhaust exposure among adolescents in in Harlem: a community driven study. Am J Public Health 1999; 89(7):998–1002.

76. Claudio L, Torres T, Sanjurjo E, Sherman LR, Landrigan PJ. Environmental health sciences education: a tool for achieving environmental equity and protecting children. Environ Health Perspect 1998; 106(suppl 3):849–855.

77. Sly RM, O'Donnell R. Stabilization of Asthma mortality. Ann Allergy Asthma Immunol 1997; 78(4):347–354.

78. Weitzman M, Gortmaker SL, Sobol AM, Perrin JM. Recent trends in the prevalence and severity of childhood asthma. J Am Med Assoc 1992; 268:2673–2677.

79. Weitzman M, Gortmaker S, Sobol A. Racial, social, and environmental risk for childhood asthma. AJDC 1990; 144:1189–1194.

80. Schwartz J, Gold D, Dockery DW, Weiss ST, Speizer FE. Predictors of asthma and persistent wheeze in a national sample of children in the United States: association with social class, perinatal events, and race. Am Rev Respir Dis 1990; 142:555–562.

81. Gold DR, Rotnitzky A, Damokosh AI, Ware JH, Speizer FE, Ferris BG, Dockery DW. Race and gender differences in respiratory illness prevalence and their rela-

tionship to environmental exposures in children 7 to 14 years of age. Am Rev Respir Dis 1993; 148:10–18.

82. Marder D, Targonski P, Orris P, et al. Effect of racial and socioeconomic factors on asthma mortality in Chicago. Chest 1992; 82:59–65.

83. Carter-Pokras OD, Gergen PJ. Reported asthma among Puerto Rican, Mexican-American, and Cuban children, 1982 through 1984. Am J Public Health 1993; 83(4):580–582.

84. Beckett WS, Belanger K, Gent JF, Holford TR, Leaderer BP. Asthma among Puerto Rican Hispanics: a multi-ethnic comparison study of risk factors. Am J Respir Crit Care Med 1996; 154(4, pt 1):894–899.

85. Ward DL. An international comparison of asthma morbidity and mortality in US soldiers, 1984 to 1988. Chest 1992; 101(3):613–620.

86. Lang DM, Polansky M. Patterns of asthma mortality in Philadelphia from 1969 to 1991. N Engl J Med 1994; 331:1542–1546.

87. Christiansen SC, Martin SB, Schleicher NC, Koziol JA, Mathews KP, Zuraw BL. Current prevalence of asthma-related symptoms in San Diego's predominantly Hispanic inner-city children. J Asthma 1996; 33(1):17–26.

88. Lin S, Fitzgerald E, Hwang SA, Munsie JP, Stark A. Asthma hospitalization rates and socioeconomic status in New York State (1987–1993). J Asthma 1999; 36(3):239–251.

89. De Palo VA, Mayo PH, Friedman P, Rosen MJ. Demographic influences on asthma hospital admission rates in New York City. Chest 1994; 106(2):447–451.

90. Hahn RA, Eaker ED, Barker ND, Teutsch SM, Sosniak WA, Krieger N. Poverty and death in the United States. Int J Health Serv 1996; 26(4):673–690.

91. Ali S, Osberg JS. Differences in follow-up visits between African American and white Medicaid children hospitalized with asthma. J Health Care Poor Underserved 1997; 8(1):83–98.

92. Blixen CE, Havstad S, Tilley BC, Zoratti E. A comparison of asthma-related healthcare use between African-Americans and Caucasians belonging to a health maintenance organization (HMO). J Asthma 1999; 36(2):195–204.

93. Murray MD, Stang P, Tierney WM. Health care use by inner-city patients with asthma. J Clin Epidemiol 1997; 50(2):167–174.

94. Brellochs C, Carter AB, Caress B, Goldman A. Building Primary Health Care Services in New York City's Low-Income Communities. Community Services Society of New York Working Papers, 1990.

95. Gilthorpe MS, Lay-Yee R, Wilson RC, Walters S, Griffiths RK, Bedi R. Variations in hospitalization rates for asthma among black and minority ethnic communities. Respir Med 1998; 92(4):642–648.

96. Zoratti EM, Havstad S, Rodriguez J, Robens-Paradise Y, Lafata JE, McCarthy B. Health services use by African Americans and Caucasians with asthma in a managed care setting. Am J Respir Crit Care Med 1998; 158(2):371–377.

10

Environmental Asthma
Diagnostic Approaches

JEFFREY R. STOKES

The Asthma & Allergy Center
Papillion, Nebraska

ROBERT K. BUSH

University of Wisconsin–
   Madison Medical School
and William S. Middleton
   Memorial Veterans Hospital
Madison, Wisconsin

I. Introduction

Asthma is the most common chronic disease of childhood, affecting 14 million to 15 million people, including 4.8 million children in the United States (1). One of the main difficulties in treating asthma is in first correctly diagnosing it. Asthma frequently is diagnosed as wheezing bronchitis, asthmatic bronchitis, bronchial asthma, recurrent bronchitis, wheezing in infancy, or reactive airways disease. There is no one test that will be diagnostic for asthma, but with a thorough history, physical exam, and specific testing aimed at the characteristic features of asthma, the correct diagnosis can be established.

II. Definition

Asthma is an extremely heterogeneous disease with a wide variety of genetic, environmental, psychosocial, and molecular biology factors contributing to the disease process. Attempts to define asthma in terms of its cause have been unsuccessful because the cause is currently unknown. Asthma can be defined in clinical terms as a disease of recurrent cough, wheeze, or shortness of breath. The pathollogist would define asthma as a disease of airway inflammation, edema, and excess mucus production. A physiologist defines asthma as a disease of airway hyperresponsiveness and reversible airway obstruction. An immunologist's definition of asthma would be related to IgE antibody specific to environmental allergens.

In an attempt to merge all the viewpoints, a working definition of asthma has been suggested (2):

> Asthma is a chronic inflammatory disorder of the airways in which many cells and cellular elements play a role, in particular mast cells, eosinophils, T lymphocytes, macrophages, neutrophils, and epithelial cells. In susceptible individuals, this inflammation causes recurrent episodes of wheezing, breathlessness, chest tightness, and coughing, particularly at night or in the early morning. These episodes are usually associated with widespread but variable airflow obstruction that is reversible either spontaneously or with treatment. The inflammation also causes an associated bronchial hyperresponsiveness to a variety of stimuli.

Environmental or "allergic" extrinsic asthma is a subclassification of asthma based upon a precipitating exogenous cause, whereas with intrinsic asthma no known external cause is identifiable (3). Allergic asthma is the most common form of asthma. About 90% of asthmatic individuals younger than 16 years of age are allergic, while 70% of asthmatic individuals younger than 30 years are allergic, and 50% of those older than 30 are allergic (4).

III. Differential Diagnosis

Due to the common symptoms of asthma such as cough and shortness of breath, the differential diagnosis can be quite extensive. The more common causes of cough and wheeze are listed in Table 1.

Testing is aimed at confirming the diagnosis of asthma based on objective measures of reversible airway obstruction and airway hyperresponsiveness. The history and physical exam are essential in the diagnosis of asthma, but without further testing physicians correctly predict pulmonary function

Table 1 Differential Diagnosis of Asthma Symptoms (Cough, Wheeze, Shortness of Breath)

Symptoms more commonly seen in children	Symptoms common in both adults and children	Symptoms more commonly seen in adults
Viral bronchiolitis	Rhinosinusitis (allergic or	COPD
Respiratory syncytial	nonallergic)	Chronic bronchitis
virus (RSV)	Gastroesophageal reflux	Emphysema (α-1 anti-
Parainfluenza virus	disease (GERD) (with/	trypsin deficiency)
Laryngotracheomalacia,	without aspiration)	Hypersensitivity pneumo-
tracheal stenosis, or	Vocal cord dysfunction	nitis
bronchostenosis	Hyperventilation	Medication-related effects
Foreign body aspiration	Cardiac disease (conges-	Angiotensin converting
Extrathoracic obstruction	tive heart failure)	enzyme (ACE)
Vascular ring or sling		inhibitor
Lymphadenopathy		associated cough
Cystic fibrosis		Carcinoid syndrome
Croup		Pulmonary embolism
Bronchopulmonary dyspla-		Bronchiectasis
sia (esp. premature infant)		Pulmonary infiltrates with
Mycoplasma infection (esp.		eosinophilia
>5 yr old)		Extrathoracic obstruction
Mechanical obstruction		Neoplasm (benign or
Tracheal stenosis		malignant)
Laryngeal or glottic web		Lymphadenopathy
		Laryngeal dysfunction

about half the time and correctly diagnose asthma only 63–74% of the time (5). The diagnosis of atopy differentiates allergic asthma from intrinsic asthma.

IV. Pulmonary Function Testing

A. Spirometry

Spirometric measurements of pulmonary function are valuable in both diagnosing asthma and assessing disease severity. This testing can been done on patients as young as 5 years old with reproducibility (2). The percent predicted is based on an individual's age, gender, and height (6). Specific ethnic groups will also have different percents predicted based on reference values of a comparable population. Centers should use values that are representative of the population to be tested.

In assessing asthma by spirometry, several measurements are of primary importance: the functional vital capacity (FVC), the forced expiratory volume in 1 sec (FEV_1), the forced expiratory flow during the middle half of the vital capacity (FEF_{25-75}), and the FEV_1/FVC ratio. The obstructive lung disease pattern of asthma can be distinguished from a nonobstructive pulmonary disease on the basis of decrease in the FEV_1/FVC ratio (6). Healthy individuals can maximally exhale approximately 80% of their forced vital capacity in 1 sec. Typically in obstructive disease the FEV_1/FVC value is less than 80%, while in restrictive pulmonary disorders, such as obesity, values may be 90% or greater. In some healthy individuals with normal values of FEV_1 and FVC, the FVC value may be relatively larger than the FEV_1, resulting in a lower FEV_1/FVC ratio despite a normal pulmonary system. If the ratio is borderline, the FEV_1 and FEF_{25-75} values may be used to confirm the presence of airway obstruction. When the FEV_1/FVC and FEV_1 values are both normal, abnormalities in the FEF_{25-75} should be interpreted with caution.

In assessing airway obstruction severity, the FEV_1 is a better measure than either the FEV_1/FVC or FEF_{25-75} (6). A decrease in FEV_1 to less than 80% predicted is indicative of significant airway obstruction (6). One example for assessing asthma severity on the basis of FEV_1 values is shown in Table 2.

B. Bronchodilator Response

The obstructive pattern of asthma noted on basic spirometry does not distinguish it from other obstructive lung diseases such as emphysema, chronic bronchitis, and cystic fibrosis. One characteristic feature of asthma is "reversible"

Table 2 Asthma Severity

Disease severity	Percent predicted FEV_1
Mild	<100 and ≥80
Moderate	<80 and ≥60
Moderately severe	<60 and ≥50
Severe	<50 and ≥34
Very severe	<34 or less than 1 L

airway obstruction. In view of abnormal initial spirometry this may be demonstrated by a positive response following the use of a short-acting beta$_2$-agonist. In evaluating a significant post-bronchodilator effect, the FEV$_1$ and FVC should be the primary indices, while FEF$_{25-75}$ should be considered secondary and the FEV$_1$/FVC ratio should not be used (6,7). An increase from pre-bronchodilator values, either FEV$_1$ or FVC, by 12% and a 200 cm^3 increase are reasonable criteria for a positive response in adults (6). A negative response to bronchodilator does not eliminate the diagnosis of asthma. The major component of obstruction in asthma is inflammation, not bronchospasm, so reversibility of obstruction may not be demonstrated unless anti-inflammatory treatment such as with oral corticosteroids is implemented.

C. Flow–Volume Loops

Displaying the values measured by spirometry may be required to fully appreciate the degree of airway obstruction. The standard expression is by spirogram (Fig. 1). This representation demonstrates the relationship between the volume, the vital capacity exhaled, and time in seconds. The relationships between asthmatic and normal lung patterns are shown in Figure 1. Normally the volume exhaled in 1 sec (FEV$_1$) is approximately 80% of the total volume, while the volume after 3 sec is equal to the FVC. In obstructive lung disease the lung volume exhaled after 1 sec is less than 80% of the total, and after 3 sec the volume exhaled is still less than the total volume.

Another useful measure is the flow–volume loop formed by plotting both the inspiratory and expiratory flow vs. volume (Fig. 2). This is compiled by initial tidal breathing followed by a maximal inspiration with a maximal forced exhalation. Small airway obstruction will demonstrate a concave expiratory loop with eventual decreases in all points along the curve depending upon the severity of the obstruction. This initial concavity is independent of the patient's effort in the maneuver. The peak expiratory flow (PEF), also known as the forced expiratory flow maximum (FEF$_{max}$), is at the apex of the expiratory curve. The FEF$_{max}$ is effort-dependent and will decrease in obstructive lung disease, but it is not as sensitive a measure of airway obstruction as FEV$_1$.

Certain pulmonary disorders will affect the flow–volume loop in characteristic ways (8) (Fig. 3). An intrathoracic lesion, such as distal tracheal stenosis, will flatten the PEF. Extrathoracic lesions will truncate the inspiratory loop but preserve the expiratory loop, as can be demonstrated with vocal cord dysfunction. A fixed lesion such as subglottic stenosis may impede both the maximum inspiratory and expiratory flows.

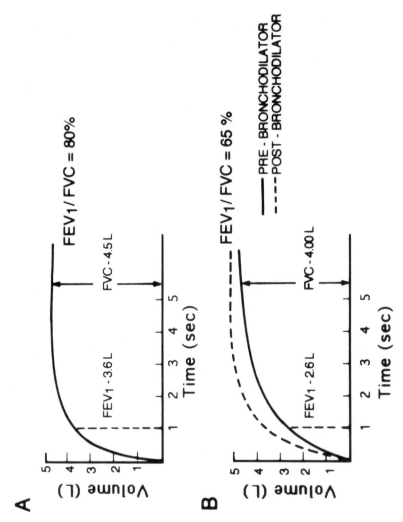

Figure 1 Spirograms plot volume exhaled over a time period measured in seconds. (A) The normal pattern seen in a healthy lung with the ratio of the volume exhaled in 1 sec (FEV_1) to the total volume exhaled forcibly (FVC) of 80%. (B) The FEV_1/FVC ratio is reduced as expiratory airflow is obstructed. This airflow obstruction reverses after bronchodilator use and can even become normal.

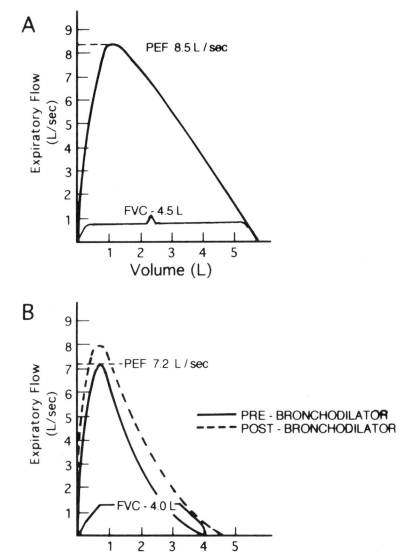

Figure 2   Flow–volume loops represent the expiratory flow plotted against lung volume exhaled. (A) A healthy person demonstrates the typical normal pattern. (B) The pattern noted in patients with asthma. Here the peak expiratory flow is diminished and the expiratory flow is concave in comparison to the normal pattern seen in (A). This obstructive pattern is improved after bronchodilator use, but still the "scooped out" appearance is apparent.

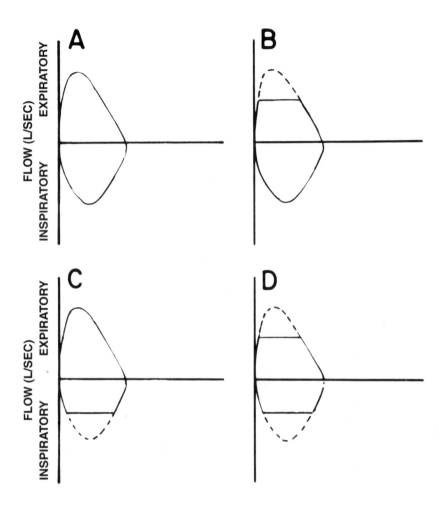

Figure 3 Typical patterns seen in inspiratory/expiratory flow volume loops. (A) Normal patterns of inspiratory and expiratory flows plotted against volume. In (B) the expiratory flow is "cut off" due to intrathoracic airflow obstruction such as tracheal stenosis. (C) Here the inspiratory flow is truncated while the expiratory loop is preserved. This is due to extrathoracic airway obstruction such as vocal cord dysfunction. (D) shows both intra- and extrathoracic airway obstruction or a fixed-airway obstruction such as a subglottic stenosis. Both the inspiratory and expiratory flow are compromized.

D. Bronchoprovocation Testing

Measuring pulmonary functions following an airway challenge with histamine, methacholine, or exercise may demonstrate significant airway obstruction when the diagnosis of asthma is in question. Bronchoprovocation testing needs to be performed under the supervision of knowledgeable individuals and is not recommended as a standard office test for the untrained due to the possibility of inducing significant bronchospasm. It is also not recommended for a patient with an FEV_1 of less than 65% of predicted. Testing for airway hyperresponsiveness is useful when a patient reports recurrent asthma-type symptoms such as chronic cough but does not demonstrate wheezing or spirometric values consistent with the diagnosis of asthma.

Airway responsiveness is assessed by the degree of drop in the FEV_1 30–180 sec after a dose of either histamine or methacholine. Two techniques are commonly used for histamine or methacholine challenge (9). The first involves counted breaths of increasing doses from some form of dosing device. This measures a provocation dose of histamine or methacholine to produce a 20% fall in FEV_1 (PD_{20}). The second method involves a period of tidal breathing from a continuous methacholine source. This measures the provocation concentration required to reduce the FEV_1 by 20% (PC_{20}). The PC_{20} can be converted to an equivalent PD_{20} value (10). The lower the PC_{20}, the greater the responsiveness.

An arbitrary PC_{20} of 8 mg/mL histamine identified 100% of 205 documented asthmatics, while 3.9% of 355 healthy controls responded to 8 mg/mL or less (10). Allergic patients without asthma are more responsive to histamine or methacholine than nonallergic patients (11). The shape of a histamine or methacholine challenge curve will vary depending on the severity of asthma, with mildly asthmatic and normal individuals demonstrating a plateau effect with increasing doses of provocation. This plateau effect is eliminated in moderate asthma, leading to continued worsening constriction with subsequent doses of stimulus (12). In the case of chronic asthma-induced cough, the positive predictive value of methacholine challenge was 74% whereas the negative predictive value was 100% (13). Other states that would lead to an increase in airway reactivity include allergic rhinitis, cystic fibrosis (CF), chronic obstructive pulmonary disease (COPD), and, in otherwise healthy patients, viral infections or recent oxidant exposure (14). A positive methacholine challenge does not definitively diagnose asthma, especially in an atopic patient, but a negative challenge makes the diagnosis of asthma unlikely.

For patients with exercise-induced bronchospasm (EIB), an exercise challenge or hyperventilation of cold dry air simulates the conditions that usually induce bronchospasm (15). The standard protocol for exercise challenge requires exercising on a treadmill to raise the subject's heart rate to 90% of predicted maximum values to increase oxygen consumption. Once this rate is maintained for 6–8 min, FEV_1 values are obtained after exercise in 5 min intervals for 20–30 min and compared to preexercise values (16). Typically in EIB the maximal fall in FEV_1 occurs within 10–15 min after completion of exercise (17). A decrease in FEV_1 of 10% from baseline is suspicious for EIB, while a drop of 15% or greater is diagnostic of exercise-induced asthma (14). Up to 40% of non-asthmatic atopic individuals may demonstrate exercise-induced bronchospasm, but in nonatopic individuals only 2–5% will have bronchospasm (18). Exercise testing is useful in differentiating asthma from some other forms of chronic disease in children (19). Tests with methacholine or histamine are more sensitive for the detection of hyperresponsiveness than exercise (9,20).

E. Lung Volumes

Measurements of lung volumes are not necessary to make the diagnosis of asthma. Lung volume measures demonstrate typical findings associated with obstructive lung disease such as a decreased vital capacity and increases in functional residual capacity (FRC), total lung capacity (TLC), and residual volume (RV) (21). An increased ratio of residual volume to total lung capacity is indicative of air trapping and may be an early indicator of obstructive lung disease. The changes seen in RV, TLC, and the RV/TLC ratio may be present prior to any decreases in normal spirometric measures (22).

F. Peak Expiratory Flow Rates

Home monitoring or measurements of lung function can be accomplished by peak flow meters. These handheld devices measure the peak expiratory flow rate (PEFR). The PEFR is measured in liters per minute, while the PEF is in liters per second, but both are representations of maximum flow during exhalation and are effort-dependent. The technique for the PEFR is slightly different and does not require prolonged exhalation, as the peak flow is reached in 1–2 sec (23).

In using PEFR it is necessary to establish personal best values and diurnal (morning to evening) variation. Normal diurnal changes can be demonstrated by monitoring PEFR twice a day for 2 weeks (24). The diurnal variation averages about 8% in healthy individuals but can approach 50% in those with severe asthma (25). More than 20% diurnal variation in PEFR is suggestive of asthma, but no specific cutoff value is diagnostic of asthma due to a continuous distribution of variability in the general population (26). The patient's weight and aerobic fitness may be explanations as well. Having a patient check peak flow rates following activity or exertion can distinguish between poor fitness and exercise-induced bronchoconstriction (27). Peak flow variability over time is associated with positive methacholine challenges, indicating underlying bronchial hyperresponsiveness (28). Well-performed serial peak flow measurements over days (or weeks) are more sensitive than either spirometry or the response to bronchodilator in the diagnosis of asthma (29).

G. Other Pulmonary Function Tests

Other pulmonary function testing is aimed at detecting nonspecific features of asthma. Due to the airway inflammation characteristic of asthma, airway resistance increases and conductance decreases directly with airway obstruction (30). The measurement of airway resistance is quite sensitive to induced airway bronchoconstriction (11).

The diffusing capacity is a measurement of gas exchange that is useful in differentiating asthma from COPD. The total diffusing capacity may be low in asthma, but once corrected for, measured alveolar volume will normalize (31). In patients with emphysema the diffusing capacity is reduced even after correction for alveolar volume.

A broad overview of the usefulness of spirometry in the diagnosis of asthma is illustrated in Figure 4.

V. Radiology

The diagnosis of asthma can not be made radiologically, but that does not decrease the importance of X-ray films in the diagnosis by excluding other causes of chest symptoms. Chest radiographs in asthma may demonstrate hyperinflation of the chest (flattened diaphragms or increased anterio-posterior diameter) and minimal interstitial abnormalities but typically are normal (32). In severe acute asthma, hyperinflation is common with bronchial wall thickening. In a few patients the X-ray findings may demonstrate more significant pulmonary abnormalities than were detected by physician assessment and alter the course of therapy (33). Chest radiographs help differentiate other causes of wheeze and breathlessness, including other pulmonary disorders or congestive heart failure. Additionally, chest radiographs in patients with asthma are valu-

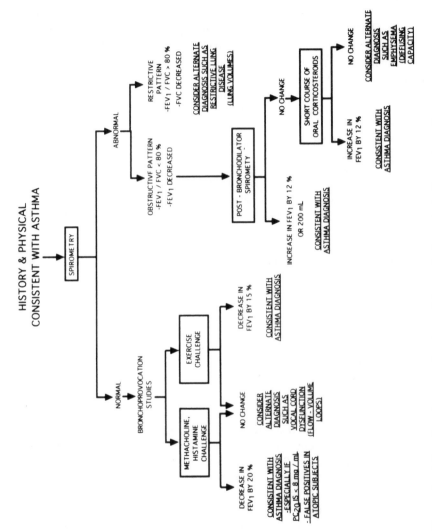

Figure 4   A flowchart demonstrating the usefulness of spirometry in diagnosing asthma.

able in evaluating complications of asthma such as rib fractures, pneumothorax, pneumomediastinum, atelectasis, and pneumonia (21).

Chest computerized tomographic (CT) scans of patients with asthma may demonstrate these same findings such as bronchial wall thickening but may also show areas of bronchiectasis (34). Generally in patients with allergic asthma the abnormalities noted on high resolution CT are not as severe as those of their nonallergic asthma counterparts (35). The CT scan may help differentiate other diseases that will give airflow obstruction such as emphysema and may also show pathognomonic findings of co-morbid diseases such as allergic bronchopulmonary aspergillosis (ABPA) with its characteristic features of central bronchiectasis. In children a chest scan by either magnetic resonance imaging (MRI) or CT is helpful in airway compression due to a vascular compression such as a pulmonary artery sling. Generally CT scans are not nearly as useful in the diagnosis of asthma as pulmonary function testing and are reserved for patients with findings consistent with either ABPA or emphysema.

Adult asthmatic patients have an increased frequency of abnormal sinus X-rays compared to asymptomatic healthy adults (36). Sinus imaging by either sinus roentgenography or computerized tomography will be sufficient to diagnose sinusitis with a corresponding history (37). Untreated sinus infection may make asthma more difficult to manage even if the patient's asthma is treated appropriately.

VI. Arterial Blood Gases

Measurements of oxygen and carbon dioxide are not helpful in the diagnosis of asthma but rather are a reflection of the severity of an acute asthma attack (38). With worsening airflow obstruction, abnormalities in the ventilation/perfusion ratio develop. Initially hypocarbia and respiratory alkalosis occur with normal oxygenation. Hypoxia develops as the carbon dioxide and pH approach normal values. As ventilation–perfusion mismatching deteriorates, the $PaCO_2$ normalizes as does the pH. As the patient tires he is unable to "blow off" the carbon dioxide, and eventually the $PaCO_2$ increases and acidosis is noted, suggesting impending respiratory failure (14).

VII. Other Testing

Gastroesophageal reflux disease (GERD) also triggers asthma symptoms, especially nighttime cough. GERD alone can cause cough and may coexist with asthma, worsening asthma symptoms despite optimal asthma therapy (39). Treatment of the esophageal reflux can decrease asthma symptoms (40,41). Diagnosis of GERD requires esophageal pH probe monitoring or a barium esophagram and may be indicated especially with symptoms of nocturnal asthma.

In patients with suspected vocal cord dysfunction the flow–volume loops may be normal if the patient is asymptomatic at the time of maneuver. The diagnosis may require direct visualization of the vocal cords by a qualified expert. Even if abnormal vocal cord movement is not noted at the time, erythema of the vocal cords secondary to GERD is suggestive of the diagnosis. In patients with diagnosed vocal cord dysfunction, approximately 50% have asthma also (42).

VIII. Atopy

In extrinsic or environmental asthma, the diagnosis of atopy is essential. Determination of sensitivity to allergens is not possible from a patient's medical history alone (43). Obvious worsening of asthma symptoms during specific times of the year, e.g., ragweed season, or with specific exposure, e.g., cat exposure, is consistent with allergic asthma. Specific concurrent physical findings such as eczema or pale swollen nasal turbinates are findings of atopic disease.

A. Eosinophilia

Generally, eosinophilia (5–15% eosinophils) is suggestive but not diagnostic of allergic disease. Not all patients with allergic disease have eosinophilia, and other causes of eosinophilia such as parasitic disease have no allergic basis. Of patients with allergic rhinitis and asthma, only 30–40% may have peripheral blood eosinophilia (4). This increase in peripheral eosinophil amount can be seen in both allergic and nonallergic asthma and cannot differentiate between them (21). There has been some association with peripheral blood eosinophilia in patients with asthma such that the higher the total peripheral blood eosinophil count, the smaller the FEV_1. In patients with marked increase in total eosinophil counts (> 3000 mm^3), other diagnoses need to be considered such as Loffler's syndrome, hypereosinophilic syndrome, allergic bronchopulmonary aspergillosis, or Churg-Strauss disease (21).

B. Total IgE Levels

The usefulness of measuring total serum IgE levels for the diagnosis of allergic asthma has been questionable (21). Only 60% of allergic asthmatic patients have elevated IgE levels, and the other 40% have levels in the normal range (4). Airway hyperresponsiveness diagnosed by methacholine challenge correlated very highly with the serum IgE level in children. The prevalence of diagnosed asthma was strongly related to the serum IgE level; 36% of children with IgE levels greater that 1000 IU/mL were reported to have asthma, and no children with IgE levels less than 32 IU/mL were diagnosed with asthma (44). Elevation of serum IgE levels as early as 9 months of age has been associated with persistent wheezing in children (45). When adjusted for age and gender, asthma has been associated with total serum IgE levels even when evaluation to common aeroallergens was negative (46). In patients with a marked elevation of IgE, concurrent diseases such as ABPA need to be considered.

C. Specific IgE Antibodies

Even though the usefulness of measuring total IgE levels is in doubt, assessment of specific IgE antibodies to aeroallergens has been helpful in managing and anticipating exacerbations of asthma. Since asthma is frequently associated with concurrent atopy, objective evidence of atopy may help identify asthma from the differential diagnosis. Skin or in vitro allergy tests are reliable in determining the presence of antigen-specific IgE, but the determination of the clinical significance of the testing requires physician interpretation (47). Skin testing or in vitro tests such as RAST (radioallergosorbent test) is used both to establish atopy and to elicit specific aeroallergen sensitivity (47).

The principal methods of immediate hypersensitivity skin testing are the prick test and the intradermal test. These test and the scratch test. All of these tests measure an in vivo IgE response to standardized allergen on the skin as demonstrated by a wheal-and-flare response. Positive (histamine) and negative (diluent) controls are used to verify normal skin reactivity (48). The size of the wheal response is proportional to the antigen potency (48). Skin testing is considered positive if the wheal response is greater than 5 mm in diameter for intradermal testing or greater than 3 mm for prick tests, surrounded by significant erythema (48,49). Erythema larger than 10 mm, regardless of wheal size, is predictive of an increased risk of asthma or allergic rhinitis in the normal population (48). A positive reaction reaches a maximum size in 10–20 min (50). Generally the prick test is done initially. Negative tests can then be followed by intradermal tests to allergens that are still suspected on the basis of clinical findings, due to their greater sensitivity (48–50). If the response is negative, IgE-mediated hypersensitivity to that allergen is excluded with a high degree of certainty (49).

Skin testing is not without risks; there is a risk of a systemic anaphylactic reaction, especially with intradermal testing (49). Pregnancy is another contraindication to skin testing because anaphylaxis may produce hypoxemia in the fetus. If an anaphylactic reaction does occur, treatment with subcutaneous epinephrine is effective in relieving symptoms. Beta-blockers may blunt the effect of epinephrine on treating an anaphylactic reaction, so they must be discontinued prior to skin testing (51). Antihistamines inhibit skin test responsiveness for variable periods of time depending on the specific antihistamine used. Oral or inhaled corticosteroids have no effect on immediate hypersensitivity skin testing. Patients with severe lung disease, congestive heart failure, or unstable asthma should not be tested until their symptoms have been stabilized.

An in vitro method for evaluation of antigen-specific IgE is the RAST (radioallergosorbent test). This is a solid-phase immunoassay in which serum to be tested is added to a specific allergen bound to insoluble carrier. The amount of antigen-specific IgE is determined by adding radiolabeled anti-IgE and measuring the radioactivity bound to the disk (50). The patient's IgE antibody specific for that antigen will bind to the antigen, while other IgE will be left unbound. Anti-IgE antibody will then bind to the IgE in the sample and be washed out, with only the bound anti-IgE remaining. The amount of radioactivity measured is directly proportional to the antigen-specific IgE in the sample. The amount of bound radioactivity is compared with a standard reference curve using five dilutions of pooled positive sera and scored accordingly: 0 (undetectable), 1 (low), through 4 (very high) (50). As an alternative to radiolabeled anti-IgE, an enzyme-linked anti-IgE can be used (ELISA, enzyme-linked immunoassay). Such tests are more expensive than skin testing, and the results are not immediately available. Prick tests are often positive when in vitro test results are negative, but in vitro test results are seldom positive when prick tests are negative (48). Comparison of skin testing to in vitro testing is shown in Table 3.

Recent studies among susceptible populations demonstrate the association between allergen sensitization and asthma. Perennial allergen sensitization is strongly associated with asthma, while exclusive seasonal outdoor allergen sensitization is typically associated with rhinitis symptoms (52). In adults less than 50 years old being evaluated in the emergency room for asthma attacks, specific IgE antibodies to aeroallergens are increased fourfold compared to control subjects (53).

In genetically susceptible children, sensitization is dependent upon the prevalent antigen in the environment. The amount of allergen-specific IgE to house dust mite has also been shown to be increased in asthmatic children compared to their peers (54). Perennial allergens such as house dust mite and cat were independent risk factors associated with the development of asthma, whereas seasonal allergens such as grass pollen were not associated with asthma (55). In the inner city, cockroach allergy is common; and in patients

Table 3 Comparison of Skin Tests Versus In Vitro Tests

Skin tests	In vitro tests
Measures in vivo response	Measures in vitro response
Less expensive than in vitro test	More expensive than skin test
Greater sensitivity than in vitro tests	Less sensitive than in vivo tests
Rapid results	Results not immediately available
Results visible to patient	Results not visible to patient
Affected by concurrent use of antihistamines	Not affected by concurrent use of antihistamines
Affected by skin disease	Not affected by skin disease
Risk of anaphylaxis	No risk of anaphylaxis
Avoid if pregnant	Safe if pregnant
Avoid if on beta-blockers	Safe if on beta-blockers
Require knowledge of skin testing technique	Do not require knowledge of skin testing technique
Require allergen extract	Do not require allergen extract
Large numbers of allergens available for testing	Small number of allergens available for testing

with asthma, cockroach allergy has been directly related to asthma-related health problems (56). In a desert environment, the major allergen is *Alternaria alternata;* house dust mites are not prevalent due to the lack of humidity required for mite reproduction (57). In children raised in a desert environment, *Alternaria* was associated with the development of asthma, which was not seen with house dust mites (58). In young asthmatics *Alternaria* sensitivity was associated with a 200-fold increase in risk of respiratory arrest compared to asthma patients not allergic to *Alternaria* (59). Seasonal asthma has been shown to be associated with exposure to pollen such as ragweed or grass pollen (60,61). Exercise-induced asthma has also been associated with both perennial and seasonal allergens (62). Reducing the exposure of allergens, specifically house dust mites, reduces asthma symptoms, nonspecific bronchial hyperresponsiveness, and evidence of active inflammation (63–65).

IX. Summary

Asthma is a common chronic disease that has been difficult to define owing to the varied presentations of the disease. No one test can be used to define asthma, but in association with a high clinical suspicion of asthma, testing can be undertaken to evaluate the characteristic features of asthma, reversible airway obstruction and airway hyperresponsiveness. Spirometric measurements are the backbone of asthma diagnosis and treatment. Obstructive measurements need to be further evaluated by either bronchodilator response or a short course of oral corticosteroids to differentiate asthma from other obstructive lung diseases. Normal spirometric measurements do not rule out asthma, and further evaluation by provocation testing is warranted if clinically indicated. Other spirometric testing and radiological evaluation are helpful to evaluate other possible concurrent diseases. The diagnosis of atopy can be suspected in a patient with an elevation of peripheral eosinophils or IgE. Definite diagnosis of atopy requires identification of specific IgE antigens by either in vivo or in vitro testing. Despite all of the testing available, asthma still is frequently misdiagnosed and therefore inappropriately treated; only through correct diagnosis can this be prevented.

References

1. Centers for Disease Control and Prevention. Asthma mortality and hospitalization among children and young adults—United States, 1980–1993. MMWR 1996; 45:350–353.
2. National Heart, Lung, and Blood Institute. Expert Panel Report 2. Guidelines for the Diagnosis and Management of Asthma (EPR-2). National Institutes of Health Pub 97-4051. Bethesda, MD: NIH, 1997.
3. Rackemann FM. A working classification of asthma. Am J Med 1947; 3:601–606.
4. Kaliner M, Lemanske R. Rhinitis and asthma. JAMA 1992; 268:2807–2829.
5. Li JT, O'Connell EJ. Clinical evaluation of asthma. Ann Allergy Asthma Immunol 1996; 76:1–13.
6. American Thoracic Society. Lung function testing: selection of reference values and interpretive strategies. Am Rev Respir Dis 1991; 144:1202–1218.
7. Light RW, Conrad SA, George RB. Clinical significance of pulmonary function tests: the one best test for evaluating the effects of bronchodilator therapy. Chest 1977; 72:512–516.
8. Hyatt RE, Black LF. The flow–volume curve: a current perspective. Am Rev Respir Dis 1973; 107:191–199.
9. Hargreave FE, Dolovich J, Boulet, LP. Inhalation provocation tests. Sem Respir Med 1983; 4:224–236.
10. Cockcroft DW. Airway responsiveness. In: Barnes PJ, Leff AR, Grunstein MM, Woolcock AJ, eds. Asthma. Philadelphia: Lippincott, 1997:1253–1266.
11. Fish JE, Rosenthal RR, Batra G, Menkes H, Summer W, Permutt P, Norman P. Airway responses to methacholine in allergic and nonallergic subjects. Am Rev Respir Dis 1976; 113:579–586.

12. Woolcock AJ, Salome CM, Yan K. The shape of the dose-response curve to histamine in asthmatic and normal subjects. Am Rev Respir Dis 1984; 130:71–75.

13. Pratter MR, Bartter T, Akers S, DuBois J. An algorithmic approach to chronic cough. Ann Intern Med 1993; 119:977–983.

14. Lemanske RF, Busse WW. Asthma. JAMA 1997; 278:1855–1873.

15. Irvin CG. Airways challenge. Respir Care 1989; 34:455–464.

16. Eggleston PA. Methods of exercise challenge. J Allergy Clin Immunol 1984; 73:666–669.

17. Eggleston PA, Guerrant JL. A standardized method of evaluating exercise-induced asthma. J Allergy Clin Immunol 1976; 58:414–425.

18. Council on Scientific Affairs. In vivo diagnostic testing and immunotherapy for allergy: report I, part I, of the allergy panel. JAMA 1987; 258:1363–1367.

19. Godfrey S, Springer C, Noviske N, Maayan Ch, Avital A. Exercise but not methacholine challenge differentiates asthma from chronic lung disease in children. Thorax 1991; 46:488–492.

20. Eliasson HH, Phillips YY, Rajagopal KR, Howard RS. Sensitivity and specificity of bronchial provocation testing: an evaluation of four techniques in exercise induced bronchospasm. Chest 1992; 102:3347–3355.

21. American Thoracic Society. Standards for the diagnosis and care of patients with chronic obstructive pulmonary disease (COPD) and asthma. Am Rev Respir Dis 1987; 136:225–244.

22. Cooper DM, Cutz E, Levison H. Occult pulmonary abnormalities in asymptomatic asthmatic children. Chest 1977; 71:361–365.

23. American Thoracic Society. Standardization of spirometry, 1994 update. Am J Respir Crit Care 1995; 152:1107–1136.

24. Quakenboss JJ, Lebowitz MD, Krzyzanowski M. The normal range of diurnal changes in peak expiratory flow rates: relationship to symptoms and respiratory disease. Am Rev Respir Dis 1991; 143:323–330.

25. Hetzel MR, Clark TJH. Comparison of normal and asthmatic circadian rhythms in peak expiratory flow rate. Thorax 1980; 35:732–738.

26. Higgins BG, Britton JR, Chinn S, Jones TD, Jenkinson D, Burney PG, Tattersfield AE. The distribution of peak expiratory flow variability in a population sample. Am Rev Respir Dis 1989; 140:1368–1372.

27. Janson-Bjerklie S, Shnell S. Effect of peak flow information on patterns of self-care in adult asthma. Heart Lung 1988; 17:543–549.

28. Neukirch F, Liard R, Segala C, Korobaeff M, Henry C, Cooreman J. Peak expiratory flow variability and bronchial responsiveness to methacholine. Am Rev Respir Dis 1992; 146:71–75.

29. Enwright PL, Lebowitz MD, Cockcroft DW. Physiologic measures: pulmonary function tests. Am J Respir Crit Care Med 1994; 149:S9–S18.

30. Woolcock AJ, Read J. Lung volumes in exacerbations of asthma. Am J Med 1966; 41:259–263.

31. Kaminsky DA, Irvin CG. Lung function in asthma. In: Barnes PJ, Leff AR, Grunstein MM, Woolcock AJ, eds. Asthma. Philadelphia: Lippincott, 1997; 1277–1299.

32. Findley LJ, Sahn SA. The value of chest roentgenograms in acute asthma in adults. Chest 1981; 80:535–536.

33. Petheram IS, Kerr IH, Collins JV. Value of chest radiographs in severe acute asthma. Clin Radiol 1981; 32:281–282.

34. Park JW, Hong YK, Kim CW, Kim DK, Choe KO, Hong CS. High-resolution computed tomography in patients with bronchial asthma: correlation with clinical features, pulmonary functions and bronchial hyperresponsiveness. J Invest Allergol Clin Immunol 1997; 7:186–192.

35. Paganin F, Seneterre E, Chanez P, Daures JP, Bruel JM, Michel FB, Bousquet J. Computed tomography of the lungs in asthma: influence of disease severity and etiology. Am J Respir Crit Care Med 1996; 153:110–114.

36. Berman SZ, Mathison DA, Stevenson DD, Usselman JA, Shore S, Tan EM. Maxillary sinusitis and bronchial asthma: correlation of roentgenograms, cultures, and thermograms. J Allergy Clin Immunol 1974; 53:311–317.

37. Kuhn JP. Imaging of the paranasal sinuses: current status. J Allergy Clin Immunol 1986; 77:6–8.

38. Corbridge TC, Hall JB. The assessment and management of adults with status asthmaticus. Am J Respir Crit Care Med 1995; 151:1296–1316.

39. Martin RJ: Nocturnal asthma: circadian rhythms and therapeutic interventions. Am Rev Respir Dis 1993; 147:S25–S28.

40. Harding SM, Richter JE, Guzzo MR, Schan CA, Alexander RW, Bradley LA. Asthma and gastroesophageal reflux: acid suppressive therapy improves asthma outcome. Am J Med 1996; 100:395–405.

41. Perrin-Fayolle M, Gormand F, Braillon G, Lonbard-Platet R, Vignal J, Azzar D, Forichon J, Adeleine P. Long term results of surgical treatment for gastroesophageal reflux in asthmatic patients. Chest 1989; 96:40–45.

42. Newman KB, Mason UG 3rd, Schmaling KB. Clinical features of vocal cord dysfunction. Am J Respir Crit Care Med 1995; 152:1382–1386.

43. Murray AB, Milner RA. The accuracy of features in the clinical history for predicting atopic sensitization to airborne allergens in children. J Allergy Clin Immunol 1995; 96:588–596.

44. Sears MR, Burrows B, Flannery EM, Herbison GP, Hewitt CJ, Holdaway MD. Relation between airway responsiveness and serum IgE in children with asthma and in apparently normal children. N Engl J Med 1991; 325:1067–1071.

45. Martinez FD, Wright AL, Taussig LM, Holberg CJ, Halonen M, Morgan WJ, Group Health Medical Associates. Asthma and wheezing in the first six years of life. N Engl J Med 1995; 332:133–138.

46. Burrows B, Martinez FD, Halonen M, Barbee RA, Cline MG. Association of asthma with serum IgE levels and skin-test reactivity to allergens. N Engl J Med 1989; 320:271–277.

47. Adinoff AD, Rosloniec DM, McCall LL, Nelson HS. Immediate skin test reactivity to Food and Drug Administration-approved standardized extracts. J Allergy Clin Immunol 1990; 86:766–774.

48. Ten RM, Klein JS, Frigas E. Laboratory medicine and pathology: allergy skin testing. Mayo Clin Proc 1995; 70:783–784.

49. American College of Physicians. Allergy testing. Ann Interm Med 1989; 110: 317–320.

50. VanArdsel PP Jr, Larson EB. Diagnostic tests for patients with suspected allergic disease: utility and limitations. Ann Interm Med 1989; 110:304–312.

51. Bush RK, Gern JE. Allergy evaluation: who, what and how. In: Schidlow DV, Smith D, eds. A Practitioners Guide to Pediatric Respiratory Disorders. Philadelphia: Hanley and Belfus, 1994:261–270.

52. Boulet LP, Turcotte H, Laprise C, Lavertu C, Bedard PM, Lavoie A, Hebert J. Comparative degree and type of sensitization to common indoor and outdoor allergens in subjects with allergic rhinitis and/or asthma. Clin Exper Allergy 1996; 27:52–59.

53. Pollart SM, Chapman MD, Fiocco GP, Rose G, Platts-Mills TAE. Epidemiology of acute asthma: IgE antibodies to common inhalant allergens as a risk factor for emergency room visits. J Allergy Clin Immunol 1989; 83:875–882.

54. Shibasaki M, Noguchi E, Takeda K, Takita H. Distribution of IgE and IgG antibody levels against house dust mites in schoolchildren, and their relation with asthma. J Asthma 1997; 34:235–242.

55. Sears MR, Herbison GP, Holdaway MD, Flannery EM, Silva PA. The relative risks of sensitivity to grass pollen, house dust mite, and cat dander in the development of childhood asthma. Clin Exp Allergy 1989; 19:419–424.

56. Rosenstreich DL, Eggleston P, Kattan M, Baker D, Slavin D, Gergen P, Mitchell H, McNiff-Mortimer K, Lynn H, Ownby D, Malveaux F. The role of cockroach allergy and exposure to cockroach allergen in causing morbidity among inner-city children with asthma. N Engl J Med 1997; 336:1382–1384.

57. Peat JK, Tovey CM, Mellis CM, Leeder SR, Woolcock AJ. Importance of house dust mite and Alternaria allergens in childhood asthma: an epidemiological study in two climatic regions of Australia. Clin Exp Allergy 1993; 23:812–820.

58. Halonen M, Stern DA, Wright AL, Taussing LM, Martinez FD. Alternaria as a major allergen for asthma in children raised in a desert environment. Am J Respir Crit Care Med 1997; 155:1356–1361.

59. O'Holleren MT, Yunginger JW, Offord KP, Somers MJ, O'Connell EJ, Ballard DJ, Sachs MI. Exposure to an aeroallergen as a possible precipitating factor in respiratory arrest in young patients with asthma. N Engl J Med 1991; 3234:359–363.

60. Creticos PS, Reed CE, Norman PS, Khoury J, Adkinson NF, Buncher CR, Busse WW, Bush RK, Gadde J, Li JT, Richerson HB, Rosenthal RR, Solomon WR, Steinberg P, Yunginger JW. Ragweed immunotherapy in adult asthma. N Engl J Med 1996; 334:501–506.

61. Reid MJ, Moss RB, Hsu YP, Kwasnicki JM, Commerford TM, Nelson BL. Seasonal asthma in northern California: allergic causes and efficacy of immunotherapy. J Allergy Clin Immunol 1986; 78:590–600.

62. Brutsche M, Britschgi D, Dayer E, Tschopp JM. Exercise-induced bronchospasm

(EIB) in relation to seasonal and perennial specific IgE in young adults. Allergy 1995; 50:905–909.

63. Peroni DG, Boner AL, Vallone G, Antolini I, Warner JO. Effective allergen avoidance at high altitude reduces allergen-induced bronchial hyperresponsiveness. Am J Respir Crit Care Med 1994; 149:1442–1446.

64. Piacentini GL, Martinati L, Fornari A, Comis A, Carcereri L, Boccagni P, Boner AL. Antigen avoidance in a mountain environment: influence on basophil releasability in children with allergic asthma. J Allergy Clin Immunol 1993; 92:644–650.

65. Simon HU, Grotzer M, Nikolaizik WH, Blaser K, Schoni MH. High altitude climate therapy reduces peripheral blood T lymphocyte activation, eosinophilia, and bronchial obstruction in children with house-dust mite allergic asthma. Pediatr Pulmonol 1994; 17:304–311.

11

Occupational Asthma
Role of High Molecular Weight Agents

JEAN-LUC MALO
and DENYSE GAUTRIN

University of Montreal
and Sacré-Coeur Hospital
Montreal, Quebec, Canada

ANDRÉ CARTIER

Sacré-Coeur Hospital
Montreal, Quebec, Canada

I. Introduction

Occupational asthma (OA) with a latency period can be due to high (protein-aceous) or low molecular weight agents. OA due to high molecular weight agents is interesting and relevant as it can be considered a satisfactory model of IgE-mediated human asthma. Indeed, the mechanism of OA due to high molecular weight agents is similar to that of common allergic asthma. Type I sensitization can be confirmed by skin testing and/or assessment of specific IgE in most instances.

II. Frequency

The list of high molecular weight products causing OA is long and extensive and appears as an Appendix to this chapter. The most relevant ones are covered under specific headings.

III. Common High Molecular Weight Agents Causing Occupational Asthma

A. Enzymes

Enzymes were of great concern in causing OA among detergent manufacturers in the 1970s. Enzyme-containing preparations can originate from foods, mammalian organs, and other, miscellaneous sources.

Proteolytic enzymes derived from *Bacillus subtilis* were described as a cause of OA almost simultaneously in 1969 by Flindt (1) and Pepys et al. (2). Evidence for IgE-mediated immunoreactivity was obtained from skin reactivity and increased specific IgE levels to alcalase and maxatase. Specific inhalation challenges confirmed the presence of immediate or dual reactions (2). Initial reports showed high rates of symptoms and skin reactivity. In a plant survey, Mitchell and Gandevia (3) showed that 50% of 98 workers had symptoms suggestive of OA, whereas 64% had immediate skin reactivity. Greenberg et al. (4) found that 40% of 121 workers had immediate skin reactivity.

It was initially thought that consumers in the general population (5,6) would be at risk of sensitization, but later reports denied that this would be the case (7). Various measures were rapidly proposed to reduce exposure to enzymatic dust. These resulted in a substantial decrease in the number of cases of sensitization (8), confirming for the first time in the case of OA that reducing exposure results in an efficient decrease in sensitization, although it cannot be completely eliminated (9).

Papain is a protease enzyme that originates from the papapya fruit, *Carica papaya*. Chymopapain, a related protein, has been used to dissolve herniated discs in patients with lumbar disc disease (10). Flindt (11) identified a subject employed in a factory where papain powder was used who developed asthma symptoms. In the same year, Tarlo et al. (12) reported on two other subjects and showed that 7 of 330 subjects who underwent routine allergy skin tests reacted to papain. Baur and Fruhmann (13) later confirmed an asthmatic reaction in seven exposed workers. Twelve of 23 subjects exposed to papain described by Novey et al. (14) had symptoms that suggested OA. Another cross-sectional evaluation showed that 17 of 33 papain workers reported asthmatic symptoms (15). Vandenplas et al. (16) recently showed a strong association between latex and papain sensitization; they indeed showed that 60% of health care professionals with allergy to latex had immediate skin reactivity to papain. Bromelin is a protease derived from pineapple, *Ananas comosus,* that can cause OA as initially shown by Baur and Fruhmann (17). Pectin obtained from fruit rinds is also a cause of OA (18). Enzymes derived from various molds, such as amylase, cellulase, lactase, and peptidase, have been incriminated (19–22). Wheat flour peroxidase has been identified as a major allergen associated with baker's asthma (23). Enzymes from animal origins can also cause OA. Pancreatic extracts have been incriminated for a long time (24), as have hog trypsin (25), and, more recently, pepsin (26) and egg lysozyme (27).

B. Flour

Handling of cereal dusts was the first hazard identified as responsible for asthma in the workplace (28). Baker's asthma is probably the oldest cause of OA and is due to respiratory sensitization to a variety of proteinaceous agents contained in flour. Work-related asthmatic symptoms are preceded by sneezing, rhinorrhea, and ocular itching as for other high molecular weight agents (29). The risk of sensitization to flour antigens as determined by skin testing increases with the number of years of exposure, the degree of airway hyperresponsiveness, FEV_1, and skin reactivity to bakery antigens (30). Successful attempts to quantify and properly characterize exposure have been realized in recent years (31,32). Many substances present in flour have been identified as potential causative allergens, the principal ones being the cereal proteins contained in flour. Allergenic cross-reactivity exists between wheat, rye, and barley as well as, to a lesser extent, oat, corn, and rice antigens. A variety of noncereal antigens have also been identified as possible causative allergens in bakers and cereal handlers (33): grain mites to which up to one-third of bakers can develop immediate sensitization (30), mold spores from *Aspergillus* and *Alternaria* (34,35), baking additives, enzymes (36) (see above) such as α-amylase and hemicellulase (37), and papain.

C. Animal-, Insect-, Fish- and Seafood-Derived Allergens

Just as domestic pets are a frequent cause of environmental asthma, laboratory animals such as rats, mice, guinea pigs, rabbits, and locusts are a common cause of OA (38). Major sources of allergens are the animal excreta and secreta that become airborne. It has been estimated that as much as one-third of animal handlers will develop ocular, nasal, or respiratory symptoms (39). In a prospective study, Gautrin and coworkers recently estimated that the risk of sensitization in animal-exposed apprentices is much higher than in flour- and latex-exposed

Table 1 Prevalence of Immunological Sensitization as Determined by Preexposure
Skin Testing and Incidence at Follow-ups

	Animal health (lab animals)	Pastry-making (cereals)	Dental hygiene (latex)	Total
Prevalence preexposure	57/413	11/222	1/122	69/757
	(13.8%)	(5.0%)	(0.8%)	(9%)
Apprentices at risk	390	183	110	683
Incidence (18–24 m)	68	10	3	81
	(17.4%)	(5.5%)	(2.7%)	(11.9%)
Incidence (person–months)	9.6×10^{-3}	4.7×10^{-3}	1.2×10^{-3}	—

Source: Gautrin D, et al., in preparation.

individuals (Table 1). Atopy is a predictive factor but is not a discriminant of sufficient power for effective preemployment screening (39,40).

The urine of rats and mice was first identified as an important source of allergen in 1977 (41). In recent years, extensive efforts have been made to efficiently collect and identify the allergen in workplaces (42–44). Immunoblotting methods have allowed for the identification of the major urinary allergens, most heavily concentrated in adult male rats and mice. The ultimate aim of these efforts is to define a threshold at which sensitization is almost unlikely. It is known that proper ventilation is efficient in reducing exposure (45). Epidemiological surveys have generally included a cross-sectional assessment followed by a longitudinal component (46).

Many insect-derived allergens (mites, weevils, mealworms, larvae, moths, butterflies, crickets, cockroaches, and locusts) can cause OA (see Appendix). Allergic reactions to cuttlefish, including asthma, have been reported in Polish crew members harvesting the fish in the South Atlantic (47). Trout processors can be affected by occupational rhinitis and asthma (48). A survey of all 291 employees of a salmon processing plant in Scotland identified 24 (8%) with OA (49).

Several agents can affect seafood processors. In 1950, oyster handlers in Hiroshima who developed work-related asthma due to a parasite (Protochordae) (hoya or sea-squirt) were described (50). A survey carried out in 1964 showed that 20% of 1416 workers had asthmatic symptoms. A survey carried out among 50 subjects exposed to prawn (Norway lobster, *Nephrops norvegicus*) showed that 18 of them had respiratory symptoms (51). Forty-six (16%) of 303 employees exposed to snow crab were found to have OA, the diagnosis being confirmed by specific inhalation challenges in 33 and by monitoring peak expiratory flow rates in the rest. In a subsequent study (52), a strong association was found between the presence of asthma due to snow crab and cutaneous reactivity to specific snow crab extracts (52).

D. Gums

Several gums have been incriminated as causing OA. Gums are derived from plants and contain carbohydrates that produce mucilages when they react with water. Psyllium is a high molecular weight gum widely used as a laxative. Nasal, ocular, and chest symptoms in subjects handling this product, mainly pharmaceutical workers and nurses, have been documented in several case reports. The prevalence of immunological sensitization in pharmaceutical workers has been estimated to vary between 28% (53) and 44% (54), whereas the prevalence of OA as confirmed by specific inhalation challenges is estimated to be 4% (53). A survey of 193 nurses employed by long-term care hospitals showed that the prevalence of immunological sensitization to psyllium varied between 5% (skin testing) and 12% (increased specific IgE levels), whereas 4% had OA as confirmed by specific inhalation challenges. There are various other types of gums that cause OA: acacia or arabic gum, tragacanth, karaya, and gums obtained from seeds such as carob and guar. The prevalence of sensitization to guar gum among 162 carpet manufacturers has been estimated to vary between 5% (skin testing) and 8% (specific IgE assessments) (55) and the prevalence of OA as confirmed by specific inhalation challenges, 2%.

IV. Asthma Caused by High Molecular Weight Agents as a Satisfactory Model for Common Asthma

Existing models of asthma have several limitations. Animal models cannot be extrapolated to humans in terms of inflammatory mechanisms and basic airway physiology such as the degree of bronchial responsiveness. Epidemiological models of common asthma also have several limitations:

1. Immunological sensitization can occur at a very early age, which makes prospective observation awkward.
2. Sensitization is generally due to several inhalants.
3. The dose and the duration of exposure are difficult to estimate.
4. Thorough control of the environment is impossible.

In the case of OA due to HMW agents,

1. Asthma develops in adulthood, making it possible to assess an individual before and at the time of sensitization, at the time he or she develops asthma, and after removal from exposure (Fig. 1).

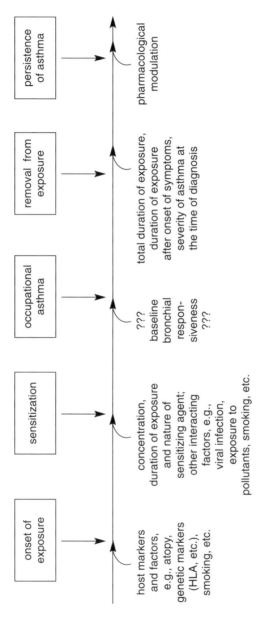

Figure 1 Natural history of asthma and occupational asthma. The steps from the start of exposure to the permanence of asthma are shown above the horizontal line, and risk factors and markers are listed below.

Table 2 Validity of an Open Physician-Based Questionnaire in the Diagnosis of Occupational Asthma

Final diagnosis	Questionnaire result		
	Occupational asthma		
	Very likely or likely[a]	Uncertain	Unlikely-absent[b]
Occupational asthma	65	6	4
Nonoccupational asthma	25	19	10
No asthma	14	10	9

[a]Of 104 subjects with a suggestive history, 65 (63%) had occupational asthma.
[b]Of 23 subjects with a nonsuggestive history, 19 (83%) had occupational asthma.
Source: Ref. 81.

2. Asthma is caused by only one agent.
3. The dose of exposure can now be assessed (56,57) and threshold limit values for lower risk of sensitization proposed (58).
4. Complete removal from exposure is possible.
5. The asthmatic reaction can be examined in the laboratory without contamination, i.e., possible exposure to common inhalants.

Using a model of OA due to HMW agents can provide relevant answers to some general questions related asthma, which are discussed in the remainder of this section.

A. What Is the Value of Questionnaires for Diagnosing Asthma?

The results of physician-based diagnosis of OA were compared with the final diagnosis obtained from specific inhalation challenges. It was shown that the questionnaire is a sensitive but not very specific tool (Table 2).

B. What Is the Usefulness of Combining Skin Tests and the Assessment of Bronchial Responsiveness in the Investigation of Asthma?

The respective roles of immunological reactivity and bronchial responsiveness in conditioning the likelihood of developing an asthmatic reaction on exposure to a specific sensitizing agent can be addressed in several ways. Tiffeneau (59) and, more recently, Cockcroft and coworkers (60), examining the results of skin testing and bronchial responsiveness to pharmacological agents, concluded that each factor is additive. Such a relationship can be examined in subjects with possible OA due to HMW agents. Eight of ten nurses (80%) with immediate skin reactivity to psyllium and nonspecific bronchial hyperresponsiveness showed an asthmatic reaction after exposure to psyllium in the laboratory (61). Seven of twelve (58%) health care professionals with immediate skin reactivity to latex and bronchial hyperresponsiveness demonstrated an asthmatic reaction after exposure to latex in the laboratory (62).

C. What Is the Validity of Serial Monitoring of Airway Caliber in the Assessment of Asthma?

Because asthma is a fluctuating condition, peak expiratory flow (PEF) monitoring was proposed for the assessment of common asthma (63,64) and, a few years later, OA (65,66). Consensus reports outlined the interest in and limitations of PEF recording in OA (67). These limitations, including the problems of compliance and adequacy of results, can also apply to common asthma (68).

D. What Is the Physiopathology of Asthma?

Several questions related to the basic mechanisms of asthma can be addressed by the model of OA due to HMW agents. Late asthmatic reactions to common agents were identified in the 1950s by Herxheimer (69). Pepys and Hutchcroft (70), in the 1970s, used the model of specific inhalation challenges in the laboratory to examine the efficacy of bronchodilator and anti-inflammatory medications. The baseline status of airway inflammation can be assessed: It was found that the inflammatory infiltrates of cells were not different for high and low molecular weight agents (71) and that airway subepithelial fibrosis correlated with the degree of bronchial hyperresponsiveness (72). Lavages, biopsies, and induced sputum can be obtained at the time of specific inhalation challenges in a laboratory setup (73) and after workplace exposure by comparison with a control period (74). The assessment of response to bronchodilator can be carried out at the time of the late reaction after laboratory challenges (75).

E. Can Asthma Be Cured?

Occupational asthma provides a unique opportunity to know whether asthma can be cured by removal from exposure and anti-inflammatory treatment, as subjects with OA have their asthma caused by a single agent found in the workplace only. Several retrospective studies summarized elsewhere have shown that a variable proportion of subjects (from 25% to 50% depending on the studies) with OA due to high and low molecular weight agents are cured after removal from exposure (76). The determinants of a less favorable outcome, i.e., the persistence of asthma, are the duration of exposure with symptoms and the severity of asthma at the time of removal. We have shown that coupling removal from exposure with an anti-inflammatory treatment, more so if treatment is administered as soon as removal is observed, can further improve the outcome but does not generally result in curing more subjects (77). Therefore, this suggests that structural changes can play a major role in the persistence of asthma.

F. Of the Genetic or Environmental Causes of Asthma, Which Are the Most Relevant in Determining the Risk for Sensitization?

Although genetic factors and exposure to a sensitizing agent each play a role in the onset of sensitization, the relative weight of each of these factors can be questioned. We examined the relative roles of atopy used as the genetic marker and the environment quantified as the total number of years of exposure in determining the risk for developing rhinoconjunctivitis symptoms in lawn cutters (78). We found that atopy, much more than the degree of exposure, was the principal determinant in the development of symptomatology, along with results of a previous study in which atopy was again found to be a stronger determinant than exposure in the development of symptomatology as a result of exposure to domestic pets (79).

G. What Is the Natural History of Asthma Due to Sensitization to Proteinaceous Aeroallergens?

Because several HMW work-related allergens have been identified as causes of OA, it is possible to study the natural history of OA in subjects starting apprenticeship or entering a workforce where exposure to such hazards is known to take place. The model of OA offers a number of advantages:

1. The characteristics of the subjects at risk, mostly atopy and nonspecific bronchial responsiveness, can be assessed before they start being exposed to specific proteinaceous agents.
2. Data on the individual medical history suggestive of susceptibility to allergens and on personal habits such as smoking, recorded through questionnaires before the start of exposure, are unlikely to be affected

by a recall bias, because they are obtained before the onset of the work-related symptoms under study.

3. Ambient exposure levels to allergens and to other air contaminants can be estimated prospectively.

4. Periodic screening for the onset of Type I immunological sensitization to the specific work-related aeroallergens, for change in the degree of bronchial responsiveness, and for the development of work-related symptoms can take place from the start of exposure.

We designed a prospective study to investigate the natural history of OA from the start of exposure to work-related HMW agents (Fig. 1). The study was set up in 14 specialized schools in Quebec. During 1993–1995, we recruited 769 subjects starting apprenticeship to become either veterinarians, animal health technicians, bakers, pastry chefs, or dental hygienists, career programs where exposure to laboratory animal-, cereal-, or latex-derived allergens occurs.

We aimed at answering the following questions:

1. What is the relationship between Type I immunological sensitization and qualitative and quantitative estimates of exposure to HMW allergens, taking into account atopy and individual and family medical history suggestive of susceptibility to allergens?

2. What is the effect of potential environmental factors (e.g., smoking) on the development of Type I immunological sensitization?

3. Are changes in bronchial responsiveness from preexposure levels greater in subjects who develop Type I immunological sensitization than in subjects who do not?

4. What is the proportion of sensitized subjects who will develop OA, what is the target organ in which symptoms will first appear (eye, nose, skin), and what are the determinants (genetic, environmental)?

Various outcome, exposure, and confounding variables were collected during visits with the study subjects at the training program's site. Specific IgE-mediated sensitization and atopy were evaluated by skin prick tests for specific and common allergens. Bronchial responsiveness was measured through nonspecific provocation tests, and respiratory symptoms were assessed using a standardized respiratory questionnaire. Ambient exposure levels to allergens were estimated following both semiquantitative and quantitative approaches, Semiquantitative estimates of exposure were obtained by means of questionnaires on individual exposure. To obtain quantitative and qualitative data, we performed fixed sampling and personal sampling on a subsample of the population and carried out immunochemical analyses.

At entry into these career programs, the prevalence of atopy was 55.2% in the whole cohort, and bronchial hyperresponsiveness (BHR) (PC_{20} < 8 mg/mL) was present in 18.1% of subjects. Skin reactivity to work-specific proteins was as follows in students in animal health technology or veterinary medicine, in pastry apprentices, and in dental hygiene students. For laboratory animal proteins, 13.8%, 14%, and 15.6%, respectively, and for flour, 1.2%, 5%, and 4.1%, respectively (80). Five subjects in the cohort reacted to latex, 1 (or 0.8%) in the group of dental hygiene students. The results from the preexposure survey suggested that students starting career programs with exposure to HMW allergens have a low but substantial frequency of specific sensitization to work-related allergens that is related to atopy and BHR.

Eighteen months on average after the start of the training program, 90% of the subjects (683/758 with preexposure skin prick test results) had been reassessed on at least one occasion (Gautrin D, et al., in preparation). Results showed that 68 students (17.4%) of the 390 students at risk in animal health technology or veterinary medicine had become sensitized to at least one work-specific allergen, 10/183 (5.5%) in pastry-making, and 3/110 (2.7%) in dental hygiene technology, for a total of 81 subjects. When expressed in person-months since the beginning of the training program, the incidence of immunological sensitization to a work-specific allergen was 9.6×10^{-3}, 4.7×10^{-3}, and 1.2×10^{-3} for students in animal health technology or veterinary medicine, pastry-making, and dental hygiene, respectively. Preliminary results from the industrial hygiene study indicate that average exposure levels, in descending order, were as follows: wheat gluten, 37,873 ng/m^3; guinea pig urinary proteins, 4001 ng/m^3; and latex, 90.7 ng/m^3 in the different training program sites (Gautrin D, et al., in preparation). These results suggest that the incidence of immunological sensitization to specific work-related allergens occurs with a short latency period. Students exposed to laboratory animals became sensitized at a higher rate than those exposed to flour or latex. The concentration levels of the aeroallergens measured do not appear to be the only relevant characteristics of exposure for the development of sensitization.

When comparing the change in bronchial responsiveness in subjects with newly detected immunological sensitization to a work-specific allergen (cases) and controls matched for atopy and baseline bronchial responsiveness, 23/78 cases (29.5%) had a significant increase in bronchial responsiveness compared to 16/78 controls (20.5%) ($p = 0.26$). In subjects with normal baseline bronchial responsiveness, onset of bronchial hyperresponsiveness was seen in the following proportions for cases and controls: 14/42 (33.3%) compared to 6/41 (14.6%) overall ($p = 0.08$), and 13/36 (36.1%) compared to 5/35 (14.3%) among students in animal health technology or veterinary medicine ($p = 0.06$)

(Gautrin D, et al., in preparation). These findings suggest that the onset of bronchial hyperresponsiveness is more than twice as frequent among students newly sensitized to work-related allergens, mostly in those exposed to laboratory animals, than in those exposed to latex or flour.

V. Conclusion

We have shown that many HMW agents can cause OA, mostly through an IgE-dependent mechanism. This makes this model relevant and interesting for examining common asthma. Research needs in that field include (1) finding the genetic markers for susceptibility, (2) assessing the threshold dose for risk of developing immunological sensititization and asthma, and (3) evaluating the efficacy of prevention through immunological screening.

Acknowledgment

We are grateful to Moira Chan-Yeung for reviewing the list of references used in the Appendix.

References

1. Flindt MLH. Pulmonary disease due to inhalation of derivatives of Bacillus subtilis containing proteolytic enzyme. Lancet 1969; 1:1177–1181.
2. Pepys J, Longbottom JL, Hargreave FE, Faux J. Allergic reactions of the lungs to enzymes of Bacillus subtilis. Lancet 1969; 1:1811–1814.
3. Mitchell CA, Gandevia B. Respiratory symptoms and skin reactivity in workers exposed to proteolytic enzymes in the detergent industry. Am Rev Respir Dis 1971; 104:1–12.
4. Greenberg M, Milne JF, Watt A. A survey or workers exposed to dusts containing derivatives of Bacillus subtilis. Br Med J 1970; 2:629–633.
5. Belin L, Hoborn J, Falsen E, André J. Enzyme sensitization in consumers of enzyme-containing washing powder. Lancet 1970; 2:1153–1157.
6. Bernstein IL. Enzyme allergy in populations exposed to long-term, low-level concentrations of household laundry products. J Allergy Clin Immunol 1972; 49:219–237.
7. Pepys J, Mitchell J, Hawkins R, Malo JL, Ashforth GK, Wilson ER. A longitudinal study of possible allergy to enzyme detergents. Clin Allergy 1985; 15: 101–116.
8. Juniper CP, How MJ, Goodwin BFJ. Bacillus subtilis enzymes: a 7-year clinical, epidemiological and immunological study of an industrial allergen. J Soc Occup Med 1977; 27:3–12.

9. Liss GM, Kominsky JR, Gallagher JS, Melius J, Brooks SM, Bernstein IL. Failure of enzyme encapsulation to prevent sensitization of workers in the dry bleach industry. J Allergy Clin Immunol 1984; 73:348–355.

10. Bernstein DI, Gallagher JS, Ulmer A, Bernstein IL. Prospective evaluation of chymopapain sensitivity in patients undergoing chemonucleolysis. J Allergy Clin Immunol 1985; 76:458–465.

11. Flindt MLH. Respiratory hazards from papain. Lancet 1978; 1:430–432.

12. Tarlo SM, Shaikh W, Bell B, Cuff M, Davies GM, Dolovich J, Hargreave FE. Papain-induced allergic reactions. Clin Allergy 1978; 8:207–215.

13. Baur X, Fruhmann G. Papain-induced asthma: diagnosis by skin test, RAST and bronchial provocation test. Clin Allergy 1979; 9:75–81.

14. Novey HS, Keenan WJ, Fairshter RD, Wells ID, Wilson AF, Culver BD. Pulmonary disease in workers exposed to papain: clinico-physiological and immunological studies. Clin Allergy 1980; 10:721–731.

15. Baur X, Konig G, Bencze K, Fruhmann G. Clinical symptoms and results of skin test, RAST and bronchial provocation test in thirty-three papain workers: evidence for strong immunogenic potency and clinically relevant "proteolytic effects of airborne papain." Clin Allergy 1982; 12:9–17.

16. Vandenplas O, Vandezande LM, Halloy JL, Delwiche JP, Jamart J, Looze Y. Association between sensitization to natural rubber latex and papain. J Allergy Clin Immunol 1996; 97:1421–1424.

17. Baur X, Fruhmann G. Allergic reactions, including asthma, to the pineapple protease bromelain following occupational exposure. Clin Allergy 1979; 9:443–450.

18. Jaakkola MS, Tammivaara R, Tuppurainen M, Lahdenne L, Tupasela O, Keskinen H. Asthma caused by occupational exposure to pectin. J Allergy Clin Immunol 1997; 100:575–576.

19. Losada E, Hinojosa M, Quirce S, Sànchez-Cano M, Moneo I. Occupational asthma caused by α-amylase inhalation: clinical and immunologic findings and bronchial response patterns. J Allergy Clin Immunol 1992; 89:118–25.

20. Losada E, Hinojosa M, Moneo I, Dominguez J, Gomez MLD, Ibanez MD. Occupational asthma caused by cellulase. J Allergy Clin Immunol 1986; 77:635–639.

21. Muir DCF, Verrall AB, Julian JA, Millman HM, Beaudin MA, Dolovich J. Occupational sensitization to lactase. Am J Ind Med 1997; 31:570–571.

22. Park HS, Nahm DH. New occupational allergen in a pharmaceutical industry: serratial peptidase and lysozyme chloride. Ann Allergy Asthma Immunol 1997; 78:225–229.

23. Sanchez-Monge R, Garcia-Casado G, Lopez-Otin C, Armential A, Salcedo G. Wheat flour peroxidase is a prominent allergen associated with baker's asthma. Clin Exp Allergy 1997; 27:1130–1137.

24. Dolan TP, Meyers A. Bronchial asthma and allergic rhinitis associated with inhalation of pancreatic extracts. Am Rev Respir Dis 1974; 110:812–813.

25. Colten HR, Polakoff PL, Weinstein SF, Strieder DJ. Immediate hypersensitivity to hog trypsin resulting from industrial exposure. N Engl J Med 1975; 292:1050–1053.

26. Cartier A, Malo J-L, Pineau L, Dolovich J. Occupational asthma due to pepsin. J Allergy Clin Immunol 1984; 73:574–577.

27. Bernstein JA, Kraut A, Berntein DI, Warrington R, Bolin T, Warren CPW, Bernstein IL. Occupational asthma induced by inhaled egg lysozyme. Chest 1993; 103: 532–535.

28. Ramazzini B. De morbis artificium diatribas 1713. WC Wright, transl. Chicago: University of Chicago Press, 1940.

29. Malo JL, Lemière C, Desjardins A, Cartier A. Prevalence and intensity of rhinoconjunctivitis in subjects with occupational asthma. Eur Respir J 1997; 10:1513–1515.

30. Musk AW, Venables KM, Crook B, Nunn AJ, Hawkins R, Crook GDW, Graneek BJ, Tee RD, Farrer N, Johnson DA, Gordon DJ, Darbyshire JH, Newman-Taylor AJ. Respiratory symptoms, lung function, and sensitisation to flour in a British bakery. Br J Ind Med 1989; 46:636–642.

31. Nieuwenhuijsen MJ, Sandiford CP, Lowson D, Tee RD, Venables KM, McDonald JC, Newman Taylor AJ. Dust and flour aeroallergen exposure in flour mills and bakeries. Occup Environ Med 1994; 51:584–588.

32. Sandiford CP, Nieuwenhuijsen MJ, Tee RD, Newman Taylor AJ. Measurement of airborne proteins involved in bakers' asthma. Clin Exp Allergy 1994; 24:450–456.

33. Alvarez MJ, Tabar AI, Quirce S, Olaguibel JM, Lizaso MT, Echechipia S, Rodriguez A, Garcia BE. Diversity of allergens causing occupational asthma among cereal workers as demonstrated by exposure procedures. Clin Exp Allergy 1996; 26:147–153.

34. Weiner A. Occupational bronchial asthma in a baker due to Aspergillus. Ann Allergy 1960; 18:1004–1007.

35. Klaustermeyer WB, Bardana EJ, Hale FC. Pulmonary hypersensitivity to Alternaria and Aspergillus in baker's asthma. Clin Allergy 1977; 7:227–233.

36. Vanhanen M, Tuomi T, Hokkanen H, Tupasela O, Tuomainen A, Holmberg PC, Leisola M, Nordman H. Enzyme exposure and enzyme sensitisation in the baking industry. Occup Environ Med 1996; 53:670–676.

37. Baur X, Fruhmann G, Haug B, Rasche B, Reiher W, Weiss W. Role of Aspergillus amylase in baker's asthma. Lancet 1986; 1:43.

38. Newman Taylor AJ, Gordon S. Laboratory animal and insect allergy. In: Bernstein IL, Chan-Yeung M, Malo JL, Bernstein DI, eds. Asthma in the Workplace 1993. New York: Marcel Dekker, 1993; 399–414.

39. Slovak AJ, Hill RN. Laboratory animal allergy: a clinical survey of an exposed population. Br J Ind Med 1981; 38:38–41.

40. Renstrom A, Malmberg P, Larsson K, Sundblad BM, Larsson PH. Prospective study of laboratory-animal allergy: factors predisposing to sensitization and development of allergic symptoms. Allergy 1994; 49:548–552.

41. Newman-Taylor A, Longbottom JL, Pepys J. Respiratory allergy to urine proteins of rats and mice. Lancet 1977; 847–849.

42. Gordon S, Tee RD, Newman Taylor AJ. Analysis of the allergenic composition of rat dust. Clin Exp Allergy 1996; 26:533–541.

43. Hollander A, Heederik D, Doekes G. Respiratory allergy to rats: exposure–response relationships in laboratory animal workers. Am J Respir Crit Care Med 1997; 155: 562–567.

44. Nieuwenhuijsen MJ, Gordon S, Harris J, Tee RD, Venables KM, Newman Taylor AJ. Determinants of airborne allergen exposure in an animal house. Occup Hyg 1995; 1:317–324.

45. Gordon S, Wallace J, Cook A, Tee RD, Newman-Taylor AJ. Reduction of exposure to laboratory animal allergens in the workplace. Clin Exp Allergy 1997; 27:744–751.

46. Cullinan P, Lowson D, Nieuwenhuijsen MJ, Gordon S, Tee RD, Venables KM, McDonald JC, Newman Taylor AJ. Work related symptoms, sensitisation, and estimated exposure in workers not previously exposed to laboratory rats. Occup Environ Med 1994; 51:589–592.

47. Tomaszunas S, Weclawik Z, Lewinski M. Allergic reactions to cuttlefish in deep-sea fishermen. Lancet 1988; 1:1116–1117.

48. Sherson D, Hansen I, Sigsgaard T. Occupationally related respiratory symptoms in trout-processing workers. Allergy 1989; 44:336–341.

49. Douglas JDM, McSharry C, Blaikie L, Morrow T, Miles S, Franklin D. Occupational asthma caused by automated salmon processing. Lancet 1995; 346:737–740.

50. Jyo T, Kohmoto K, Katsutani T, Otsuka T, Oka SD, Mitsui S. Hoya (sea-squirt) asthma. Occupational Asthma. London: Von Nostrand Reinhold, 1980; 209–228.

51. Gaddie J, Legge JS, Friend JAR, Reid TMS. Pulmonary hypersensitivity in prawn workers. Lancet 1980; 2:1350–1353.

52. Cartier A, Malo JL, Ghezzo H, McCants M, Lehrer SB. IgE sensitization in snow crab-processing workers. J Allergy Clin Immunol 1986; 78:344–348.

53. Bardy JD, Malo JL, Séguin P, Ghezzo H, Desjardins J, Dolovich J, Cartier A. Occupational asthma and IgE sensitization in a pharmaceutical company processing psyllium. Am Rev Respir Dis 1987; 135:1033–1038.

54. Goransson K, Michaelson N, Gunnar. Ispagula powder. An allergen in the work environment. Scand J Work Environ Health 1979; 5:257–261.

55. Malo JL, Cartier A, L'Archevêque J, Ghezzo H, Soucy F, Somers J, Dolovich J. Prevalence of occupational asthma and immunological sensitization to guar gum among employees at a carpet-manufacturing plant. J Allergy Clin Immunol 1990; 86:562–569.

56. Reed CE, Swanson MC, Li JTC. Environmental monitoring of protein aeroallergens. in: Bernstein IL, Chan-Yeung M, Malo JL, Bernstein DI, eds. Asthma in the Workplace 1993. New York: Marcel Dekker, 1993:249–275.

57. Nieuwenhuijsen MJ, Sandiford CP, Lowson D, Tee RD, Venables KM, Newman Taylor AJ. Peak exposure concentrations of dust and flour aeroallergen in flour mills and bakeries. Ann Occup Hyg 1995; 39:193–201.

58. Houba R, Heederik DJJ, Doekes G, Run PEM van. Exposure-sensitization relationship for α-amylase allergens in the baking industry. Am J Respir Crit Care Med 1996; 154:130–136.

59. Tiffeneau R. Hypersensibilité cholinergo-histaminique pulmonaire de l'asthmatique. Relation avec l'hypersensibilité allergénique pulmonaire. Acta Allergol 1958; suppl V:187–221.

60. Cockcroft DW, Ruffin RE, Frith PA, Cartier A, Juniper EF, Dolovich J, Hargreave FE. Determinants of allergen-induced asthma: dose of allergen, circulating IgE antibody concentration, and bronchial responsiveness to inhaled histamine. Am Rev Respir Dis 1979; 120:1053–1058.

61. Malo JL, Cartier A, L'Archevêque J, Ghezzo H, Lagier F, Trudeau C, Dolovich J. Prevalence of occupational asthma and immunologic sensitization to psyllium among health personnel in chronic care hospitals. Am Rev Respir Dis 1990; 142:1359–1366.

62. Vandenplas O, Delwich JP, Evrard G, Aimont P, Brempt X van der, Jamart J, Delaunois L. Prevalence of occupational asthma due to latex among hospital personnel. Am J Respir Crit Care Med 1995; 151:54–60.

63. Epstein SW, Fletcher CM, Oppenheimer EA. Daily peak flow measurements in the assessment of steroid therapy for airway obstruction. Br Med J 1969; 1:223–225.

64. Turner-Warwick M. On observing patterns of airflow obstruction in chronic asthma. Br J Dis Chest 1977; 71:73–86.

65. Burge PS, O'Brirn IM, Harries MG. Peak flow rate records in the diagnosis of occupational asthma due to isocyanates. Thorax 1979; 34:317–323.

66. Burge PS, O'Brien IM, Harries MG. Peak flow rate records in the diagnosis of occupational asthma due to colophony. Thorax 1979; 34:308–316.

67. Moscato G, Godnic-Cvar J, Maestrelli P, Malo JL, Burge PS, Coifman R. Statement on self-monitoring of peak expiratory flows in the investigation of occupational asthma. J Allergy Clin Immunol 1995; 96:295–301.

68. Verschelden P, Cartier A, L'Archevêque J, Trudeau C, Malo JL. Compliance with and accuracy of daily self-assessment of peak expiratory flows (PEF) in asthmatic subjects over a three month period. Eur Respir J 1996; 9:880–885.

69. Herxheimer H. The late bronchial reaction in induced asthma. Int Arch Allergy Appl Immunol 1952; 3:323–328.

70. Pepys J, Hutchcroft BJ. Bronchial provocation tests in etiologic diagnosis and analysis of asthma. Am Rev Respir Dis 1975; 112:829–859.

71. Boulet LP, Boutet M, Laviolette M, Dugas M, Milot J, Leblanc C, Paquette L, Côté J, Cartier A, Malo JL. Airway inflammation after removal from the causal agent in occupational asthma due to high and low molecular weight agents. Eur Respir J 1994; 7:1567–1575.

72. Boulet LP, Laviolette M, Turcotte H, Cartier A, Dugas M, Malo JL, Boutet M. Bronchial subepithelial fibrosis correlates with airway responsiveness to methacholine. Chest 1997; 112:45–52.

73. Fabbri LM, Boschetto P, Zocca E, Milani G, Pivirotto F, Plebani M, Burlina A, Licata B, Mapp CE. Bronchoalveolar neutrophilia during late asthmatic reactions induced by toluene diisocyanate. Am Rev Respir Dis 1987; 136:36–42.

74. Lemière C, Efthimiadis A, Hargreave FE. Occupational eosinophilic bronchitis without asthma: an unknown occupational airway disease. J Allergy Clin Immunol 1997; 100:852–854.

75. Malo JL, Perrin B, L'Archevêque J, Ghezzo H, Cartier A. Effet d'un agent bêta-2-adrénergique inhalé administré au moment des réactions bronchiques retardées après exposition à des agents professionnels. Rev Mal Respir 1994; 11:479–484.

76. Chan-Yeung M, Malo JL. Natural history of occupational asthma. In: Bernstein IL, Chan-Yeung M, Malo JL, Bernstein DI, eds. Asthma in the Workplace 1993. New York: Marcel Dekker, 1993: 299–322.

77. Malo JL, Cartier A, Côté J, Milot J, Leblanc C, Paquette L, Ghezzo H, Boulet LP. Influence of inhaled steroids on the recovery of occupational asthma after cessation of exposure: an 18-month double-blind cross-over study. Am J Crit Care Respir Med 1996; 153:953–960.

78. Gautrin D, Vandenplas O, DeWitte JD, L'Archevêque J, Leblanc C, Trudeau C, Paulin C, Arnoud D, Morand S, Comtois P, Malo JL. Allergenic exposure, IgE-mediated sensitization and related symptoms in lawn cutters. J Allergy Clin Immunol 1994; 93:437–445.

79. Desjardins A, Benoit C, Ghezzo H, L'Archevêque J, Leblanc C, Paquette L, Cartier A, Malo JL. Exposure to domestic animals and risk of immunologic sensitization in subjects with asthma. J Allergy Clin Immunol 1993; 91:979–986.

80. Gautrin D, Infante-Rivard C, Dao TV, Magnan-Larose M, Desjardins D, Malo JL. Specific IgE-dependent sensitization, atopy and bronchial hyperresponsiveness in apprentices starting exposure to protein-derived agents. Am J Respir Crit Care Med 1997; 155:1841–1847.

81. Malo JL et al. Am Rev Respir Dis 1991; 143:528–532.

Appendix: High Molecular Weight Agents Causing Occupational Asthma

Agent	Occupation	Ref.	Subjects (n)	Prevalence (%)	Skin test	Specific IgE	Other immunological test	Broncho-provocation test	Other evidence
Animal-derived antigens									
Laboratory animal	Laboratory worker	1	296	13	17%+	34% of 255+	ND	ND	
		2	5	NA	100%+	100%+	Neg precipitin	100%+	
Cow dander	Agricultural worker	3	49	NA	100%	ND	Immunoblotting	ND	
Monkey dander	Laboratory worker	4	2	NA	2+	2+	ND	ND	
Deer dander	Farmer	5	1	NA	+	ND	ND	+	
Mink urine	Farmer	6	1	NA	+	–	ND	+	
Chicken	Poultry worker	7, 8		NA	79%+	79%+	ND	1/1+	
Pig	Butcher	9	1	NA	ND	+	ND	ND	PEF
Frog	Frog catcher	10	1	NA	+	+	Neg precipitin	ND	
Lactoserum	Dairy industry	11	1	NA	+	ND	Basophil degranulation	+	
Bovine serum albumin	Laboratory technician	12	1	NA	+	ND	ND	+	
Lactalbumin	Chocolate candy maker	13	1	NA	+	+	ND	+	+ Conjunctival
Casein (cow's milk)	Tanner	14	1	NA	ND	+	ND	+	
Egg protein	Egg producer	15	188	7	34%+	29%	ND	ND	PEF
Endocrine glands	Pharmacist	16	1	NA	+	ND	ND	+	
Bat guano	Various	17	7	NA	+	+	RAST inhibition	ND	
Ivory dust	Ivory worker	18	1	NA	Neg	ND	ND	+	FEV$_1$ at work
Nacre dust	Nacre button maker	19	1	NA	+	ND	Neg precipitin	+	
Sericin	Hairdresser	20	2	NA	1/1+	ND	ND	ND	

Crustacea, seafoods, fish

Crab	Snow crab processor	21	303	16	22%+	ND	ND	72% of 46+	PEF, PC20
Prawn	Prawn processor	22	50	36	26%+	16%+	ND	2/2+	
Hoya	Oyster farm	23	1413	29	82% of 511 with asthma+	89% of ~180 with asthma+	ND	ND	
Clam and shrimp	Food processor	24	2	4%	+	+	RAST inhibition	+	PC20
Lobster and shrimp	Fishmonger shop	25	1	NA	+	+	ND	+	
Cuttlefish	Deep-sea fisherman	26	66	1%/yr	ND	ND	ND	ND	
Cuttlefish bone	Jewelery polisher	27	1	NA	+	ND	ND	+	
Salmon	Processing plant	28	291	24 (8%)	ND	25 (9%)	Spec IgG (33%)	ND	PEF
Trout (?)	Trout processor	29	5	NA	ND	100% neg	100% +	ND	
Shrimp meal	Technician	30	1	NA	+	+	ND	+	
Red soft coral	Fisherman	31	74	9	2/2+	ND	ND	ND	
Marine sponge	Laboratory grinder	32	1	NA	+	ND	Precipitins	ND	Asthma attack at work
Various fishes	Fish processor	33	2	NA	+	+	ND	+	PEF
Arthropods									
Grain mite	Farmer	34	290	12	21%+	19% of 219+	ND	ND	
	Grain store worker	35	133	33	25%+	23% of 128+	ND	1/1+	21% of 116 with + PC$_{20}$
Locust	Laboratory worker	36	118	26	32% of 113+	done	Specific IgG	ND	Reduced FEV$_1$
		37	15	60	77%+	53%	RAST inhibition	ND	ND

Appendix (Continued)

Agent	Occupation	Ref.	Subjects (n)	Prevalence (%)	Skin test	Specific IgE	Other immunological test	Broncho-provocation test	Other evidence
Screw worm fly	Flight crew	38	182	25	91% of 11+	ND	ND	ND	
Cricket	Laboratory worker	39	2	NA	+	+	Passive transfer	+	PEF
Insect larvae	Fish bait breeder	40	14	NA	+	+	RAST inhibition	+	
Moth, butterfly	Entomologist	41	2	NA	+	ND	ND	ND	
Mexican bean weevil	Seed house worker	42	2	NA	+	ND	Passive transfer	ND	
Fruit fly	Laboratory worker	43	22	32	27%+	27%+	RAST inhibition	21% of 14+	
Honeybee	Honey processor	44	1	NA	+	+	ND	+	
L. caesar larvae	Angler	45	14	NA	13/14	13/14	RAST inhibition	7/7+	
Lesser mealworm	Entomologist	46	3	NA	neg	100% of 3+	RAST inhibition	ND	
Mealworm larvae (Tenibrio molitor)	Fish bait handler	47	5	NA	4/5	2/5	RAST inhibition	2/2	
Fowl mite	Poultry worker	48	13	NA	77%+	60%	ND	1/1+	
Barn mite	Farmer	49	38	NA	100%+	~100%	ND	ND	
Mites and parasites	Flour handler	50	12	NA	ND	+	ND	ND	
Acarian (Panonychus ulmi)	Apple grower	51	4	NA	+	ND	Neg precipitins	ND	
Tetranychus macdanieli	Vine grower	52	35	4/35 (11%)	100%	ND	ND	ND	
T. urticae	Farmer	53	16	16/46 (35%)	100%	100%	ND	ND	
Daphnia	Fish market worker	54	2	NA	+	+	ND	2/2+	
Sheep blowfly	Technician	55	53	24	ND	67% of 15+	ND	ND	
Grasshopper	Laboratory worker	56	16	4 (25%)	7 (44%)	ND	ND	+ in one	

Sewer fly (Psychoda alternata)	Sewage plant worker	57	1	NA	+	+	Histamine-rel.; PK+	+	
Chironimid midge	Aquarist, fish food	58	225	45%	80%	34%	ND	ND	
Beetles (Coleoptera)	Museum curator	59	1	NA	+	ND	passive transfer	ND	
Silkworm	Silk worker	60	53	34%	ND	ND	ND	ND	
Larva of silkworm	Sericulture	61	5519	0.2	100% of 9 (?)+	1/1 (?)+	P-K reaction	100% of 9+	PEF
Fish feed									
(Echinodorus larva)	Aquarium keeper	62	1	NA	+	+	ND	+	
Arthropod	Technician	63	3	23%	ND	+	ND	ND	
Ground bug	Bottler	64	1	NA	+	+	ND	ND	PEF
Molds									
Dictyostelium discoideum (mold)	Technician	65	1	NA	+	+	ND	Workplace+	
Aspergillus niger	Technician	66	3	1%	3+	ND	ND	ND	
Aspergillus	Beet sugar worker	67	1	1%	+	+	ND	ND	
Aspergillus	Baker	68	1	NA	+	ND test	Neg precipitins	+	
Alternaria	Baker	69	1	NA	+ test	ND test	Neg precipitins	+	
Trichoderma koningii	Sawmill worker	69	1	NA	ND	ND	Precipitin-spec. IgG	ND	PEF
Plasmopara viticola	Agriculturist	70	1	NA	+	+	Various	+	
Neurospora	Plywood factory worker	71	1	NA	+	+	ND	+	
Chrysonilia sitophila	Logging worker	72	1	NA	+	+	ND	ND	PEF
Rhizopus nigricans	Coal miner	73	1	NA	+	+	ND	+	
Algae									
Chlorella	Pharmacist	74	1	NA	+	ND	ND	+	PEF

Appendix (Continued)

Agent	Occupation	Ref.	Subjects (n)	Prevalence (%)	Skin test	Specific IgE	Other immunological test	Broncho-provocation test	Other evidence
Plants									
Grain dust	Grain elevator worker	75	610	~40	9%+	ND	Neg precipitins	ND	Spirometry pre post shift
		76, 77	502	47	~50% of 51 exposed+	ND	ND	ND	FEV_1, volumes
Wheat, rye, and soy flour	Baker, miller	78	22	NA	0%+	ND	Neg precipitins	27%+	50% PC_{20}+
		79	279	35	9%+ (cereals)	ND	ND	ND	FEV_1, PC_{20}
Lathyrus sativus	Flour handler	80	7	100	100%+	100%+	100% neg	57%+	
		81	9	100	ND	100%+	Western blot, etc.	ND	
Lathyrus odoratus	Greenhouse worker	82	1	NA	+	ND	Precipitins	+	
Saccharomyces cerevisiae	Baker	83	1	NA	+	+	ND	ND	PEF
		84	1	NA	+	+	ND	+	PEF
Vicia sativa	Farmer	85	1	NA	+	+	+ Precipitins, passive transfer	+	
Buckwheat	Baker	86	3	NA	100%+	ND	ND	ND	
Gluten	Baker	87	1	NA	+	+	RAST inhibition	+	
Coffee bean	Food processor	88	372	34	24%+	12%+	ND	ND	Lung function
		89	45	9	9–40%+	ND	ND	ND	Spirometry
		90	22	NA	82%+	50%+	ND	67% of 12+	PC_{20}+ in 14
Castor bean	Oil industry	91	14	NA	100%+	100%+	ND	ND	
Green bean (*Phaseolus multiflorus*)	Homemaker	92	1	NA	+	+	Histamine	+	
Carob bean	Jam factory worker	93	1	NA	–	+	ND	+	

Material	No.	Occupation	n						
Tea	94	Tea processor	3	NA	+	+	+PCA with catechin	+	
Herbal tea	95	Herbal tea processor	1	NA	ND	neg	ND	+	
Tobacco	96	Tobacco manufacturer	1	NA	+	+	ND	+	Tobacco leaf
Hops	97	Brewery chemist	16	69	ND	ND	ND	ND	PEF
Baby's breath (Gypsophila paniculata)	98	Florist	1	NA	+	ND	ND	ND	
	99		1	NA	+	+	Histamine release	+	
Freesia and paprika	100	Horticulture	2	NA	+	+	Histamine release	ND	
Amaryllis	101	Greenhouse worker	1	NA	+	+	ND	+	PEF
Limonium tataricum	102	Floral worker	1	NA	+	+	ND	ND	PEF
Decorative flowers	103	Floral worker	4	NA	+2/4	+2/4	ND	+3/4	
Spathe flowers	104	Floral worker	1	NA	+	+	Immunoblott	neg (done 8 months later)	
Herb material	105	Herbal worker	1	NA	+	+	Ident 3 protein fractions	+	
Sarsaparilla root	106	Herbal tea worker	1	NA	+	+	ND	+	
Soybean lecithin	107	Bakers	2	NA	+	+	ND	+	
Olive oilcake	108	Oil industry	1	NA	+	ND	ND	+	
Brazil ginseng (Pfaffia paniculata)	109	Medicinal plant processor	1	NA	+	+	Neg precipitins	+	
Voacanga africana	110	Chemist's spouse	1	NA	+	+	Neg precipitins	+	
Onion	111	Homemaker	3	NA	+	+	ND	+	
Onion seeds (Allium cepa, red onion)	112	Seed packing	1	NA	+	+	Immunoblot	+	

Appendix (Continued)

Agent	Occupation	Ref.	Subjects (n)	Prevalence (%)	Skin test	Specific IgE	Other immunological test	Broncho-provocation test	Other evidence
Fennel seed	Sausage processing	113	1	NA	ND	+	Immunoblot	ND	
Sesame seeds	Baker	114	1	NA	+	+	Immunoblot	+	
Grass juice	Gardener	115	1	NA	+	+	Immunoblot	+	
Potato	Homemaker	116	2	NA	+	+	Histamine release	+	
Swiss chard (Beta vulgaris L. cycla)	Homemaker	117	1	NA	+	+	Histamine release	+	
Mushroom	Mushroom soup processors	118	8	NA	+	ND	ND	50% of 8+	
	Mushroom producers	119	1	NA	ND	+	Immunoblot	ND	PEF
Mushroom (Boletus edulis)	Office worker, cook hotel manager	120	3	NA	+	+	ND	2+	
Cacoon seed	Decorator	121	1	NA	+	ND	ND	ND	
Chicory	Vegetable wholesaler	122	1	NA	+	+	Immunoblot	ND	
Rose hips	Pharmaceutical	123	9	NA	67%+	67%+	ND	50% of 4+	
Sunflower	Laboratory worker	124	1	NA	+	+	RAST inhibition	+	
Phoenix canariensis	Gardener	125	1	NA	+	+	ND	+	
Garlic dust	Food packager	126	1	NA	+	+	ND	+	
		127	1	NA	+	+	RAST inhibition	+	
Spices	Spices processor	128	1	NA	+	+	ND	ND	
Saffron spice (Crocus sativus)	Saffron processor	129	5	10%	6%+	26%	Immunoblot RAST inhibition	+ in 1	
Aromatic herbs	Butcher	130	1	NA	+	+	ND	+	PEF

Lycopodium	Powder	131	30	7	ND	ND	ND	2/2+	PC20
Weeping fig	Plant keepers	132	84	7	21%+	21%	ND	100% of 6+	
Pectin	Christmas candy maker	133	1	NA	+	−	Spec IgG4	+	
Henna (conchiolin?)	Hairdresser	134	2	NA	+	+	ND	1/2+	
Fenugreek	Food industry	135	1	NA	+	+	ND	ND	
Aniseed	Food industry	136	1	NA	+	+	ND	+	
Kapok	Sewer	137	1	NA	−	−	ND	+	
Latex	Glove manufacturer	138	81	6	11% +	ND	ND	ND	Lung function PEF
Latex	Health professional	139	72.5%	4.7% +	ND	ND	+	+	
Latex	Health professional	139	72.5%	4.7% +	ND	ND	+	+	
Biological enzymes									
B. subtilis	Detergent industry	140	1642	3.2 (over 7 years)	4.5–75% +	26% of 248 +	ND	ND	Lung function
		141	38	NA	66% +	ND	Passive transfer 100% of 5 + precipitin (nonspec)	90% +	Lung function
Trypsin	Plastic, pharmaceutical	142	14	29	+	+	ND	75% of 4 +	
Papain	Pharmaceutical	143	29	45	34% +	34% +	ND	89% of 9 +	
Pepsin	Pharmaceutical	144	1	NA	+	+		+	
Pancreatin	Pharmaceutical	145	14	NA	93% +	100% of 3 +	ND	100% of 8 +	Lung function
Flaviastase	Pharmaceutical	146	3	NA	+	+	+ Precipitin	ND	
Bromelin	Pharmaceutical	147	76	11	25% +	ND	ND	ND	
	Pharmaceutical	148	2	NA	+	ND	ND	2/2 +	
Egg lysosyme	Pharmaceutical	149	1	NA	+	+	ND	+	PEF

Appendix (Continued)

Agent	Occupation	Ref.	Subjects (n)	Prevalence (%)	Skin test	Specific IgE	Other immunological test	Broncho-provocation test	Other evidence
Fungal amylase	Baker	150	118	NA	100% of 10 +	2% exposed + 34% occup. asthma +	ND	ND	
		151	1	NA	+	+	ND	+	
Fungal amyloglucosidase and hemicellulase	Bakers	152	140	NA	ND	5–24%	ND	ND	
Serratial peptidase and lysozyme	Pharmaceutical	153	1	NA	ND	+	Immunoblot	+	
Esperase	Detergent industry	154	667	NA	ND	5%	ND	ND	
Xylanase	Laboratory worker	155	2	NA	2	2	ND	ND	PFR
Pectinase	Enzyme factory	156	1	NA	1	neg	ND	+	
Lactase	Pharmaceutical	157	207	4%	31% +	ND	ND	ND	
Vegetable gums									
Acacia	Printer	158	63	19% of 31 (selection)	ND	ND	ND	ND	
		159	10	NA	+	ND	Passive transfer (3 +)	ND	
Tragacanth	Gum importer	160	1	NA	+	ND	ND	ND	
Karaya	Hairdresser	161	9	4	+	ND	ND	ND	
Guar	Carpet manufacturer	162	162	2	5% +	8% +	Passive transfer	67% of 3 +	PC_{20}
Gutta-percha	Dental hygienist	163	1	NA	+	ND	ND	ND	

NA = not applicable; ND = not done; neg = negative. The number of subjects tested is not specified if it included all subjects; otherwise it is mentioned. * = Based on challenge data; ** = presence of bronchial hyperresponsiveness; † = subjects with symptoms; PCA = passive cutaneous anaphylaxis; PPI = polymethylene polyphenylisocyanate. All proportions including 3 or more as the denominator are expressed as percent.

Appendix References

1. Venables KM, Tee RD, Hawkins ER, Gordon DJ, Wale CJ, Farrer NM, Lam TH, Baxter PJ, Newman-Taylor AJ. Laboratory animal allergy in a pharmaceutical company. Br J Ind Med 1988; 45:660–666.

2. Newman Taylor A, Longbottom JL, Pepys J. Respiratory allergy to urine proteins of rats and mice. Lancet 1977; 847–849.

3. Mäntyjärvi J, Ylönen R, Taivainen A, Virtanen T. IgG and IgE antibody responses to cow dander and urine in farmers with cow-induced asthma. Clin Exp Allergy 1992; 22:83–90.

4. Petry RW, Voss MJ, Kroutil LA, Crowley W, Bush RK, Busse WW. Monkey dander asthma. J Allergy Clin Immunol 1985; 75:268–271.

5. Nahm DH, Park JW, Hong CS. Occupational asthma due to deer dander. Ann Allergy Asthma Immunol 1996; 76:423–426.

6. Jiménez Gomez I, Anton E, Picans I, Jerez J, Obispo T. Occupational asthma caused by mink urine. Allergy 1996; 51:364–365.

7. Bar-Sela S, Teichtahl H, Lutsky I. Occupational asthma in poultry workers. J Allergy Clin Immunol 1984; 73:271–275.

8. Lutsky I, Teichtahl H, Bar-Sela S. Occupational asthma due to poultry mites. J Allergy Clin Immunol 1984; 73:56–60.

9. Brennan NJ. Pig butcher's asthma: case report and review of the literature. Irish Med J 1985; 78:321–322.

10. Armentia A, Martin-Santos J, Subiza J, Pla J, Zapata C, Valdivieso R, Losada E. Occupational asthma due to frogs. Ann Allergy 1988; 60:209–210.

11. Moneret-Vautrin DA, Pupil P, Courtine D, Grilliat JP. Asthme professionnel aux protéines du lactosérum. Rev Fr Allergol 1984; 24:93–95.

12. Joliat TL, Weber RW. Occupational asthma and rhinoconjunctivitis from inhalation of crystalline bovine serum albumin powder. Ann Allergy 1991; 66:301–304.

13. Bernaola G, Echechipia S, Urrutia I, Fernandez E, Audicana M, Fernandez de Corres L. Occupational asthma and rhinoconjunctivitis from inhalation of dried cow's milk caused by sensitization to alpha-lactalbumin. Allergy 1994; 49:189–191.

14. Olaguibel JM, Hernandez D, Morales P, Peris A, Basomba A. Occupational asthma caused by inhalation of casein. Allergy 1990; 45:306–308.

15. Smith A Blair, Bernstein DI, London MA, Gallagher J, Ornella GA, Gelletly SK, Wallingford D. Newman MA. Evaluation of occupational asthma from airborne egg protein exposure in multiple settings. Chest 1990; 98:398–404.

16. Breton JL, Leneutre F, Esculpavit G, Abourjaili M. Une nouvelle cause d'asthme professionnel chez un préparateur en pharmacie. Presse Méd 1989; 18:433.

17. El-Ansary EH, Gordon DJ, Tee RD, Newman-Taylor AJ. Respiratory allergy to inhaled bat guano. Lancet 1987; 1:316–318.

18. Armstrong RA, Neill P, Mossop RT. Asthma induced by ivory dust: a new occupational cause. Thorax 1988; 43:737–738.

19. Zedda S. A case of bronchial asthma from inhalation of nacre dust. Med Lavoro 1967; 58:459–464.

20. Charpin J, Blanc M. Une cause nouvelle d'allergie professionnelle chez les coiffeuses: l'allergie à la séricine. Marseille Méd 1967; 104:169–170.

21. Cartier A, Malo JL, Forest F, Lafrance M, Pineau L, St Aubin JJ, Dubois JY. Occupational asthma in snow crab-processing workers. J Allergy Clin Immunol 1984; 74:261–269.

22. Gaddie J, Legge JS, Friend JAR, Reid TMS. Pulmonary hypersensitivity in prawn workers. Lancet 1980; 2:1350–1353.

23. Jyo T, Kohmoto K, Katsutani T, Otsuka T, Oka SD, Mitsui S. Hoya (sea-squirt) asthma. Occupational Asthma London: Von Nostrand Reinhold, 1980:209–228.

24. Desjardins A, Malo JL, L'Archevêque J, Cartier A, McCants M, Lehrer SB. Occupational IgE-mediated sensitization and asthma due to clam and shrimp. J Allergy Clin Immunol 1995; 96:608–617.

25. Lemière C, Desjardins A, Lehrer S, Malo JL. Occupational asthma to lobster and shrimp. Allergy 1996; 51:272–273.

26. Tomaszunas S, Weclawik Z, Lewinski M. Allergic reactions to cuttlefish in deep-sea fishermen. Lancet 1988; 1:1116–1117.

27. Beltrami V, Innocenti A, Pieroni MG, Civai R, Nesi D, Bianco S. Occupational asthma due to cuttlefish bone dust. Med Lav 1989; 80:425–428.

28. Douglas JDM, McSharry C, Blaikie L, Morrow T, Miles S, Franklin D. Occupational asthma caused by automated salmon processing. Lancet 1995; 346: 737–740.

29. Sherson D, Hansen I, Sigsgaard T. Occupationally related respiratory symptoms in trout-processing workers. Allergy 1989; 44:336–341.

30. Carino M, Elia G, Molinini R, Nuzzaco A, Ambrosi L. Shrimpmeal asthma in the aquaculture industry. Med Lav 1985; 76:471–475.

31. Onizuka R, Inoue K, Kamiya H. Red soft coral-induced allergic symptoms observed in spiny lobster fishermen. Aerugi 1990; 39:339–347.

32. Baldo BA, Krilis S, Taylor KM. IgE-mediated acute asthma following inhalation of a powdered marine sponge. Clin Allergy 1982; 12:179–186.

33. Rodriguez J, Reano M, Vives R, Canto G, Daroca P, Crespo JF, Vila C, Villarreal O, Bensabat Z. Occupational asthma caused by fish inhalation. Allergy 1997; 52:866–869.

34. Cuthbert OD, Jeffrey IG, McNeill HB, Wood J, Topping MD. Barn allergy among Scottish farmers. Clin Allergy 1984; 14:197–206.

35. Blainey AD, Topping MD, Ollier S, Davies RJ. Allergic respiratory disease in grain workers: the role of storage mites. J Allergy Clin Immunol 1989; 84: 296–303.

36. Burge PS, Edge G, O'Brien IM, Harries MG, Hawkins R, Pepys J. Occupational asthma in a research centre breeding locusts. Clin Allergy 1980; 10:355–363.

37. Tee RD, Gordon DJ, Hawkins ER, Nunn AJ, Lacey J, Venables KM, Cooter RJ, McCaffery AR, Newman Taylor AJ. Occupational allergy to locusts: an investigation of the sources of the allergen. J Allergy Clin Immunol 1988; 81:517–525.

38. Gibbons HL, Dille JR, Cowley RG. Inhalant allergy to the screwworm fly. Arch Environ Health 1965; 10:424–430.

39. Bagenstose AH, Mathews KP, Homburger HA, Saaveard-Delgado AP. Inhalant allergy due to crickets. J Allergy Clin Immunol 1980; 65:71–74.

40. Stevenson DD, Mathews KP. Occupational asthma following inhalation of moth particles. J Allergy 1967; 39:274–283.

41. Randolph H. Allergic reaction to dust of insect origin. JAMA 1934; 103:560–562.

42. Wittich FW. Allergic rhinitis and asthma due to sensitization to the Mexican bean weevil (*Zabrotes subfasciatus boh.*). J Allergy 1940; 12:42–45.

43. Spieksma FTM, Vooren PH, Kramps JA, Dijkman JH. Respiratory allergy to laboratory fruit flies (*Drosophila melanogaster*). J Allergy Clin Immunol 1986; 77:108–113.

44. Ostrom NK, Swanson MC, Agarwal MK, Yunginger JW. Occupational allergy to honeybee-body dust in a honey-processing plant. J Allergy Clin Immunol 1986; 77:736–740.

45. Siracusa A, Bettini P, Bacoccoli R, Severini C, Verga A, Abbritti G. Asthma caused by live fish bait. J Allergy Clin Immunol 1994; 93:424–430.

46. Schroeckenstein DC, Meier-Davis S, Graziano FM, Falomo A, Bush RK. Occupational sensitivity to *Alphitobius diaperinus* (Panzer) (lesser mealworm). J Allergy Clin Immunol 1988; 82:1081–1088.

47. Bernstein DI, Gallagher JS, Bernstein IL. Mealworm asthma: clinical and immunologic studies. J Allergy Clin Immunol 1983; 72:475–480.

48. Lutsky I, Bar-Sela S. Northern fowl mite (*Ornithonyssus sylviarum*) in occupational asthma of poultry workers. Lancet 1982; 2:874–875.

49. Cuthbert OD, Brostoff J, Wraith DG, Brighton WD. "Barn allergy": asthma and rhinitis due to storage mites. Clin Allergy 1979; 9:229–236.

50. Granel-Tena C, Cistero-Bahima A, Olive-Perez A. Allergens in asthma and baker's rhinitis. Alergia 1985: 32:69–73.

51. Michel FB, Guin JJ, Seignalet C, Rambier A, Martier JC, Caula F, Laveil G. Allergie à Panonychus ulmi (Koch). Rev Franç Allergol 1977: 17:93–97.

52. Carbonnelle M, Lavaud F, Bailly R. Les acariens de la vigne sont-ils susceptibles de provoquer une allergie respiratoire? Rev Fr Allergol 1986: 26:171–178.

53. Astarita C, Franzese A, Scala G, Sproviero S, Raucci G. Farm workers' occupational allergy to *Tetranychus urticae*: clinical and immunologic aspects. Allergy 1994; 49:466–471.

54. Meister W. Professional asthma owing to Daphnia-allergy. Allergy Immunol (Leipz) 1978; 24:191–193.

55. Kaufman GL, Gandevia BH, Bellas TE, Tovey ER, Baldo BA. Occupational allergy in an entomological research centre. I. Clinical aspects of reactions to the sheep blowfly Lucilia cuprina. Br J Ind Med 1989; 46:473–478.

56. Soparkar GR, Patel PC, Cockcroft DW. Inhalant atopic sensitivity to grasshoppers in research laboratories. J Allergy Clin Immunol 1993; 92:61–65.

57. Gold BL, Mathews KP, Burge HA. Occupational asthma caused by sewer flies. Am Rev Respir Dis 1985: 131:949–952.

58. Liebers V, Hoernstein M, Baur X. Humoral immune response to the insect allergen Chi t1 in aquarists and fish-food factory workers. Allergy 1993; 48: 236–239.

59. Sheldon JM, Johnston JH. Hypersensitivity to beetles (*Coleoptera*). J Allergy 1941; 12:493–494.

60. Uragoda CG, Wijekoon PMB. Asthma in silk workers. J Soc Occup Med 1991; 41:140–142.

61. Kobayashi S. Different aspects of occupational asthma in Japan. Frazier CA, ed. Occupational Asthma. New York: Van Nostrand Reinhold, 1980:229–244.

62. Resta O, Foschino-Barbaro MP, Carnimeo N, Di Napoli PL, Pavese I, Schino P. Occupational asthma from fish-feed. Med Lavoro 1982; 3:234–236.

63. Lugo G, Cipolla C, Bonfiglioli R, Sassi C, Maini S, Cancellieri MP, Raffi GB, Pisi E. A new risk of occupational disease: allergic asthma and rhinoconjunctivitis in persons working with beneficial arthropods. Int Arch Occup Environ Health 1994; 65:291–294.

64. Garcia Lazaro MA, Muela RA, Irigoyen JA, Higuero NC, Alguacil PV, Gregorio AM de, Senent CJ. Occupational asthma caused by hypersensitivity to ground bugs. J Allergy Clin Immunol 1997; 99:267–268.

65. Gottlieb SJ, Garibaldi E, Hutcheson PS, Slavin RG. Occupational asthma to the slime mold *Dictyostelium discoideum*. J Occup Med 1993; 35:1231–1235.

66. Seaton A, Wales D. Clinical reactions to Aspergillus niger in a biotechnology plant: an eight-year follow up. Occup Environ Med 1994; 51:54–56.

67. Jensen PA, Todd WF, Hart ME, Mickelsen RL, O'Brien DM. Evaluation and control of worker exposure to fungi in a beet sugar refinery. Am Ind Hyg Assoc J 1993; 54:742–748.

68. Klaustermeyer WB, Bardana EJ, Hale FC. Pulmonary hypersensitivity to *Alternaria* and *Aspergillus* in baker's asthma. Clin Allergy 1977; 7:227–233.

69. Halpin DMG, Graneek BJ, Turner-Warwick M, Newman Taylor AJ. Extrinsic allergic alveolitis and asthma in a sawmill worker: case report and review of the literature. Occup Environ Med 1994; 51:160–164.

70. Schaubschlager WW, Becker WM, Mazur G, Godde M. Occupational sensitization to *Plasmopara viticola*. J Allergy Clin Immunol 1994; 93:457–463.

71. Côté J, Chan H, Brochu G, Chan-Yeung M. Occupational asthma caused by exposure to *Neurospora* in a plywood factory worker. Br J Ind Med 1991; 48:279–282.

72. Tarlo SM, Wai Y, Dolovich J, Summerbell R. Occupational asthma induced by *Chrysonilia sitophila* in the logging industry. J Allergy Clin Immunol 1996; 97:1409–1413.

73. Gamboa PM, Jauregui I, Urrutia I, Antépara I, Gonzalez G, Mugica V. Occupational asthma in a coal miner. Thorax 1996; 51:867–868.

74. Ng TP, Tan WC, Lee YK. Occupational asthma in a pharmacist induced by *Chlorella*, a unicellular algae preparation. Respir Med 1994; 88:555–557.

75. Chan-Yeung M, Schulzer M, MacLean L, Dorken E, Grzybowski S. Epidemiologic health survey of grain elevator workers in British Columbia. Am Rev Respir Dis 1980; 121:329–338.

76. Williams N, Skoulas A, Merriman JE. Exposure to grain dust. I. A survey of the effects. J Occup Med 1964; 6:319–329.

77. Skoulas A, Williams N, Merriman JE. Exposure to grain dust. II. A clinical study of the effects. J Occup Med 1964; 6:359–372.

78. Chan-Yeung M, Wong R, MacLean L. Respiratory abnormalities among grain elevator workers. Chest 1979; 75:461–467.

79. Musk AW, Venables KM, Crook B, Nunn AJ, Hawkins R, Crook GDW, Graneek BJ, Tee RD, Farrer N, Johnson DA, Gordon DJ, Darbyshire JH, Newman-Taylor AJ. Respiratory symptoms, lung function, and sensitisation to flour in a British bakery. Br J Ind Med 1989; 46:636–642.

80. Block G, Tse KS, Kijek K, Chan H, Chan-Yeung M. Baker's asthma. Clin Allergy 1983; 13:359–370.

81. Sutton R, Skerritt JH, Baldo BA, Wrigley CW. The diversity of allergens involved in bakers' asthma. Clin Allergy 1984; 14:93–107.

82. Valdivieso R, Quirce S, Sainz T. Bronchial asthma caused by *Lathyrus sativus* flour. Allergy 1988; 43:536–539.

83. Jansen A, Vermeulen A, van Toorenenbergen AW, Dieges PH. Occupational asthma in horticulture caused by *Lathyrus odoratus*. Allergy Proc 1995; 16:135–139.

84. Belchi-Hernandez J, Mora-Gonzalez A, Iniesta-Perez J. Baker's asthma caused by *Saccharomyces cerevisiae* in dry powder form. J Allergy Clin Immunol 1996; 97:131–134.

85. Picon SJ, Carmona JGB, Sotillos MDMG. Occupational asthma caused by vetch (*vicia sativa*). J Allergy Clin Immunol 1991; 88:135–136.

86. Ordman D. Buckwheat allergy. S Afr Med J 1947; 21:737–739.

87. Lachance P, Cartier A, Dolovich J, Malo J-L. Occupational asthma from reactivity to an alkaline hydrolysis derivative of gluten. J Allergy Clin Immunol 1988; 81:385–390.

88. Jones RN, Hughes JM, Lehrer SB, Butcher BT, Glindmeyer HW, Diem JE, Hammad YY, Salvaggio J, Weill H. Lung function consequences of exposure and hypersensitivity in workers who process green coffee beans. Am Rev Respir Dis 1982; 125:199–202.

89. Zuskin E, Valic F, Kanceljak B. Immunological and respiratory changes in coffee workers. Thorax 1981; 36:9–13.

90. Osterman K, Johansson SGO, Zetterstrom O. Diagnostic tests in allergy to green coffee. Allergy 1985; 40:336–343.

91. Panzani R, Johansson SGO. Results of skin test and RAST in allergy to a clinically potent allergen (castor bean). Clin Allergy 1986; 16:259–266.

92. Igea JM, Fernandez M, Quirce S, de la Hoz B, Gomez MLD. Green bean hypersensitivity: an occupational allergy in a homemaker. J Allergy Clin Immunol 1994; 94:33–35.

93. vanderBrempt X, Ledent C, Mairesse M. Rhinitis and asthma caused by occupational exposure to carob bean flour. J Allergy Clin Immunol 1992; 90:1008–1010.

94. Shirai T, Sato A, Hara Y. Epigallocatechin gallate. The major causative agent of green tea-induced asthma. Chest 1994; 106:1801–1805.

95. Blanc PD, Trainor WD, Lim DT. Herbal tea asthma. Br J Ind Med 1986; 43:137–138.

96. Gleich GJ, Welsh PW, Yunginger JW, Hyatt RE, Catlett JB. Allergy to tobacco: an occupational hazard. N Engl J Med 1980; 302:617–619.

97. Lander F, Gravesen S. Respiratory disorders among tobacco workers. Br J Ind Med 1988; 45:500–502.

98. Newmark FM. Hops allergy and terpene sensitivity: an occupational disease. Ann Allergy 1978; 41:311–312.

99. Twiggs JT, Yunginger JW, Agarwal MK, Reed CE. Occupational asthma in a florist caused by the dried plant, baby's breath. J Allergy Clin Immunol 1982; 69:474–477.

100. van Toorenenbergen AW, Dieges PH. Occupational allergy in horticulture: demonstration of immediate-type allergic reactivity to freesia and paprika plants. Int Arch Allergy Appl Immunol 1984; 75:44–47.

101. Jansen APH, Visser FJ, Nierop G, Jong NW De, Waanders-De Lijster De Raadt J, Vermeulen A, van. Toorenenbergen AW. Occupational asthma to amaryllis. Allergy 1996; 51:847–849.

102. Quirce S, Garcia-Figueroa B, Olaguibel JM, Muro MD, Tabar AI. Occupational asthma and contact urticaria from dried flowers of Limonium tataricum. Allergy 1993; 48:285–290.

103. Piirila P, Keskinen H, Leino T, Tupasela O, Tuppurainen M. Occupational asthma caused by decorative flowers: review and case reports. Int Arch Occup Environ Health 1994; 66:131–136.

104. Kanerva L, Makinen-Kijunen S, Kiistala R, Granlund H. Occupational allergy caused by spathe flower (Spathiphyllum wallisii). Allergy 1995; 50:174–178.

105. Park HS, Kim MJ, Moons HB. Occupational asthma caused by two herb materials, Dioscorea batatas and Pinellia ternata. Clin Exp Allergy 1994; 24:575–581.

106. Vandenplas O, Depelchin S, Toussaint G, Delwiche JP, Vande Weyer R, Saint-Remy JM. Occupational asthma caused by sarsaparilla root dust. J Allergy Clin Immunol 1996; 97:1416–1418.

107. Lavaud F, Perdu D, Prévost A, Vallerand H, Cossart C, Passemard F. Baker's asthma related to soybean lecithin exposure. Allergy 1994; 49:159–162.

108. Benzarti M, Tlili MS, Klabi N, Hassayoun H, Ammar M Ben, Jerray M, Djenayah F. Asthma aux tourteaux d'olives. Rev Fr Allergol 1986; 26:205–207.

109. Subiza J, Subiza JL, Escribano PM, Hinojosa M, Garcia R, Jerez M, Subiza E. Occupational asthma caused by Brazil ginseng dust. J Allergy Clin Immunol 1991; 88:731–736.

110. Hinojosa M, Moneo I, Cuevas M, Diaz-Mateo P, Subiza J, Losada E. Occupational asthma caused by Voacanga africana seed dust. J Allergy Clin Immunol 1987; 79:574–578.

111. Valdivieso R, Subiza J, Varela-Losada S, Subiza JL, Narganes MJ, Martinez-Cocera C, Cabrera M. Bronchial asthma, rhinoconjunctivitis, and contact dermatitis caused by onion. J Allergy Clin Immunol 1994; 94:928–930.

112. Navarro JA, Pozo MD del, Gastaminza G, Moneo I, Audicana MT, Corres LD de. *Allium cepa* seeds: a new occupational allergen. J Allergy Clin Immunol 1995; 96:690–693.

113. Schwartz HJ, Jones RT, Rojas AR, Squillace DL, Yunginger JW. Occupational allergic rhinoconjunctivitis and asthma due to fennel seed. Ann Allergy Asthma Immunol 1997; 78:37–40.

114. Alday E, Curiel G, Lopez-Gil MJ, Carreno D. Occupational hypersensitivity to sesame seeds. Allergy 1996; 51:69–70.

115. Subiza J, Subiza JL, Hinojosa M, Varela S, Cabrera M, Marco F. Occupational asthma caused by grass juice. J Allergy Clin Immunol 1995; 96:693–695.

116. Quirce S, Diez Gomez ML, Hinojosa M, Cuevas M, Urena V, Rivas MF, Puyana J, Cuesta J, Losada E. Housewives with raw potato-induced bronchial asthma. Allergy 1989; 44:532–536.

117. Parra FM, Lazaro M, Cuevas M, Ferrando MC, Martin JA, Lezaun A, Alonso MD, Sanchez-Cano M. Bronchial asthma caused by two unrelated vegetables. Ann Allergy 1993; 70:324–327.

118. Symington IS, Kerr JW, McLean DA. Type I allergy in mushroom soup processors. Clin Allergy 1981; 11:43–47.

119. Michils A, De Vuyst P, Nolard N, Servais G, Duchateau J, Yernault JC. Occupational asthma to spores of *Pleurotus cornucopiae*. Eur Respir J 1991; 4:1143–1147.

120. Torricelli R, Johansson SGO, Wuthrich B. Ingestive and inhalative allergy to the mushroom *Boletus edulis*. Allergy 1997; 52:747–751.

121. Rubin JM, Duke MB. Unusual cause of bronchial asthma. Cacoon seed used for decorative purposes. NY State J Med 1974; 538–539.

122. Cadot P, Kochuyt AM, Deman R, Stevens EAM. Inhalative occupational and ingestive immediate-type allergy caused by chicory (*Cichorium intybus*). Clin Exp Allergy 1996; 26:940–944.

123. Kwaselow A, Rowe M, Sears-Ewald D, Ownby D. Rose hips: a new occupational allergen. J Allergy Clin Immunol 1990; 85:704–708.

124. Bousquet OJ, Dhivert H, Clauzel AM, Hewitt B, Michel FB. Occupational allergy to sunflower pollen. J Allergy Clin Immunol 1985; 75:70–75.

125. Blanco C, Carrillo T, Wuiralte J, Pascual C, Esteban MM, Castillo R. Occupational rhinoconjunctivitis and bronchial asthma due to Phoenix canariensis pollen allergy. Allergy 1995; 50:277–280.

126. Falleroni AE, Zeiss CR, Levitz D. Occupational asthma secondary to inhalation of garlic dust. J Allergy Clin Immunol 1981; 68:156–160.

127. Lybarger JA, Gallagher JS, Pulver DW, Litwin A, Brooks S, Bernstein IL. Occupational asthma induced by inhalation and ingestion of garlic. J Allergy Clin Immunol 1982; 69:448–454.

128. van Toorenenbergen AW, Dieges PH. Immunoglobulin E antibodies against coriander and other spices. J Allergy Clin Immunol 1985; 76:477–481.

129. Feo F, Martinez J, Martinez A, Galindo PA, Cruz A, Garcia R, Guerra F, Palacios R. Occupational allergy in saffron workers. Allergy 1997; 52:633–641.

130. Lemière C, Cartier A, Lehrer SB, Malo JL. Occupational asthma caused by aromatic herbs. Allergy 1996; 51:647–649.

131. Catilina P, Chamoux A, Gabrillargues D, Catilina MJ, Royfe MH, Wahl D. Contribution à l'étude des asthmes d'origine professionnelle: l'asthme à la poudre de lycopode. Arch Mal Prof 1988; 49:143–148.

132. Axelsson IGK, Johansson SGO, Zetterstrom O. Occupational allergy to weeping fig in plant keepers. Allergy 1987;42:161–167.

133. Kraut A, Peng Z, Becker AB, Warren CPW. Christmas candy maker's asthma. IgG4-mediated pectin allergy. Chest 1992; 102:1605–1607.

134. Starr JC, Yunginger J, Brahser GW. Immediate type I asthmatic response to henna following occupational exposure in hairdressers. Ann Allergy 1982; 48: 98–99.

135. Dugue J, Bel J, Figueredo M. Le fenugrec responsable d'un nouvel asthme professionnel. Presse Mé 1993; 22:922.

136. Fraj J, Lezaun A, Colas C, Duce F, Dominguez MA, Alonso MD. Occupational asthma induced by aniseed. Allergy 1996; 51:337–339.

137. Kern DG, Kohn R. Occupational asthma following kapok exposure. J Asthma 1994; 31:243–250.

138. Tarlo SM, Wong L, Roos J, Booth N. Occupational asthma caused by latex in a surgical glove manufacturing plant. J Allergy Clin Immunol 1990; 85:626–631.

139. Vandenplas O, Delwiche JP, Evrard G, Aimont P, Van der Brempt X, Jamart J, Delaunois L. Prevalence of occupational asthma due to latex among hospital personnel. Am J Respir Crit Care Med 1995; 151:54–60.

140. Juniper CP, How MJ, Goodwin BFJ. Bacillus subtilis enzymes: a 7-year clinical, epidemiological and immunological study of an industrial allergen. J Soc Occup Med 1977; 27:3–12.

141. Franz T, McMurrain KD, Brooks S, Bernstein IL. Clinical, immunologic, and physiologic observations in factory workers exposed to B. subtilis enzyme dust. J Allergy 1971; 47:170–179.

142. Colten HR, Polakoff PL, Weinstein SF, Strieder DJ. Immediate hypersensitivity to hog trypsin resulting from industrial exposure. N Engl J Med 1975; 292: 1050–1053.

143. Baur X, Konig G, Bencze K, Fruhmann G. Clinical symptoms and results of skin test, RAST and bronchial provocation test in thirty-three papain workers: evidence for strong immunogenic potency and clinically relevant "proteolytic effects of airborne papain." Clin Allergy 1982; 12:9–17.

144. Cartier A, Malo J-L, Pineau L, Dolovich J. Occupational asthma due to pepsin. J Allergy Clin Immunol 1984; 73:574–577.

145. Wiessmann KJ, Baur X. Occupational lung disease following long-term inhalation of pancreatic extracts. Eur J Respir Dis 1985; 66:13–20.

146. Pauwels R, Devos M, Callens L, Van der Straeten M. Respiratory hazards from proteolytic enzymes. Lancet 1978; 1:669.

147. Cortona G, Beretta F, Traina G, Nava C. Preliminary investigation in a pharmaceutical industry: bromelin-induced pathology. Med Lavoro 1980; 1:70–75.

148. Galleguillos F, Rodriguez JC. Asthma caused by bromelin inhalation. Clin Allergy 1978; 8:21–24.

149. Bernstein JA, Kraut A, Warrington RJ, Bolin T, Bernstein DI. Clinical and immunologic evaluation of a worker with occupational asthma from exposure to egg lysozyme. J Allergy Clin Immunol 1991; 87:201 (abstract).

150. Baur X, Fruhmann G, Haug B, Rasche B, Reiher W, Weiss W. Role of Aspergillus amylase in baker's asthma. Lancet 1986; 1:43.

151. Birnbaum J, Latil F, Vervloet D, Senft M, Charpin J. Rôle de l'alpha-amylase dans l'asthme du boulanger. Rev Mal Respir 1988; 5:519–521.

152. Baur X, Weiss W, Sauer W, Fruhmann G, Kimm KW, Ulmer WT, Mezger VA, Woitowitz HJ, Steurich FK. Baking components as a contributory cause of baker's asthma. Deut Med Wochschr 1988; 113:1275–1278.

153. Park HS, Nahm DH. New occupational allergen in a pharmaceutical industry: serratial peptidase and lysozyme chloride. Ann Allergy Asthma Immunol 1997; 78:225–229.

154. Zachariae H, Høegh-Thomsen J, Witmeur O, Wide L. Detergent enzymes and occupational safety. Observations on sensitization during Esperase production. Allergy 1981; 36:513–516.

155. Tarvainen K, Kanerva L, Tupasela O, Grenquist-Norden B, Jolanki R, Estlander T, Keskinen H. Allergy from cellulase and xylanase enzymes. Clin Exp Allergy 1991; 21:609–615.

156. Merget R, Stollfuss J, Wiewrodt R, Fruhauf H, Koch U, Bolm-Audorff U, Bienfait HG, Hiltl G, Schultze-Werninghaus G. Diagnostic tests in enzyme allergy. J Allergy Clin Immunol 1993; 92:264–277.

157. Muir DCF, Verrall AB, Julian JA, Millman HM, Beaudin MA, Dolovich J. Occupational sensitization to lactase. Am J Ind Med 1997; 31:570–571.

158. Fowler PBS. Printers' asthma. Lancet 1952; 2:755–757.

159. Bohner CB, Sheldon JM, Trenis JW. Sensitivity to gum acacia, with a report of ten cases of asthma in printers. J Allergy 1941; 12:290–294.

160. Gelfand HH. The allergenic properties of vegetable gums: a case of asthma due to tragacanth. J Allergy 1943; 14:203–219.

161. Feinberg SM, Schoenkerman BB. Karaya and related gums as causes of atopy. Wiscomsin Med J 1940; 39:734.

162. Malo JL, Cartier A, L'Archevêque J, Ghezzo H, Soucy F, Somers J, Dolovich J. Prevalence of occupational asthma and immunological sensitization to guar gum among employees at a carpet-manufacturing plant. J Allergy Clin Immunol 1990; 86:562–569.

163. Boxer MB, Grammer LC, Orfan N. Gutta-percha allergy in a health care worker with latex allergy. J Allergy Clin Immunol 1994; 93:943–944.

12

The Role of Low Molecular Weight Agents in Environmental Asthma

LESLIE C. GRAMMER

Northwestern University Medical School
and Northwestern Memorial Hospital
Chicago, Illinois

I. Introduction

Low molecular weight agents have been identified as a cause of asthma for more than six decades (1). In almost all instances, the asthma develops due to occupational exposure to the low molecular weight agent. Occupational asthma is defined as a disease characterized by variable airflow limitation and/or bronchial hyperresponsiveness due to causes and conditions attributable to a particular working environment and not to stimuli encountered outside the workplace (2).

There are two types of occupational asthma: immunologically mediated asthma, which appears after a latency period, and nonimmunologically mediated asthma, which appears without a latency period. Reactive airways dysfunction syndrome (RADS) is most illustrative of the latter type of occupational asthma.

A variety of low molecular weight reactive chemical substances have been reported to cause immunologically mediated asthma. The most common respiratory sensitizers are diisocyanates and acid anhydrides (3). Many other chemicals have been documented to cause asthma in smaller case series or in case reports. The immunogenicity of low molecular weight agents is due to their ability to chemically react with human airway proteins. Once this reaction occurs, the proteins are haptenized by the chemical. The hapten–protein complexes can then be recognized as foreign by the host's immunological system (4). As a result of the immunological response, several different forms of respiratory hypersensitivity syndromes can occur, the most common of which is occupational asthma.

II. Nonimmunological Asthma: Reactive Airways Dysfunction Syndrome

The acronym RADS for reactive airways dysfunction syndrome was first published in 1985 in a case series of 10 individuals who developed irritant-induced nonimmunological asthma without a latency period (5), RADS was initially defined as asthma that occurred after a single exposure to very high levels of an irritating fume, vapor, or smoke. In general, the irritants that cause RADS are low molecular weight chemicals such as ammonia, chlorine gas, or sulfuric acid. The criteria for diagnosis of RADS are listed in Table 1.

Initial symptoms of RADS develop within minutes or hours of high level airborne irritant exposure. The symptoms—cough, wheeze, and dyspnea—are those of asthma. They must persist for at least 3 months; in the majority of cases, the symptoms are still present at 1 year. Individuals with RADS also have increased nonspecific bronchial hyperreactivity (NSBH), which also tends to persist for at least 1 year. Other pulmonary diseases such as byssinosis and bronchiolitis obliterans must be excluded in order to invoke the diagnosis of RADS. Subsequent to the initial description of RADS there have been several other reported case series (6–8). In a study of 71 individuals exposed to high levels of chlorine in a pulpmill operation, 58 had respiratory symptoms, 29 had NSBH, and 16 had obstructed pulmonary functions after 3–6 months of follow-up (9).

Table 1   Criteria for Diagnosis of Reactive Airways Dysfunction Syndrome (RADS)

1. Absence of preexisting respiratory symptoms.
2. High level exposure to respiratory irritant (e.g., chlorine gas, sulfuric acid).
3. Cough and other asthma-like symptoms begin within 24 hr of exposure.
4. Increased NSBH.
5. Other diagnoses excluded.

The pathogenesis of RADS has not been entirely elucidated. In bronchial biopsies from individuals with RADS, denuded epithelium, chronic submucosal inflammation, and deposition of collagen below the basement membrane were reported (10). Why the inflammation persists rather than resolving is not clear; however, the persistent inflammation is presumably responsible for the NSBH and respiratory symptoms. It has been suggested that measurement of NSBH is useful for following the course of the disease and that significant reduction in NSBH is a good omen for recovery from RADS (10).

III. Immunological Asthma

Immunological asthma begins after a period of workplace exposure to a causative agent; this time that precedes the development of asthma is the latency period. More than 140 low molecular weight agents have been described to cause asthma. Since low molecular weight allergens are not of sufficient size to be recognized by the immunological system, they must conjugate with airway proteins, rendering the hapten–protein complex immunogenic. Most commonly, allergic sensitization occurs during a latency period of 1–3 years and results in production of allergen-specific IgE. Subsequent inhalational exposure to the allergen will result in immediate mediator release as well as cytokine production and delayed inflammatory reactions. The clinical result is asthma. In the case of high molecular weight agents, rhinoconjunctivitis often precedes the development of asthma. In the case of low molecular weight agents, rhinitis is not as likely to precede the development of asthma (11).

Mechanisms of hypersensitivity responses can be classified according to the Gell and Coombs rubric with modifications published by Janeway and Travers (12) and further modified by Kay (13). Type I is immediate IgE-mediated anaphylactic hypersensitivity that results in immediate-type allergic reactions. Type IIa reactions are cytotoxic, whereas Type IIb are stimulating responses. Type III is immune complex response. Type IV reactions involving interaction of allergen and T-cell surface receptor can be divided into three subcategories. Type IVa1 is delayed-type hypersensitivity mediated by Th1 CD4[+] cells. Type IVa2 is cell-mediated eosinophilic hypersensitivity involving Th2 CD4[+] cells; this mechanism is believed to account for the late phase of allergic reactions. There is also evidence that CD8[+] Tc2 type cells may be the initiating cell in some Type IVa2 reactions. Type IVb reactions are cytotoxic, mediated by CD8[+] Tc1 type cells.

Most high molecular weight agents as well as many low molecular weight agents are thought to induce asthma via a Type I IgE-mediated mecha-

Table 2 Low Molecular Weight Agents That Cause Immunological Occupational Asthma

Class	Agent	Industry
Metals	Platinum salts	Platinum refining
	Nickel	Nickel plating
	Chromium	Chromium plating
Acid anhydrides	Phthalic anhydride	Plastic manufacture
	Trimellitic anhydride	Epoxy resins
	Hexahydrophthalic anhydride	Epoxy resins
	Pyromellitic anhydride	Epoxy resins
Wood dust	Western red cedar (plicatic acid)	Lumber, carpentry
Azo compounds	Reactive dyes	Textile
	Diazonium	Photocopy, fluorine polymers
Pharmaceuticals	Antibiotics (penicillins, spiramycin, isoniazid, tetracycline)	Pharmaceutical, hospital
	Others (methyldopa, penicillamine)	Pharmaceutical
Diisocyanates	Toluene diisocyanate	Urethane manufacture
	Hexamethylene diisocyanate	Vehicle spray paint
	Diphenylmethylene diisocyanate	Urethane manufacture
Miscellaneous	Ethylenediamine	Shellac, cosmetics
	Chloramine T	Disinfectant
	Colophony	Electronics
	Persulfate	Beauty salon
	Acrylates	Health care, artificial nails
	Hexachlorophene chlorohexidine	Disinfectant

nism that accounts for immediate-type symptoms. Low molecular weight allergens are also recognized as being able to induce late-phase responses. Histological examination of tissue biopsies during late-phase responses shows a Type IVa2 response, eosinophilic cell-mediated hypersensitivty, and a predominance of cells expressing mRNA for Th2 type cytokines (14,15).

The immunopathogenesis of asthma caused by some low molecular weight allergens, for instance diisocyanates, has not been well defined. In many cases, humoral mechanisms do not appear to be operative. From analyses of bronchial biopsies and bronchoalveolar lavage from individuals with diisocyanate asthma, it appears that CD8[+], IFN-γ, and IL-5 producing cells may be the initiating cells (16,17). This could possibly represent a cellular immunological response mediated by CD8[+] Tc2 cells.

A. Metals

Metals that have been reported to have induced immunologically mediated asthma include platinum, nickel, chromium, and cobalt. Asthmatic responses to aluminum (potroom asthma), vanadium, uranium, and metal fumes have also been described, but the mechanism is not defined as immunological. Because each metal is unique in the characteristics of the asthma it produces, each metal is discussed separately here.

Platinum is a rare inert metal. In order to extract platinum from other metals with which it is alloyed in nature, the use of acids, resulting in production of platinum salts, is generally necessary. Platinum salts are also used for electroplating and in some photographic processes.

Platinum salt exposure was first reported to cause asthma and rhinitis in 1945 (18). The platinum salts that have been implicated as sensitizers include tetrachloroplatinate salts as well as hexachloroplatinate salts. The number of chlorine atoms in the salt is related to its sensitizing potential (19). Positive skin tests, in vitro tests for IgE, and positive specific and nonspecific inhalation challenges have been reported (20–22). The degree of specific bronchial hyperresponsiveness to platinum is correlated with the degree of positive cutaneous tests but does not correlate well with nonspecific bronchial responsiveness (23). Palladium salts have been reported to have similar sensitizing potential (22). Smoking appears to be a risk factor for the development of platinum asthma, but atopy does not (24). The treatment of choice for occupational asthma due to low molecular weight agents such as platinum salts is avoidance of further exposure. It is important to identify these sensitized individuals early in order to avoid the potential of permanent asthma (25).

Nickel was initially reported to cause asthma in 1973 (26). The patient was employed in a metal plating process and had a positive inhalation challenge and positive antibodies to nickel. Almost a decade later two other metal workers were reported to have nickel-induced asthma (27,28). One individual was a metal polisher who had a positive skin test and a positive inhalation challenge test (27). The other worker, in a metal plating factory, had a positive skin test, positive RAST, and positive inhalation challenge (28). Another metal plate employee was described to have positive inhalation challenges and positive RAST to both nickel and chromium. Inexplicably, the employee's skin tests were negative (29). Subsequently, a small case series of seven individuals was described with positive challenges to chrome and nickel (30). There is a case report of a nickel casting grinder who developed allergic contact dermatitis as well as urticaria, rhinitis, and asthma due to nickel; that individual had positive RAST and patch tests to nickel (31). A small case series of 21 workers with hard metal asthma included six individuals with allergic asthma to both cobalt and nickel; those individuals had a positive RAST to Ni-HSA (32). In review, individuals with nickel asthma generally have evidence of specific antibody either by skin test or by in vitro assay. Specific bronchoprovocation testing in the workplace or the laboratory may be useful diagnostically (25).

Cobalt has been reported to be a cause of occupational asthma. In a report of four individuals with positive bronchial provocation, all had positive skin tests with 10 mg/mL $Cr_2(SO_4)$. With removal from exposure, two of three improved remarkably (33). In a series of eight individuals with positive specific bronchial challenge to cobalt, all but one were removed from exposure and evaluated at 1 and 3 years. Two were asymptomatic, five were improved, and one was unchanged. The subject with continued exposure deteriorated (34). In a cross-sectional survey of 706 individuals exposed to cobalt, there was no association between cigarette smoking and asthma. There was a correlation between cobalt exposure and RAST against Co-HSA, leading the authors to conclude that antibody level could serve as a biological marker of exposure (35).

Several metal exposures have been reported to cause symptoms of asthma and NSBH after a latency period, but no immunological mechanism has been elucidated. Those metal exposures include aluminum (potroom asthma), vanadium, uranium, and metal fumes (25).

B. Acid Anhydrides

Acid anhydrides are highly reactive low molecular weight chemicals that are used as curing agents in the manufacture of epoxy resins and surface coatings. The first report of acid anhydride asthma was in 1939 in an individual exposed to phthalic anhydride (PA) (36). A large series of 118 PA-exposed employees was reported; of those, two had positive skin tests and positive specific bronchial provocation (37). Since the appearance of that first report of anhydride asthma, a variety of clinical and immunological studies have been published relative to hypersensitivity reactions to acid anhydrides (38–53).

Several of the Gell and Coombs hypersensitivity responses have been demonstrated or implicated in acid anhydride immunological respiratory diseases, one of which is asthma. The acid anhydride to which immunological response has been best characterized is trimellitic anhydride (TMA) (39–42). As described in Section I, the antigen is the acid anhydride conjugated to a human airway protein such as human serum albumin (HSA). Immediate-type asthma and rhinitis are mediated by a Type I IgE mechanism, whereas late asthma is mediated by a Type IVa2 mechanism. Late respiratory systemic syndrome (LRSS) is likely due, at least in part, to a Type III mechanism. Pulmonary disease anemia syndrome (PDA), which consists of pulmonary infiltrates, hemoptysis, and anemia, involves both Type IIa and Type III mechanisms.

Specific IgE and immediate-type asthma and rhinitis have been reported to occur as a result of exposure to a number of different anhydrides (38). As with asthma caused by other low molecular weight agents, it appears that early removal of the individuals with TMA asthma from the source will generally result in disappearance of the disease (43).

The association between MHC Class II alleles and sensitization to acid anhydrides has been studied. In one report, the association between development of specific IgE against acid anhydrides and HLA-DR3 was strong; this association was especially significant for TMA (44). In another study of 100 individuals exposed to hexahydrophthalic anhydride (HHPA) and methyltetrahydrophthalic anhydride (MTHPA), there was no HLA association between specific IgE and HLA type; there was a trend toward a protective effect of HLA-A25 and HLA-A32 (45).

A case series of 27 individuals exposed to HHPA was reported in 1985. Twelve of the 27 had IgE against HHPA-HSA, and four of these had occupational asthma, resulting in the conclusion that HHPA is a potent sensitizer. HHPA can also cause immunologically mediated hemorrhagic rhinitis (47). Antibody against HHPA-HSA is a good predictor of which exposed individuals will develop disease (48). As with TMA, once asthma is diagnosed, early removal from the presence of the agent will generally result in disappearance of the disease (49).

Just as HHPA is a potent sensitizer, so is MTHPA (50). Both agents can cause contact urticaria as well as asthma in subjects with positive prick tests to acid anhydride protein conjugates (51). A number of other acid anhydrides such as pyromellitic anhydride (PDMA) (52) have been reported to cause asthma, allergic rhinitis, and hemorrhagic rhinitis (53).

C. Western Red Cedar and Plicatic Acid

Reports of sawdust inducing asthma span more than half a century (54,55). The species that has been most studied is western red cedar, first reported to cause occupational asthma in 1926 (54). The chemical composition of western red cedar has been extensively studied (56). Structurally, it is made up of cellulose and lignins, just as other trees are. One lignin, the low molecular weight agent plicatic acid, is somewhat unique in that it has a carboxylic acid group on an aromatic ring structure. Whether plicatic acid is a hapten that is the causative agent in all western red cedar asthma is somewhat controversial (57). There could be other constituents in western red cedar that are responsible, at least in some individuals. Moreover, plicatic acid may act as an irritant in asthmatics.

Doig (58) reported two small epidemics of western red cedar asthma. Some of these individuals were studied using extract from sawdust. The individuals with asthma had large cutaneous reaction, while smaller reactions were reported in controls (59). The clinical history of cedar asthma has been fairly well characterized and begins with a long latency (60). The initial symptoms are generally those of rhinitis. After some period of time, cough develops followed by wheezing and dyspnea. Partial symptom relief occurs over weekends and vacations.

Chan-Yeung and her colleagues (61) reported their initial three cases of western red cedar asthma in 1971. They prepared crude and purified extracts to which two individuals had positive skin tests and all three had positive bronchial challenge. Two years later, they reported a series of 22 western red cedar exposed individuals with respiratory symptoms (62). These patients were challenged with an extract that was dialyzed to remove all protein; all challenges were negative. They were then challenged with plicatic acid; four had an immediate response, eight had a late asthmatic response, six had dual responses, and four had no response. Three individuals were skin test positive to plicatic acid. From this, the authors concluded that plicatic acid was the etiological agent for western red cedar asthma. Subsequently, Tse et al. (63) were able to detect, by in vitro methods, specific IgE against plicatic acid in about half of the challenge-positive individuals. None of the challenge-negative individuals had specific IgE. Plicatic acid has also been reported to cause histamine release from basophils of individuals with western red cedar asthma but not from normal or atopic individuals (64).

In later studies Chan-Yeung and coinvestigators (65) reported that atopy was not a risk factor for asthma but that it was for rhinoconjunctivitis. Smoking appeared to be a risk factor for chronic bronchitis. The prevalence of western red cedar asthma among those exposed appeared to be about 5%. Another epidemiological study of 73 individuals exposed to western red cedar and other wood dusts was reported by Brooks et al. (66). The prevalence of occupational asthma was 14%. Magnitude of dust exposure was a risk factor for developing occupational asthma.

In long-term follow-up studies, it has been reported that permanent asthma occurs in individuals who are not removed from exposure in a timely fashion (67). In those who continue exposure after diagnosis, significant deterioration in lung function occurs in spite of increased medication use (68). In BAL and bronchial biopsy studies of individuals with western red cedar asthma, there are increased numbers of $CD4^+$ T cells and $EG2^+$ activated eosinophils. The histology was very similar to that of atopic asthma (69).

D. Reactive Dyes and Related Azo Compounds

Low molecular weight textile dyes have been reported to cause occupational asthma. The chemical structures of these agents are similar; each contains a dye moiety that is usually an azo group, a hydrophilic group, and reactive groups to form covalent bonds with amino or hydroxyl groups in the textile fibers (70). These reactive dyes can therefore be conjugated to human serum albumin for a diagnostic reagent for in vitro or in vivo tests (71). In a study of 309 exposed employees, 13 had positive challenges after inhalation of one of four types of dye. Twenty-five subjects had positive skin tests to Black GR dye and 21 to Orange 3R dye; 53 had specific IgE against one or both dyes (72). Atopy was not a risk factor for occupational asthma in this study. In another cross-sectional study of 162 individuals exposed to remazol dyes, five had allergy to the reactive dye; four of those individuals had a positive RAST (73). Other low molecular weight reactive dyes such as bromoacrylamide have been reported to cause occupational asthma (74).

Another group of azo compounds are used in industries as expanding agents for resins. Azodicarbonamide is a yellow powder that releases large volumes of gas at high temperatures. It has been reported in case series to cause occupational asthma (75,76). Azo compounds are also used in the photocopying industry, in which four cases of occupational asthma due to diazonium chloride have been reported (77). Yet another azo compound, diazonium tetrafluoroborate, which is produced during the manufacture of fluorine polymers, was reported to induce specific IgE in 8 of 43 exposed individuals (78). Two of those individuals also had positive bronchial provocation tests.

E. Antibiotics and Other Pharmaceuticals

Employees at highest risk of developing occupational asthma from pharmaceuticals are those in the manufacturing facilities with significant airborne dust exposure. However, those employed in health care may also develop occupational asthma due to pharmaceutical agents.

Although beta-lactam antibiotics came into widespread use a half-century ago, there were no reports of occupational asthma until 1974, when Pepys and coworkers (79) described four employees with positive bronchial challenges to penicillins. None of those individuals had positive cutaneous tests to ampicillin, benzyl penicillin, or 6-amino penicillanic acid. In a study reported by Moller et al. a decade later (80), eight beta-lactam exposed employees were scratch and RAST negative to several penicillin antigens, but five had positive basophil histamine release (80).

A macrolide antibiotic, spiramycin, was reported as a cause of occupational asthma. The subject had a positive inhalation challenge and improved after discontinuing his employment (81). A cross-sectional study of 51 exposed pharmaceutical workers was performed by Malo and Cartier. Three had positive spiramycin challenges; skin test results could not be interpreted due to irritant effect (82). Two other antibiotics, tetracycline (83,84) and isoniazid (85), have also been reported to cause occupational asthma. Positive challenges and cutaneous tests were reported in these cases.

An antihelminthic used primarily by veterinarians, piperazine, has been reported to cause rhinitis and asthma after inhalation challenge. Cutaneous tests with piperazine were negative (86). Occupational asthma and a positive inhalation challenge have also been reported with methyldopa powder (87). Finally, penicillamine has been reported to induce occupational asthma (88). A positive bronchial challenge was reported in a pharmaceutical worker who also had occupational asthma to guar gum. In vivo and in vitro tests for specific IgE were negative.

F. Diisocyanates

The isocyanate group ($-N=C=O$) is chemically very reactive. The isocyanates are used primarily in the polyurethane industry, and annual production exceeds 3 million tons (89). With exposures exceeding 100 ppb, respiratory reactions are due to toxicity, while hypersensitivity reactions can occur at levels less than 10 ppb. The most common hypersensitivity reaction is asthma, but others, including hypersensitivity pneumonitis and hemorrhagic pneumonitis, have been reported. The prevalence of asthma among exposed individuals has been estimated to be 5–10% (90). Sensitization can occur at levels as low as 20 ppb, but characteristically sensitization is believed to occur at higher levels. Unlike many other occupational sensitizers, isocyanates do not result in specific IgE production in the majority of individuals with positive bronchial challenges (90). Toluene diisocyanate (TDI) is the most common isocyanate to cause asthma, but hexamethylene diisocyanate (HDI) and diphenyl-methane diisocyanate (MDI) have also been reported to cause asthma as well as hypersensitivity pneumonitis (91). In a report by Venables and colleagues of 221 TDI exposed subjects, symptoms of occupational asthma were present in approximately 10% (92). Only two individuals had bronchial challenge; both were positive. The average latency period was 3 years, and 40% of employees still had symptoms 1 year after removal. While most sensitized individuals have only isocyanate-induced asthma, a small number have both asthma and hypersensitivity pneumonitis (92). There is immunological and clinical cross-reactivity among isocyanates; therefore, an individual sensitized to one isocyanate may also react to another (93).

Isocyanate asthma has many characteristics of an immunological disease. There is a latency period, only a small percentage of exposed individuals are affected, and a very low exposure results in disease. While many immunological associations have been reported with isocyanate asthma, the responsible immunopathological process has not yet been conclusively identified. A small percentage of individuals with positive isocyanate bronchial challenge have specific IgE by either in vivo or in vitro assay (90,94). Although the presence of IgE or IgG against isocyanates does not invariably occur in subjects with positive isocyanate inhalation challenge, the prevalence of specific positive IgG or IgE is higher in challenge-positive individuals than in challenge-negative individuals (94). After positive inhalation challenge with isocyanates there is no change in plasma histamine, total complement, or split complement products (95). Peripheral blood mononuclear cells from individuals with isocyanate asthma have increased production of antigen-specific histamine-releasing factor (HRF) activity and monocyte chemoattractant protein (MCP-1) (96,97). More evidence for the immunological basis of isocyanate asthma comes from immunogenetic studies. Some HLA class II alleles have been associated with the development of isocyanate-induced asthma (98). In those same studies some MHC class II markers have been associated with protection against the development of occupational asthma due to isocyanates. An aspartic acid residue at position 57 has been identified as the crucial element that confers susceptibility to isocyanate asthma by the MHC class II allele, HLA-DQB1 (99). Other evidence of the immunological basis of isocyanate asthma comes from postpositive inhalational challenge studies in which high levels of eosinophilic cationic protein (ECP) are detected (100). In those studies, neither histamine nor tryptase elevations were detected. The percent of $V\beta 1$ and $V\beta 5$ expression has been reported to be selectively increased after in vitro stimulation with isocyanate–protein conjugates (101). From these studies, it is postu-

Table 3 Immunology of Diisocyanate Asthma

Immunological observation	Ref.
Low prevalence of specific IgE.	90
Positive antibody, especially IgG, more likely in challenge-positive individuals.	94
No change in plasma histamine or complement in challenge-positive individuals.	95
Peripheral blood mononuclear cells from those with isocyanate asthma have increased production of antigen-specific HRF and MCP-1.	96, 97
HLA MHC class II alleles associated with development of and protection from isocyanate asthma; aspartic acid at position 57 may be key in HLA-DQB1.	98, 99
ECP increased in peripheral blood after positive TDI challenge.	100
Preferential Vbeta expression in isocyanate asthma.	101
Bronchial biopsies from isocyanate asthma contain CD8$^+$ cells that produce IL-5 and IFN-γ.	102
Bronchial biopsies from isocyanate asthma have increased CD25, VLA-4, TNF-α, and IL-1β.	103
Bronchial biopsies from isocyanate asthma have thickened basement membrane, increased eosinophils, and increased CD3$^+$CD45$^+$ cells.	104

lated that antigen-specific T-cell subpopulations may be sequestered in the lungs of individuals with isocyanate asthma.

Several studies of bronchial biopsies of subjects with isocyante asthma have been reported that add evidence for immunological causation. Bronchial biopsies of such subjects contain CD8$^+$ cells that produce both IL-5 and IFN-γ (102). In addition, subjects with isocyanate asthma have increased CD25, VLA-4, and expression of TNF-α and IL-1 β (103). Following inhalation challenge, individuals with isocyanate asthma demonstrate increased thickness of basement membrane and increased number of cells such as eosinophils and CD3$^+$ CD45$^+$ T cells (104).

Several studies of isocyanate-exposed individuals have been published. Many isocyanate exposures result in essentially no disease. For instance, in a clinical and immunological evaluation of 96 employees exposed to aliphatic isocyanates, TMXDI, and TMI, no diseased individuals could be identified (105). On the other hand, an epidemic of isocyanate asthma was reported among employees exposed to MDI (106). As has been reported with other causes of occupational asthma, seven subjects who were removed from exposure had improvement in NSBH and reduction in airway inflammation (107). In another study of removed employees, 10 had decreased sensitivity to TDI challenge, fewer subepithelial fibroblasts, fewer mast cells, fewer lymphocytes, and reduced thickness of subepithelial fibrosis (108). Unfortunately, if sensitized subjects continue isocyanate exposure, potentially fatal outcomes may ensue (108).

G. Other Low Molecular Weight Chemicals

A variety of other chemicals have been described to cause asthma, generally in the occupational setting. Rather than large cross-sectional or longitudinal studies, these reports tend to be of single cases or small case series.

Amines

Numerous amines—secondary, tertiary, and quarternary; aliphatic, heterocyclic, and aromatic—have been described to cause asthma (109,110). Exposure to these products can occur in primary manufacturing as well as in secondary use industries such as rubber, cosmetics, shellac, epoxy resins, and photographic development (109). Specific inhalation challenges have been positive in those subjects with asthma; cutaneous testing and in vitro assay results were not reported. Environmental controls and reduced workplace exposure reportedly resulted in disappearance of symptoms and improvement of pulmonary function in affected employees (111,112). Chloramine T, an organic, highly reactive bactericidal agent, has been described to cause occupational asthma. It is used in the food and beverage industry as a sterilizing agent. Recent case reports have been from Spain (113) and Finland (114). Both in vivo and in vitro tests have implicated an IgE-mediated mechanism (115,116).

Colophony

Colophony is the resin from pine trees. An important constituent is abietic acid, which is believed to be the low molecular weight etiological agent in the asthma and alveolitis that have been described to result from colophony exposure. In the electronics industry, colophony is used as a "flux" to prevent corrosion. Burge et al. (117) described 21 individuals with positive inhalation challenges to colophony. Some reactions were immediate, some late, but the majority were dual asthmatic responses. In cross-sectional surveys of exposed individuals, approximately 20% report respiratory symptoms, and they are an important reason for turnover in exposed individuals (118). Atopy is only a weak predictor, and smoking has no association with the development of asthma in colophony-exposed subjects. In addition to having positive bronchial challenges with colophony, affected subjects have been reported to have positive challenges with abietic acid (119). Specific antibody has not been reported in the majority of affected individuals, and therefore the mechanism remains unknown. In some individuals who have been removed from exposure, persistent symptoms and NSBH have been reported (120).

Persulfate

Ammonium persulfate is a known cause of occupational asthma among those who are employed in beauty salons; a high molecular weight agent, henna, has also been reported to cause occupational asthma in this group (121). Positive inhalational challenges with ammonium persulfate have been reported (122). Positive cutaneous reactivity to ammonium persulfate has been reported in some, but not all, affected individuals. Persulfates have also been reported to cause occupational asthma in some industrial settings.

Formaldehyde and Glutaraldehyde

Formaldehyde is a low molecular weight agent with many chemical and industrial applications. It is used in hospitals as a sterilizing and fixative agent; it is also used in the manufacture of paper, textiles, furniture, plywood, and cosmetics. Two decades ago, when urea formaldehyde foam insulation was installed in many indoor environments, a variety of problems with indoor air quality were reported. Because formaldehyde was considered to be a possible causative factor, many reports of formadehyde as an irritant and potential immunogen have been published (123). Initially a level of 3.0 ppm was promulgated as the threshold for irritation of mucous membranes. Subsequently, this was revised to 1.0 ppm.

Challenging formaldehyde-exposed employees with 2.0 ppm was reported not to cause positive challenges (124). Although positive inhalation challenge has been reported, Frigas et al. (125) were unable to demonstrate positive challenges in any of 13 formaldehyde-exposed individuals with work-related asthma. A closed-circuit challenge apparatus was reported to generate chemicals such as formaldehyde in vapor form (126). Only one of four challenged individuals was positive in that report; no immunological studies were reported. While positive antibodies can be detected in some exposed individuals, attempts to relate them causally to symptomatology have generally been unsuccessful (127).

Another aldehyde, glutaraldehyde, has been reported to cause occupational asthma (128). In a case series of 21 glutaraldehyde-exposed individuals, eight had occupational asthma; seven of the eight had positive bronchial challenges with glutaraldehyde. Several of those individuals also had positive RAST using glutaraldehyde conjugated to HSA as the allergen (129). While RAST was negative in unexposed individuals, RAST percent binding did not distinguish well between exposed individuals with asthma and exposed individuals without occupational asthma.

Acrylates

The initial report of acrylate-induced asthma concerned an individual who used an acrylate-based glue in his hobby of building model airplanes (130). Other investigators reported individual cases as well (131). A case series of six individuals with occupational asthma and positive bronchial challenges was reported (132). Subsequently, there was a larger series of 10 cases of occupational asthma due to cyanoacrylates, four due to methacrylates, and two to other acrylates (133). The mechanism responsible for the occupational asthma is unclear. Health care and artificial nail making are the occupations most likely to be exposed to the sensitizing acrylate glues.

Miscellaneous Low Molecular Weight Agents

Numerous other agents have been described in single case reports or small case series to induce occupational asthma. A chemical factory employee was reported to have immediate positive bronchial challenge and rhinitis due to 1,2-benzisothiazolin-3-one (134). Immunological studies were not performed. Similarly, ninhydrin has been reported to induce rhinitis, positive bronchial challenge, and increased specific IgE (135). An individual who was employed spraying polyester powder paints was reported to have a positive bronchial challenge to triglycidyl isocyanurate, an epoxy compound used as a hardener (136).

In detergent-manufacturing employees, specific inhalation challenge to sodium isononanoyl oxybenzene sulfonate (SINOS) was reported (137). Positive inhalation challenge to tetrazene, a powder used by detonator manufacturers, was also reported (138). Two different topical disinfectants used in hospitals were reported to induce occupational asthma and positive bronchial challenge. One disinfectant is chlorhexidine (139), and the other is hexachlorophene (140). Finally, organophosphate insecticides were reported to induce occupational asthma (141). Presumably the mechanism of this type of occupational asthma is pharmacological.

IV. Summary

Low molecular weight agents are well-recognized causes of environmental asthma, primarily in the occupational setting. Two types of asthma, one immunological with a latency period and the other nonimmunological without a latency period, are recognized. The prototype of the latter is reactive airways dysfunction syndrome (RADS). In the case of immunological asthma, low molecular weight agents act as haptens, combining with human proteins in the respiratory tract to become complete immunogens. In many instances, specific IgE appears to be the operative mechanism, just as is the case for high molecular weight agents. In some cases, notably diisocyanates, the operative mechanism has not been defined, but it is almost certainly immunological.

Acknowledgments

This work was supported by The Ernest S. Bazley Grant to Northwestern Memorial Hospital and Northwestern University Medical School.

References

1. Bernstein DI. Allergic reactions to workplace allergens. J Am Med Assoc 1997; 278:1907–1913.
2. Chan-Yeung M. Assessment of asthma in the workplace. ACCP consensus statement. American College of Chest Physicians. Chest 1995; 108:1084–1117.
3. Grammer LC. Occupational immunologic lung disease. In: Patterson R, Grammer LC, Greenberger PA, eds. Allergic Diseases: Diagnosis and Management. 5th ed. Philadelphia: Lippincott-Raven, 1997:579–590.
4. Grammer LC, Patterson R. Trimellitic anhydride. In: Rom WN, ed. Environmental and Occupational Medicine. 2nd ed. Boston: Little, Brown, 1992:987–991.
5. Brooks S, Weiss MA, Bernstein IL. Reactive airways dysfunction syndrome: persistent asthma syndrome after high-level irritant exposure. Chest 1985; 88:376–384.
6. Boulet LP. Increases in airway responsiveness following acute exposure to respiratory irritants. Reactive airway dysfunction syndrome or occupational asthma. Chest 1988; 94:47–81.

7. Moisan T. Prolonged asthma after smoke inhalation: a report of three cases and a review of previous reports. J Occup Med 1991; 33:458–461.
8. Bernstein IL, Bernstein DI, Weiss M, Campbell GP. Reactive airways disease syndrome (RADS) after exposure to toxic ammonia fumes. J Allergy Clin Immunol 1989; 83:173.
9. Bherer L, Cushman R, Courteau JP, Quevillon M, Cote G, Bourbeau J, L'Archeveque J, Cartier A, Malo J-L. Survey of construction workers repeatedly exposed to chlorine over a three to six month period in a pulpmill. II. Follow up of affected workers by questionnaire, spirometry, and assessment of bronchial responsiveness 18 to 24 months after exposure ended. Occup Environ Med 1994; 51:225–228.
10. Brooks SM, Bernstein IL. Reactive airways dysfunction syndrome or irritant-induced asthma. In: Bernstein IL, Chan-Yeung M, Bernstein DI, eds. Asthma in the Workplace. New York: Marcel Dekker, 1993:533–550.
11. Malo J-L, Lemière C, Desjardins A, Cartier A. Prevalence and intensity of rhinoconjunctivitis in subjects with occupational asthma. Eur Respir J 1997; 10:1513–1515.
12. Janeway C, Travers P. Immunobiology. 2nd ed. London: Garland Press, 1995, Chap. 11.
13. Kay AB. Concepts of allergy and hypersensitivity. In: Kay AB, ed. Allergy and Allergic Disease. Oxford: Blackwell Science, 1997:23–35.
14. Azzawi M, Bradley B, Jeffery PK, Frew AJ, Wardlaw AJ, Knowles G, Assoufi B, Collins JV, Durham S, Kay AB. Identification of activated T lymphocytes and eosinophils in bronchial biopsies in stable atopic asthma. Am Rev Respir Dis 1990; 142:1410–1413.
15. Ying S, Durham SR, Corrigan CJ, Hamid Q, Kay AB. Phenotype of cells expressing mRNA for Th2-type (interleukin-4 and interleukin-5) cytokines in bronchoalveolar lavage and bronchial biopsies from atopic asthmatics and normal control subjects. Am J Respir Cell Mol Biol 1995; 12:477–487.
16. Maestrelli P, Del Prete GF, De Carli M, D'Elios MM, Saetta M, DiStefano A, Mapp CE, Romagnani S, Fabbri LM. CD8 T-cell clones producing interleukin-5 and interferon-gamma in bronchial mucosa of patients with asthma induced by toluene diisocyanate. Scan J Work Environ Health 1994; 20:376–381.
17. Maestrelli P, DiStefano A, Occari P, Turato G, Milani G, Pivirotto F, Mapp CE, Fabbri LM, Saetta M. Cytokines in the airway mucosa of subjects with asthma induced by toluene diisocyanate. Am J Respir Crit Care Med 1995; 151:607–612.
18. Hunter D, Milton R, Perry KMA. Asthma caused by the complex salts of platinum. Br J Ind Med 1945; 2:92–98.
19. Freedman SO, Kruupey J. Respiratory allergy caused by platinum salts. J Allergy 1968; 42:233–237.
20. Dally MB, Hunter JV, Hughes EG, Stewart M, Newman Taylor AJ. Hypersensitivity to platinum salts: a population study. Am Rev Respir Dis 1980; 4 (suppl):121 (abstract).

21. Cromwell O, Pepys J, Parish WE, Hughes EG. Specific IgE antibodies to platinum salts in sensitized workers. Clin Allergy 1979; 9:109–117.

22. Biagini RE, Bernstein IL, Gallagher JS, Moorman WJ, Brooks S, Gann PH. The diversity of reaginic immune responses to platinum and palladium metallic salts. J Allergy Clin Immunol 1985; 76:794–802.

23. Merget R, Dierkes A, Rueckmann A, Bergmann E-M, Schultze-Werninghaus G. Absence of relationship between degree of nonspecific and specific bronchial responsiveness in occupational asthma due to platinum salts. Eur Respir J 1996; 9:211–216.

24. Venables KM, Dally MB, Nunn AJ, Stevens JF, Stephens R, Farrer N, Hunter JV, Stewart M, Hughes EG, Newman Taylor AJ. Smoking and occupational allergy in workers in a platinum refinery. Br Med J 1989; 299:939–942.

25. O'Hollaren MT. Asthma due to metals and metal salts. In: Bardana EJ, Montanaro A, O'Hollaren MT, eds. Occupational Asthma. St Louis: Mosby, 1997:179–188.

26. McConnell LH, Fink JN, Schlueter DP, Schmidt MG Jr. Asthma caused by nickel sensitivity. Ann Intern Med 1973; 78:888–890.

27. Block GT, Yeung M. Asthma induced by nickel. J Am Med Assoc 1982; 247:1600–1602.

28. Malo J-L, Cartier A, Doepner M, Nieboer E, Evans S, Dolovich J. Occupational asthma caused by nickel sulfate. J Allergy Clin Immunol 1982; 69:55–59.

29. Novey HS, Habib M, Wells ID. Asthma and IgE antibodies induced by chromium and nickel salts. J Allergy Clin Immunol 1983; 72:407–412.

30. Bright P, Burge PS, O'Hickey PS, Gannon PFG, Robertson AS, Boran A. Occupational asthma due to chrome and nickel electroplating. Thorax 1997; 52:28–32.

31. Bernstein IL, Brooks SM. Metals. In: Bernstein IL, Chan-Yeung M, Malo J-L, Bernstein DI, eds. Asthma in the Workplace. New York: Marcel Dekker, 1993: 459–479.

32. Shirakawa T, Kusakay, Morimoto K. Metals specific IgE antibodies to nickel in workers with known reactivity to cobalt. Clin Exp Allergy 1992; 22:213–218.

33. Shirakawa T, Kusaka Y, Fujimura N, Kato M, Heki S, Morimoto K. Hard metal asthma: cross immunologic and respiratory reactivity between cobalt and nickel. Thorax 1990; 45:267–271.

34. Pisati G, Zedda S. Outcome of occupational asthma due to cobalt hypersensitivity. Sci Total Environ 1994; 150:167–171.

35. Shirakawa T, Morimoto K. Interplay of cigarette smoking and occupational exposure on specific immunoglobulin E antibodies to cobalt. Arch Environ Health 1997; 52:124–128.

36. Kern RA. Asthma and allergic rhinitis due to sensitization to phthalic anhydride; report of a case. J Allergy 1939; 10:164–165.

37. Wernfors M, Nielsen J, Schutz A, Skerfving S. Phthalic anhydride-induced occupational asthma. Int Arch Allergy Appl Immunol 1986; 79:77–82.

38. Bernstein DI, Gallagher JS, D'Souza L, Bernstein IL. Heterogeneity of specific IgE responses in workers sensitized to acid anhydride compounds. J Allergy Clin Immunol 1984; 94:794–801.

39. Zeiss CR, Patterson R, Pruzansky JJ, Miller MM, Rosenberg M, Levitz D. Trimellitic anhydride-induced airway syndromes: clinical and immunologic studies. J Allergy Clin Immunol 1977; 60:96–103.

40. Patterson R, Zeiss CR, Pruzansky JJ. Immunopathology of trimellitic anhydride pulmonary reactions. J Allergy Clin Immunol 1982; 70:19–23.

41. Zeiss CR, Wolkansky P, Pruzansky JJ, Patterson R. Clinical and immunologic evaluation of trimellitic anhydride workers in multiple industrial settings. J Allergy Clin Immunol 1982; 70:15–18.

42. Zeiss CR, Wolkansky P, Chacan R, Tuntland PA, Levitz D, Pruzansky JJ, Patterson R. Syndromes in workers exposed to trimellitic anhydride. Ann Intern Med 1983; 98:8–12.

43. Grammer LC, Shaughnessy MA, Henderson J, Zeiss CR, Kavich DE, Collins MJ, Pecis KM, Kenamore BD. A clinical and immunologic study of workers with trimellitic anhydride-induced immunologic lung disease after transfer to low exposure jobs. Am Rev Respir Dis 1993; 148:54–57.

44. Young RP, Barker RD, Pile KD, Cookson WOCM, Taylor AJN. The association of HLA-DR3 with specific IgE to inhaled acid anhydrides. Am J Respir Crit Care Med 1995; 151:219–221.

45. Nielsen J, Johnson U, Welinder H, Bensryd I, Rylander L, Skerfving S. HLA and immune nonresponsiveness in workers exposed to organic acid anhydrides. J Occup Environ Med 1996; 38:1087–1090.

46. Moller DR, Gallagher JS, Bernstein DI, Wilcox TG, Burroughs HE, Bernstein IL. Detection of IgE-mediated respiratory sensitization in workers exposed to hexahydrophthalic anhydride. J Allergy Clin Immunol 1985; 75:663–672.

47. Grammer LC, Shaughnessy MA, Lowenthal M. Hemorrhagic rhinitis: an immunologic disease due to hexahydrophthalic anhydride. Chest 1993; 104:1792–1794.

48. Grammer LC, Shaughnessy MA, Hogan MB, Berggruen SM, Watkins DM, Yarnold PR. Value of antibody level in diagnosing anhydride induced immunologic respiratory disease. J Lab Clin Med 1995; 125:650–653.

49. Grammer LC, Shaughnessy MA, Hogan MB, Lowenthal M, Yarnold PR, Watkins DM, Berggruen SM. Study of employees with anhydride-induced respiratory disease after removal from exposure. J Occup Environ Med 1995; 37:820–825.

50. Zeiss CR, Patterson R. Acid anhydrides. In: Bernstein IL, Chan-Yeung M, Malo J-L, Bernstein DI, eds. Asthma in the Workplace. New York: Marcel Dekker, 1993: 439–458.

51. Tarvainen K, Jolanki R, Estlander T, Tupasela O, Pfaffli P, Kanerva L. Acid anhydrides. Immunologic contact urticaria due to airborne methydrophthalic and methyltetrahydrophthalic anhydrides. Contact Derm 1995; 32:204–209.

52. Baur X, Czuppon AB, Rauluk I, Zimmermann FB, Schmitt B, Egen-Korthaus M, Tenkhoff N, Degens PO. A clinical and immunological study on 92 workers occupationally exposed to anhydrides. Int Arch Occup Environ Health 1995; 67: 395–403.

53. Zeiss CR. Reactive chemicals in industry. J Allergy Clin Immunol 1991; 87:755–761.

54. Seki K. American cedar-induced asthma. J Jpn Soc Intern Med 1926; 13:884.

55. Ordman D. Bronchial asthma caused by inhalation of wood dust. Ann Allergy 1949; 7:492–496.

56. Hillis W. Wood Extractives and Their Significance to the Pulp and Paper Industry. New York: Academic Press, 1962.

57. Bardana EJ Jr. Western red cedar asthma and asthma secondary to other wood dusts and wood or plant-related products. In: Bardana EJ Jr, Montanaro A, O'Hollaren MT, eds. Occupational Asthma. St. Louis: Mosby, 1992:87–106.

58. Doig AT. Other lung diseases due to dust. Postgrad Med J 1949; 25:639.

59. Aoki M. Asthma due to western red cedar among carpenters making furniture. J Allergy 1968; 17:428–430.

60. Gandevia B, Miline J. Occupational asthma due to western red cedar (*Thuja plicata*) with special reference to bronchial reactivity. Br J Ind Med 1970; 27:235–244.

61. Chan-Yeung M, Barton GM, McLean L. Bronchial reactions to western red cedar (*Thuja plicata*). Can Med Assoc J 1971; 105:56–58.

62. Chan-Yeung M. Maximal expiratory flow and airway resistance during induced bronchoconstriction in patients with asthma due to western red cedar (*Thuja plicata*). Am Rev Respir Dis 1973; 108:1103–1110.

63. Tse KS, Chan H, Chan-Yeung M. Specific IgE antibodies in workers with occupational asthma due to western red cedar. Clin Allergy 1982; 12:249–258.

64. Chan-Yeung M. Mechanism of occupational asthma due to western red cedar (*Thuja plicata*). Am J Ind Med 1994; 25:13–18.

65. Chan-Yeung M, Ashley MJ, Corey P, Willson G, Dorken E, Grzybowski S. A respiratory survey of cedar millworkers. I. Prevalence of symptoms and pulmonary function abnormalities. J Occup Med 1978; 20:323–327.

66. Brooks SM, Edwards JJ Jr, Apol A, Edwards FH. An epidemiologic study of workers exposed to western red cedar and other wood dusts. Chest 1981; 80(1 suppl):30–32.

67. Chan-Yeung M, Lam S, Koener S. Clinical features and natural history of occupational asthma due to western red cedar (*Thuja plicata*). Am J Med 1982; 72: 411–415.

68. Marabini A, Dimich-Ward H, Kwan Sy, Kennedy SM, Waxler-Morrison N, Chan-Yeung M. Clinical and socioeconomic features of subjects with red cedar asthma. A follow-up study. Chest 1993; 104:821–824.

69. Frew AJ, Chan H, Lam S, Chan-Yeung M. Bronchial inflammation in occupational asthma due to western red cedar. Am J Respir Crit Care Med 1995; 151: 340–344.

70. Alanko K, Keskinen H, Bjorksten F, Ojanen S. Immediate type hypersensitivity to reactive dyes. Clin Allergy 1978; 8:25–31.

71. Luczynska CM, Topping MD. Specific IgE antibodies to reactive dye-albumin conjugates. J Immunol Methods 1986; 95:177–186.

72. Park HS, Lee MK, Kim BO. Clinical and immunologic evaluations of reactive dye-exposed workers. J Allergy Clin Immunol 1991; 87:639–649.

73. Nilsson R, Nordlinder R, Wass U, Meding B, Belin L. Asthma, rhinitis, and dermatitis in workers exposed to reactive dyes. Br J Ind Med 1993; 50:65–70.

74. Romano C, Sulotto F, Pavan I, Chiesa A, Scansetti G. A new case of occupational asthma from reactive dyes with severe anaphylactic responses to the specific challenge. Am J Ind Med 1992; 21:209–216.

75. Malo J-L, Pineau L, Cartier A. Occupational asthma due to azobisformamide. Clin Allergy 1985; 15:261–264.

76. Normand JC, Grange F, Hernandez C, Ganay A, Davezies P, Bergeret A, Prost G. Occupational asthma after exposure to azodicarbonamide: report of four cases. Br J Ind Med 1989; 46:60–62.

77. Graham VA, Coe MJ, Davies RJ. Occupational asthma after exposure to a diazonium salt. Thorax 1981; 36:950–951.

78. Luczynska CM, Hutchcroft BJ, Harrison MA, Dornan JD, Topping MD. Occupational asthma and specific IgE to a diazonium salt intermediate used in the polymer industry. J Allergy Clin Immunol 1990; 85:1076–1082.

79. Davies RJ, Hendrick DJ, Pepys J. Asthma due to inhaled chemical agents: ampicillin, benzyl penicillin, 6 amino penicillanic acid and related substances. Clin Allergy 1974; 4:227–247.

80. Moller NE, Skov PS, Norm S. Allergic and pseudoallergic reactions caused by penicillins, coca and peppermint additives in factory workers examined by basophil histamine release. Acta Pharm Toxicol 1984; 55:139–144.

81. Davies RJ, Pepys J. Asthma due to inhaled chemical agents: the macrolide antibiotic spiramycin. Clin Allergy 1975; 1:99–107.

82. Malo J-L, Cartier A. Occupational asthma in workers of a pharmaceutical company processing spiramycin. Thorax 1988; 43:371–377.

83. Fawcett IW, Pepys J. Allergy to a tetracycline preparation: a case report. Clin Allergy 1976; 6:301–306.

84. Menon NPS, Das AK. Tetracycline asthma: a case report. Clin Allergy 1977; 7:285–290.

85. Asai S, Shimoda T, Hara K, Fujiwara K. Occupational asthma caused by isonicotinic acid hydrazide inhalation. J Allergy Clin Immunol 1987; 80:578–582.

86. Pepys J, Pickering CAC, Loudon HW. Asthma due to inhaled chemical agents: piperazine dihydrochloride. Clin Allergy 1972; 2:189–196.

87. Harries MG, Newman Taylor AJ, Wooden J, MacAuslan A. Bronchial asthma due to alpha methyldopa. Br Med J 1979; 2:1461.

88. Lagier F, Cartier A, Dolovich J, Malo J-L. Occupational asthma in a pharmaceutical worker exposed to penicillamine. Thorax 1989; 44:157–158.

89. Baur X. Occupational asthma due to isocyanates. Lung 1996; 174:23–30.

90. Butcher BT, Salvaggio JE, Weill H, Ziskind M. Toluene diisocyanate pulmonary disease: immunologic and inhalational challenge studies. J Allergy Clin Immunol 1976; 58:89–100.

91. Zammit-Tabona M, Sherkin M, Kijek K, Chan H, Chan-Yeung M. Asthma caused by diphenylmethane diisocyanate in foundry workers: clinical, bronchial provocation and immunologic studies. Am Rev Respir Dis 1983; 128:226–230.

92. Venables KM, Dally MB, Burge PS, Pickering CA, Newman Taylor AJ. Occupational asthma in a steel coating plant. Br J Ind Med 1985; 42:517–524.

93. Malo J-L, Ouimet G, Cartier A, Levitz D, Zeiss CR. Combined alveolitis and asthma due to hexamethylene diisocyanate (HDI) with demonstration of crossed respiratory and immunologic reactivities to diphenylmethane diisocyanate (MDI). J Allergy Clin Immunol 1983; 72:413–419.

94. Grammer LC, Harris KE, Malo J-L, Cartier A, Patterson R. The use of immunoassay index for antibodies against isocyanate human protein conjugate and application to human isocyanate disease. J Allergy Clin Immunol 1990; 86:94–98.

95. Butcher BT, Karr RM, O'Neil CE, Wilson MR, Dharmarajan V, Salvaggio JE, Weill H. Inhalation challenge and pharmacologic studies of toluene diisocyanate (TDI)-sensitive workers. J Allergy Clin Imunol 1979; 64:146–152.

96. Bernstein DI, Herd ZL. Antigen-specific stimulation of histamine releasing factor in diisocyanate-induced occupational asthma. Am J Respir Crit Care Med 1994; 150:988–994.

97. Lummus ZL, Alam R, Bernstein JA, Bernstein DI. Characterization of histamine releasing factors in diisocyanate-induced occupational asthma. Toxicology 1996; 111:191–206.

98. Bignon JS, Aron Y, Ju LY, Kopferschmitt MC, Garnier R, Mapp C, Fabbri LM, Pauli G, Lockhart A, Charron D, Swierczewski E. HLA class II alleles in isocyanate-induced asthma. Am J Respir Crit Care Med 1994; 149:71–75.

99. Balboni A, Baricordi OR, Fabbri LM, Gandini E, Ciaccia A, Mapp CE. Association between toluene diisocyanate-induced asthma and DQB1 markers: a possible role for aspartic acid at position 57. Eur Respir J 1996; 9:207–210.

100. Mapp CE, Plebani M, Faggian D, Maestrelli P, Saetta M, Calcagni P, Borghesan F, Fabbri M. Eosinophil cationic protein (ECP), histamine and tryptase in peripheral blood before and during inhalation challenge with toluene diisocyanate (TDI) in sensitized subjects. Clin Exp Allergy 1994; 24:730–736.

101. Bernstein JA, Munson J, Lummus ZL, Balakrishnan K, Leikauf G. T-cell receptor Vβ gene segment expression in diisocyanate-induced occupational asthma. J Allergy Clin Immunol 1997; 99:245–250.

102. Maestrelli P, Del Prete GF, DeCarli M, D'Elios MM, Saetta M, DiStefano A, Mapp CE, Romagnani S, Fabbri LM. CD8 T-cell clones producing interleukin-5 and interferon-gamma in bronchial mucosa of patients with asthma induced by toluene diisocyanate. Scan J Work Environ Health 1994; 20:376–381.

103. Maestrêlli P, DiStefano A, Occari P, Turato G, Milani G, Pivirotto F, Mapp CE,

Fabbri LM, Saetta M. Cytokines in the airway mucosa of subjects with asthma induced by toluene diisocyanate. Am J Respir Crit Care Med 1995; 151: 607–612.

104. Redlich CA, Homer RJ, Smith BR, Wirth JA, Cullen MR. Immunologic responses to isocyanates in sensitized asthmatic subjects. Chest 1996; 109:6S–8S.

105. Grammer LC, Shaughnessy MA, Davis RA. Exposure to $TMXDI_R$ (meta) aliphatic isocyanate and TMI_R (meta) unsaturated aliphatic isocyanate. Clinical and immunologic evaluation of 96 workers. J Occup Med 1993; 35:287–290.

106. Woellner RC, Hall S, Greaves I, Schoenwetter WF. Epidemic of asthma in a wood products plant using methylene diphenyl diisocyanate. Am J Ind Med 1997; 31: 56–63.

107. Lemiere C, Cartier A, Dolovich J, Chan-Yeung M, Grammer L, Ghezzo H, L'Archeveque J, Malo J-L. Outcome of specific bronchial responsiveness to occupational agents after removal from exposure. Am J Respir Crit Care Med 1996; 154:329–333.

108. Carino M, Aliani M, Licitra C, Sarno N, Ioli F. Death due to asthma at workplace in a diphenylmethane diisocyanate-sensitized subject. Respiration 1997; 64:111–113.

109. Hagmar L, Nielsen J, Skerfving S. Clinical features and epidemiology of occupational obstructive respiratory disease caused by small molecular weight organic chemicals. In: Schlumberger HD, ed. Epidemiology of Allergic Diseases. Monographs in Allergy, Vol. 21. Basel: Karger, 1987:42–58.

110. Dernehl CU. Clinical experiences with exposures to ethylene diamines. Ind Med Surg 1951; 20:541–546.

111. Brubaker RE, Muranko HJ, Smith DB, Beck GJ, Scovel G. Evaluation and control of a respiratory exposure to 3-(dimethylamino) propylamine. J Occup Med 1979; 21:688–690.

112. Vallieres M, Cockcroft DW, Taylor DM, Dolovich J, Hargreave FE. Dimethyl ethanolamine-induced asthma. Am Rev Respir Dis 1977; 115:867–871.

113. Blasco A, Joral A, Fuente R, Rodriguez M, Garcia A, Dominguez A. Bronchial asthma due to sensitization to chloramine T. J Invest Allergol Clin Immunol 1992; 2:167–170.

114. Kujala VM, Reijula KE, Ruotsalainen EM, Heikkinen K. Occupational asthma due to chloramine-T solution. Respir Med 1995; 89:693–695.

115. Kramps JA, Van Toorenenbergen AW, Vooren PH, Dijkman JH. Occupational asthma due to inhalation of chloramine-T. II. Demonstration of specific IgE antibodies. Int Arch Allergy Appl Immunol 1981; 64:428–438.

116. Wass U, Belin L, Eriksson NE. Immunological specificity of chloramine-T-induced IgE antibodies in serum from a sensitized worker. Clin Allergy 1989; 19:463–471.

117. Burge PS, Harries MG, O'Brien IM, Pepys J. Respiratory disease in workers exposed to solder flux fumes containing colophony (pine resin). Clin Allergy 1978; 8:1–14.

118. Burge PS, Perks W, O'Brien IM, Hawkins R, Green M. Occupational asthma in an electronics factory, Thorax 1979; 34:13–18.
119. Burge PS. Occupational asthma in electronics workers caused by colophony fumes: follow-up of affected workers. Thorax 1982; 37:348–353.
120. Keira T, Aizawa Y, Karube H, Niituya M, Shinohara S, Kuwashima A, Harada H, Takata T. Adverse effects of colophony. Ind Health 1997; 35:1–7.
121. Pepys J, Hutchcroft BJ, Breslin ABX. Asthma due to inhaled chemical agents: persulphate salts and henna in hairdressers. Clin Allergy 1976; 6:399–404.
122. Blainey AD, Ollier S, Cundell D, Smith RE, Davies RJ. Occupational asthma in a hairdressing salon. Thorax 1986; 41:42–50.
123. Malo J-L, Bernstein L. Other chemical substances causing occupational asthma. In: Bernstein IL, Chan-Yeung M, Malo J-L, Bernstein DI, eds. Asthma in the Workplace. New York: Marcel Dekker, 1993:481–502.
124. Witek TJ, Schachter EN, Tosun T, Beck GJ, Leaderer BP. An evaluation of respiratory effects following exposure to 2.0 ppm formaldehyde in asthmatics: lung function, symptoms, and airway reactivity. Arch Environ Health 1987; 42:230–237.
125. Frigas E, Filley WV, Reed CE. Bronchial challenge with formalehyde gas: lack of bronchoconstriction in 13 patients suspected of having formaldehyde-induced asthma. Mayo Clin Proc 1984; 59:295–299.
126. Lemière C, Cloutier Y, Perrault G, Drolet D, Cartier A, Malo J-L. Closed-circuit apparatus for specific inhalation challenges with an occupational agent, formaldehyde, in vapor form. Chest 1996; 109:1631–1635.
127. Patterson R, Grammer LC, Harris KE, Shaughnessy MA. Immunotoxicology of formaldehyde. Comments Toxicol 1992; 4:305–314.
128. Chan-Yeung M, McMurren T, Catonio-Begley F, Lam S. Occupational asthma in technologist exposed to glutaraldehyde. J Allergy Clin Immunol 1993; 91:974–978.
129. Curran AD, Burge PS, Wiley K. Clinical and immunologic evaluation of workers exposed to glutaraldehyde. Allergy 1996; 51:826–832.
130. Kopp SK, McKay RT, Moller DR, Cassedy K, Brooks SM. Asthma and rhinitis due to ethylcyanoacrylate instant glue. Ann Intern Med 1985; 102:613–615.
131. Nakazawa T. Occupational asthma due to alkyl cyanoacrylate. J Occup Med 1990; 32:709–710.
132. Lozewicz S, Davison AG, Hopkirk A, Burge PS, Boldy D, Riordan JF, McGivern DV, Platts BW, Davies D, Newman Taylor AJ. Occupational asthma due to methyl methacrylate and cyanoacrylates. Thorax 1985; 40:836–839.
133. Savonius B, Keskinen H, Tuppurainen M, Kanerva L. Occupational respiratory disease caused by acrylates. Clin Exp Allergy 1993; 23:416–424.
134. Moscato G, Omodeo P, Dellabianca A, Colli MC, Pugliese F, Locatelli C, Scibilia J. Occupational asthma and rhinitis caused by 1,2-benzisothiazolin-3-one in a chemical worker. Occup Med 1997; 47:249–251.

135. Piirilä P, Estlander T, Hytönen M, Keskinen H, Tupasela O, Tuppurainen M. Rhinitis caused by ninhydrin develops into occupational asthma. Eur Respir J 1997; 10:1918–1921.

136. Piirilä P, Estlander T, Keskinen H, Jolanki R, Laakkonen A, Pfäffli P, Tupasela O, Tuppurainen M, Nordman H. Occupational asthma caused by triglycidyl isocyanurate (TGIC). Clin Exp Allergy 1997; 27:510–514.

137. Hendrick DJ, Connolly MJ, Stenton SC, Bird AG, Winterton IS, Walters EH. Occupational asthma due to sodium iso-nonanoyl oxybenzene sulphonate, a newly developed detergent ingredient. Thorax 1988; 43:501–502.

138. Burge PS, Hendy M, Hodgson ES. Occupational asthma, rhinitis and dermatitis due to tetrazene in a detonator manufacturer. Thorax 1984; 39:470–471.

139. Waclawski ER, McAlpine LG, Thomson NC. Occupational asthma in nurses caused by chlorhexidine and alcohol aerosols. Br Med J 1989; 298:929–930.

140. Nagy L, Orosz M. Occupational asthma due to hexachlorophene. Thorax 1984; 39:630–631.

141. Bryant DH. Asthma due to insecticide sensitivity. Aust NZ J Med 1985; 15:66–68.

13

Occupational Asthma

Diagnostic Approaches and Treatment

JONATHAN A. BERNSTEIN and DAVID I. BERNSTEIN

University of Cincinnati College of Medicine
Cincinnati, Ohio

I. Introduction

The prevalence of occupational asthma appears to be increasing worldwide (1). It is estimated that 5–15% of all newly diagnosed cases of asthma are occupationally related (2). Therefore, the clinician should have a firm understanding of a rational approach to the diagnosis and management of occupational asthma. The diagnosis of occupational asthma (OA) requires an accurate and comprehensive occupational history, which can be facilitated by using specifically designed occupational lung disease questionnaires (3). The history should include information regarding the onset of the worker's symptoms, severity of symptoms, the work process, and correlation of symptoms to exposures in the workplace (3). Material safety data sheets (MSDSs) should be reviewed to identify potential causative agents in the workplace. The diagnosis of OA requires certain confirmatory and adjunctive testing, depending on the nature of the suspected inciting agent. When appropriate, specific skin testing for the suspected agent (especially natural proteins) should be conducted to confirm specific sensitization. Allergen skin testing to common seasonal and perennial allergens should be performed to investigate nonoccupational allergen triggers and to define atopic status (4). If valid tests are available for suspected inciting agents, specific serological testing can be useful. Assessment of obstructive lung changes should be performed by measuring changes in FEV_1 before and after the use of bronchodilators. Nonspecific bronchial hyperresponsiveness is determined by using methacholine or histamine bronchoprovocation protocols (3,4). Finally, correlation between exposure to the specific causative agent in the workplace and asthma should either be confirmed by serial peak expiratory flow rate (PEFR) monitoring at and away from the workplace or by a controlled laboratory bronchoprovocation challenge to the specific agent. This chapter discusses each element of the diagnostic evaluation of OA (3). Finally, a structured algorithmic approach is presented that is intended to provide the clinician with an organized approach to establishing or excluding a diagnosis of OA.

II. Occupational History

The diagnosis of OA requires a detailed and comprehensive history. An inadequate history can often delay the diagnosis of OA for months or years (3). To prevent omission of important historical data, administration of a physician-directed history in conjunction with a structured questionnaire is recommended. Table 1 outlines the key elements that should be included in the occupational history (3). The occupational history should elicit comprehensive demographic data about the worker; present and past employment history; the nature, duration, and temporal pattern of symptoms; and finally any potential risk factors for OA (3). It is essential that the physician be familiar with most of the known causative agents of OA (Table 2). (Also see Chaps. 11 and 12.)

Although questionnaires are essential, they have limitations. Malo and Cheung (5) reported that occupational questionnaires are sensitive but not specific and therefore cannot be used to make a diagnosis of OA without confirmatory objective testing. Table 3 summarizes the validity of occupational questionnaires used in several epidemiological surveys. The poor correlation between a history of OA and OA confirmed by specific challenge testing emphasizes the limitations of the medical history (5). While several itemized questionnaires have been used for obtaining an occupational history by different investigators, there is as yet no standardized instrument available for this purpose. However, several groups of experienced investigators have developed

Table 1 Key Elements of the Occupational History in the Evaluation of Occupational Asthma

---

I. Demographic information
  A. Identification and address.
  B. Personal data including sex, race, and age.
  C. Educational background with quantitation of the number of school years completed.
II. Employment history
  A. Current department and job description including dates begun, interrupted, and ended.
  B. List all other work processes and substances used in the employee's work environment. A schematic diagram of the workplace is helpful to identify indirect exposure to substances emanating from adjacent workstations.
  C. List prior jobs at current workplace with description of job, duration, and identification of material used.
  D. Work history describing employment preceding current workplace. Job descriptions and exposure history must be included.
III. Symptoms
  A. Categories
    1. Chest tightness, wheezing, cough, shortness of breath.
    2. Nasal rhinorrhea, sneezing, lacrimation, ocular itching.
    3. Systemic symptoms such as fever, arthralgias, and myalgias.
  B. Duration should be quantitated.
  C. Duration of employment at current job prior to onset of symptoms.
  D. Identify temporal pattern of symptoms in relationship to work.
    1. Immediate onset beginning at work with resolution soon after coming home.
    2. Delayed onset beginning 4–12 hr after starting work or after coming home.
    3. Immediate onset followed by recovery with symptoms recurring 4–12 hr after initial exposure to suspect agent at work.
  E. Improvement away from work.
IV. Identify potential risk factors
  A. Obtain a smoking history along with current smoking status and quantitate number of pack years.
  B. Asthmatic symptoms preceding current work exposure.
  C. Atopic status
    1. Identify consistent history of seasonal nasal or ocular symptoms.
    2. Family history of atopic disease.
    3. Confirmation by epicutaneous testing to a panel of common aeroallergens.
  D. History of accidental exposures to substances such as heated fumes or chemical spills.

Source: Ref. 2.

Table 2 Etiological Agents of Occupational Asthma and Reported Immunological Tests

Agent	In vivo	In vitro
Azodicarbonamide	Prick tests with 0.1, 1, and 5% azodicarbonamide	Not done
Baby's breath	Intradermal titration testing	RAST/histamine release
Bacillus subtilis enzymes	Prick tests with 0.05, 0.5, 5, and 10 mg/mL	RAST/radial immunodiffusion
Buckwheat flour	Prick test with 10 mg/mL	Reverse enzyme immunoassay/histamine release
Carmine dye	Skin test with *Coccus cactus*	RAST to dyes
Castor bean	Prick test with 1:100 extract	Not done
Chloramine-T, halazone	Scratch test at 10^{-5} dilution	Not done
Chromate	Prick test at 10, 5, 1, and 0.1 mg/mL $Cr_2(SO_4)_3$	RAST to HSA-chromium sulfate
Cobalt	Patch tests	
Coffee bean	Intradermal titration to coffee bean extract	RAST to coffee bean extract
Diazonium tetrafluoroborate (DTFB)	Not done	RAST to HSA-DTFB
Dimethylethanolamine	Prick tests to dimethylethanolamine undiluted at 1:10, 1:100, and 1:1000	Not done
Douglas fir tussock moth	Cutaneous tests with 1:25 extract	Histamine release
Dyes, textiles	Prick or scratch tests to dyes at 10 mg/mL in 50% glycerine	HSA-dye
Egg proteins	Prick tests with 1:10 w/v egg white, egg yolk, whole egg; prick tests to 10 mg/mL egg white fractions	RAST to egg proteins
Ethylenediamine	Intracutaneous test to 1:100 ethylenediamine	Not done
Furan binder	Not done	RAST to catalyst, sand, and furfuryl alcohol

Table 2 (*Continued*)

Agent	In vivo	In vitro
Garlic	Prick test titrations beginning at 10^{-5} garlic extract	PTRIA for IgE against garlic extract
Grain dust, grain dust mite	Prick and intracutaneous tests with grain dust and grain mite	Not done
Grain weevil	Skin test to weevil extract	Not done
Gum acacia	Skin tests with gum arabic	Not done
Guar gum	Prick tests with 1 mg/mL guar gum	RAST with guar gum
Hexamethylene-diisocyanate (HDI)	Prick tests to HSA-HDI	ELISA to HSA-HDI
Hexahydrophthalic anhydride (HHPA)	Not done	RAST to HSA-HHPA
Hog trypsin	Skin test to trypsin	Histamine release
Laboratory animals	Skin tests with serum and urine extracts from animals	ELISA
Latex	Prick test using low ammonia latex solution	Not done
Locusts	Prick tests with locust extract at 0.1, 1, and 10 mg/mL	ELISA
Mealworm	Prick test titration beginning at 1:20 w/v *Tenibrio molitor* (TM) extract	RAST to TM extract
Diphenol methane diisocyanate (MDI)	Prick test with 5 mg/mL HSA-MDI; intradermal test with 1 and 10 μg/mL	ELISA to HSA-MDI
Mushroom	Prick test with mushroom extract	Not done
Nickel	Prick tests with $NiSO_4$ at 100, 10, 5, 1, and 0.1 mg/mL	RAST to HSA-$NiSO_4$
Papain	Skin test with papain at 1.25–20 mg/mL	RAST to papain
Pancreatic extract	Prick tests with 1:100 and 1:1000 extracts	Not done

Table 2 (*Continued*)

Agent	In vivo	In vitro
Penicillin	Prick tests to ampicillin at 10^{-3} – 10^{-2} mol/L, benzyl penicilloyl polylysine at 10^{-6} mol/L, and minor determinants at 10^{-2} mol/L	Not done
Penicillamine	Prick tests with penicillamine, major and minor penicillin determinants at 0.01, 0.1, and 1 mg/mL	Not done
Phthalic anhydride (PA) and tetrachlorophthalic anhydride (TCPA)	Prick and intradermal tests to HSA-PA and HSA-TCPA	ELISA; PTRIA to HSA-PA only
Platinum	Prick tests with complex platinum salts from $10m^{-3}$ to 10^{-11} g/mL	RAST to $(NH_4)_2PtCl_2$, RAST to HSA-platinum, and histamine release
Poultry mites	Skin tests with 1:10 w/v northern fowl mite (NFM)	RAST to NFM
Protease bromelain	Prick test with bromelain at 10 mg/mL	RAST to bromelain
Redwood	Prick test to redwood sawdust extract	Not done
Spiramycin	Prick tests with 10 and 100 mg/mL spiramycin	Not done
Tobacco	Skin tests with green tobacco extract 10 mg/mL	RAST with green tobacco extract
Toluene diisocyanate (TDI)	Prick test to 5 mg/mL HSA-TDI	RAST and ELISA to HSA-TDI, histamine release
Trimellitic anhydride (TMA)	Prick tests to 3.4 mg/mL HSA-TMA and TMA in acetone	PTRIA with HSA-TMA
Western red cedar (WRC)	Prick tests with 25 mg/mL WRC extract; intracutaneous testing with 2.5 mg/mL WRC	Not done
Wheat flour	Prick tests with 10% w/v extract	RAST to wheat flour and wheat flour components

Source: Ref. 11.

questionnaires that have been validated by repeated use in cross-sectional or longitudinal studies (5).

The basic components of a structured occupational questionnaire include an employment history and medical history (5). The employment history should ascertain information regarding the individual's work process, including all jobs that could be related to specific exposures, work processes in adjacent areas, workshift hours, and previous jobs where the worker may have been exposed to similar or identical agents. The medical history should determine any relationship of symptoms experienced before, during, or after work to a specific exposure in the workplace, duration of symptoms after leaving the workplace, improvement of symptoms on weekends or vacations, associated upper respiratory and dermatological symptoms, systemic symptoms such as fever, chills, or temperature, smoking history, preexisting allergy/asthma history, and previous chemical spill exposure (3,5).

The classic presentation of a worker with OA often consists of symptoms that begin at work, resolve, or improve either shortly after leaving the workplace at night, during weekends, or while on vacation. However, a worker with OA may not improve away from the workplace because of chronic airway inflammation as a result of persistent workplace exposure to an agent for months or years after the initial onset of symptoms (6–8). In addition, patients with reactive airways dysfunction syndrome (RADS) typically do not improve away from work (9). Therefore, the diagnosis of OA should not be overlooked because of the apparent lack of correlation of symptoms to workplace exposure.

Material safety data sheets (MSDSs) are an essential part of the occupational history (3,4). They provide valuable information regarding generic chemical names and specific constituents of raw materials being used in the workplace. They also provide standard information about threshold limit values (TLVs) and permissible exposure levels (PELs) of potentially toxic and/or sensitizing agents (6). When available, assistance from industrial hygienists or safety officers familiar with the workplace and the worker's exposure history should be sought.

III. Differential Diagnosis

A diagnosis of OA can be incorrectly assigned to an individual with preexisting asthma or allergic asthma due to non-workplace allergens. In these cases, symptoms are aggravated by exposure to irritants, physical factors (e.g., cold air), or common indoor allergens (e.g., dust mites) in the workplace. However, it should be emphasized that preexisting asthma does not preclude the development of OA. At times, OA must also be distinguished from other diseases such as chronic obstructive lung disease, pneumoconiosis, bronchiolitis obliterans, and endotoxin-induced asthmalike syndromes such as grain fever or byssinosis (3,4). These disorders are differentiated from OA by history, chest X-ray, chest CAT scan, and lung volumes with diffusion capacity and, if necessary, by open lung biopsy. Chest X-rays and diffusing capacity for carbon monoxide (DLco) are usually normal in workers with OA (3–5).

IV. Immunological Assessment

Immunological mechanisms have been defined in many forms of OA. Therefore, it is important to attempt to measure specific immune responses to suspected agents that have allergenic potential. Identification of an immunological response to a specific agent is not diagnostic of OA (10). Such a response may only reflect exposure. Cutaneous sensitization to an offending agent indicates a high risk for OA but lacks the specificity needed to diagnose OA. Several types of immune responses have been associated with high molecular weight (HMW) and low molecular weight (LMW) agents that cause OA. Type I, IgE-mediated immune responses have been identified for the majority of HMW proteins derived from a variety of plant and animal sources known to cause OA. IgE-mediated immune responses have also been identified as the underlying mechanism for several LMW chemical agents such as acid anhydrides. Although Type II cytotoxic, Type III immune-complex, and Type IV cell-mediated immune responses have been linked to certain causes of OA, measures of specific IgE are the only tests that are useful in the diagnosis of OA (10).

High molecular weight antigens are considered complete allergens, because they do not require structural modification to induce and elicit a specific immune response (4,10). These allergens have been routinely used in performing in vivo skin testing and in vitro immunoassays in order to identify sensitized individuals. High molecular weight allergens include proteins from animal dander, insect scales, food products, and enzymes used in the food and pharmaceutical industries (4,10). Low molecular weight chemical agents require structural modification to act as complete antigens (4,10). Traditionally, these reactive chemicals are coupled to a carrier molecule such as an autologous human protein [e.g., human serum albumin (HSA)]. The chemical hapten–protein conjugate forms new antigenic determinants that are capable of binding of IgE (4,10).

It is important that the test reagents used in the diagnosis of OA be characterized and standardized. Standardization of an allergen extract requires identification of the allergen source, the extraction procedure, and its biochemical composition (10). The allergen source should be fresh and free of contaminants. The extraction process should record characteristics such as temperature, the medium used for extraction, the extraction time period, and the filtration methods utilized (10). Proper characterization should include total protein content, molecular weight range of proteins, isoelectric points of each protein, and identification of immunological and allergenic components (10). The latter can be determined by a variety of techniques such as RAST or ELISA inhibition assays, Western blotting, leukocyte histamine release assays, and endpoint skin test titration techniques (10).

Low molecular weight chemicals can be conjugated to a carrier protein and used as an antigen for use in immunodiagnostic tests (4,10). Platinum chloride salts and sulfonechloramide represent two examples where LMW agents have been directly used as skin test reagents without prior conjugation to proteins (11–13). The most common protein carrier used is human serum albumin (HSA). Successful hapten–protein conjugation depends on the buffers used, the amounts of protein and chemicals used, and the duration and temperature of the reaction (10). To determine the degree of chemical linkage to protein, the molecular ratio of chemical ligand to protein carrier must be established (4,10). This analysis is essential, because antigenicity and allergenicity of the final conjugate may vary with ligand density (4,10). The method of analysis depends on the chemical structure of the compound. For example, spectrophotometric analysis is used to assess aromatic compounds, and free amino analysis is used for chemicals that bind to carrier amines (10). Gas chromatography and mass spectroscopy are the preferred methods for analysis of aliphatic chemical–protein antigens. The ideal range of ligand binding should fall between 10 and 20 molecules of chemical per molecule of protein. Over- or underconjugation of ligand to protein binding can result in poor test antigens (10). The methods described for biochemical composition of HMW complete proteins can also be used for analysis of hapten–protein conjugates.

Clinical immunological assessment of workers suspected of having OA should include in vivo and in vitro tests when they are available. The skin prick test is the most commonly used in vivo test to assess IgE-mediated hypersensitivity responses to occupational protein allergens (3,4,10). The prick test concentration usually ranges between 0.1 and 10 mg/mL (10).

In vitro tests can detect specific IgG and IgE antibody responses to a suspected causative occupational agent (10). Radioallergosorbent tests (RAST) require binding of the specific allergen to a solid-phase material that is then incubated with the subject's serum and radiolabeled anti-human IgE (10). The number of radioisotopic counts bound is directly proportional to the amount of serum-specific IgE. The RAST test has been largely supplanted by the enzyme-linked immunosorbent assay (ELISA) because the latter does not require use of radioisotopes (10). This assay differs from the RAST in that the allergen is bound to a plastic well with high binding avidity and then incubated with the subject's serum and anti-human IgE conjugated to alkaline phosphatase. This results in a colorimetric change that is measured by spectrophotometry. The optical density is proportional to the amount of specific IgE in the subject's serum (10).

For natural protein allergens such as enzymes, ELISA IgE assays are specific assays albeit less sensitive than skin prick testing. False positive reactions can occur in the presence of high serum total IgE levels due to nonspecific binding, and false negatives can occur as the result of binding of a specific isotypic antibody other than IgE (10).

ELISA assays are also used to measure specific IgG antibodies. The significance of elevated specific IgG antibodies to a workplace allergen is not entirely clear. There is some evidence to suggest that it could represent a biological marker to chemicals such as MDI (14,15). Specific IgG antibodies to TMA-HSA conjugated antigens have been found in trimellitic anhydride-exposed workers with hemolytic anemia and pulmonary hemorrhage as well as in workers with late systemic symptoms, suggesting that such antibodies may have a mechanistic role in cytotoxic or immune complex mediated responses (16).

The proper interpretation of an immunological test used in the diagnosis of OA requires validation against an accepted benchmark such as the specific bronchoprovocation test (SBPT). Proper standardization of an immunoassay requires the use of well-established positive and negative control sera (17).

Other in vitro assays such as lymphocyte proliferation and leukocyte histamine release have been used primarily as research tools in the investigation of workers with OA (10). Table 2 lists several high and low molecular weight agents known to induce OA in workers and the reported immunological tests that have been performed as part of their assessment (10). It should be emphasized that skin test responses and in vitro specific antibody responses can decline within months or years after removal from exposure from the causative agent, which may limit their clinical utility in the evaluation of workers remotely exposed to an incriminated agent (18,19).

V. Physiological Assessment

Many approaches have been used in measuring lung function in workers suspected of OA. Ideally, lung function should be monitored in the workplace during a known exposure to a suspected causative agent (5). However, this may present logistical problems when conditions in the workplace are not suitable for pulmonary function testing. Often, personnel experienced in proper performance of pulmonary function testing are not readily available to conduct serial testing of lung function (5).

Spirometry should include the forced expiratory volume in 1 sec (FEV_1), forced vital capacity (FVC), and the maximum midexpiratory flow rate (FEF_{25-75}). Assessment of cross-shift lung function (i.e., pre- and post-shift FEV_1) has been used to assess correlation of asthma symptoms to the workplace, but this approach lacks sensitivity for confirming OA. Multiple assessments of PEFR during a workday (four or five times a day) are more likely to capture enough data to diagnose or exclude OA (5). Cross-shift changes in a worker's lung function have been found to be directly proportional to the levels of exposure to the sensitizing agent (20).

Serial measurements of peak expiratory flow rates (PEFRs), when performed properly and reliably, have been demonstrated to correlate moderately well with results of specific bronchoprovocation testing in the diagnosis of OA (21,22). Serial PEFR measurements should be interpreted with caution due to patient noncompliance or the potential for falsification of measurements (5,23). These problems may be circumvented by using computerized peak flow meters or spirometers that record the exact measurement and time of the reading.

Although not diagnostic, nonspecific bronchial hyperresponsiveness (NSBH) testing with agonists such as methacholine or histamine may be used for confirming the presence or absence of asthma (3–5). A positive methacholine challenge test alone is not diagnostic of OA. Subjects with a positive methacholine test and evidence of specific IgE to an HMW agent are more likely to exhibit a positive SBPT to that agent (24,25). Negative tests of NSBH are most useful in excluding a current diagnosis of OA in a symptomatic currently exposed worker (3–5).

The specific bronchoprovocation test is the gold standard for confirming a diagnosis of OA. These tests should be administered only in specially equipped centers and supervised by expert physicians (5). Specific provocation testing is time-consuming and expensive. If performed properly, the SBPT can be performed with minimal risk (5). Several patterns of airway responses may be elicited in workers with OA. An isolated early asthmatic response (EAR) is characterized by the immediate onset of asthma symptoms after exposure to an agent. This response is usually, but not exclusively, associated with IgE-mediated OA (4,26). An isolated late asthmatic response (LAR), which occurs 4–12 hr after exposure to the challenge agent, is characteristic of nonimmunological

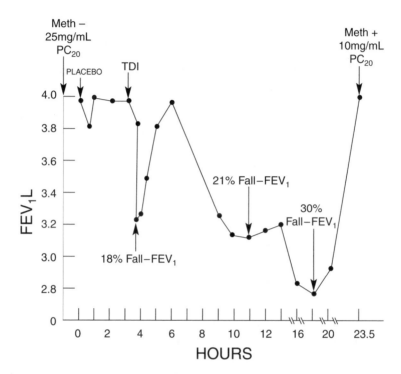

Figure 1 A dual asthmatic response in a polyurethane foam worker after bronchoprovocation to toluene diisocyanate (TDI). The early asthmatic response is followed by spontaneous recovery and then a late asthmatic response. The concentration of methacholine required to reduce the forced expiratory volume in 1 sec (FEV_1) by 20% (PC_{20}) fell from a baseline of 25 mg/mL to 10 mg/mL the day after the TDI challenge. (From Ref. 4.)

OA induced by LMW chemical agents (26). Finally, workers with OA may exhibit a dual asthmatic response (DAR) characterized by an EAR followed by a recovery period and then an LAR. Figure 1 is an example of a DAR in a worker diagnosed with diisocyanate-induced OA (4). Multiple patterns have been observed in OA caused by chemicals. For example, workers with diisocyanate-induced OA present with DARs in 30–50% of cases and an isolated LAR in the remainder of the cases. An isolated EAR is rarely encountered (26).

Asthma occurring in the workplace in the absence of a latency period is characteristic of reactive airways dysfunction syndrome (RADS), also referred to as irritant-induced OA (27,28). RADS typically occurs after one or repetitive large inhalational exposures to a toxic chemical agent such as ammonia gas, acidic fumes, smoke, or spray paints. RADS must be differentiated from the irritant symptoms that occur in patients with preexistent asthma (28). Irritant symptoms disappear promptly after cessation of exposure and are not associated with prolonged bronchoconstriction or bronchial hyperresponsiveness, which is characteristic of RADS. Workers with RADS typically do not manifest airway response patterns seen with OA induced by HMW and LMW agents. Familiarity with the different airway responses that occur with various agents known to cause OA can greatly facilitate the assessment of OA.

VI. Clinical Assessment of Occupational Asthma

Figure 2 summarizes an algorithmic approach for the clinical assessment of OA (3). This guideline can be used only for those workers with work-related symptoms who are currently exposed to suspect causative agents at work. The first step is a careful physician-administered history. As mentioned, an occupational questionnaire is useful in capturing the necessary clinical and exposure information (3). Workers with OA may present with dyspnea, chest tightness, wheezing, and/or cough. Upper airway symptoms such as rhinorrhea, nasal congestion, or ocular pruritus preceding the onset of asthmatic symptoms are characteristic of IgE-mediated sensitization to HMW agents (3). Symptoms may begin either immediately after starting a workshift (within 1–2 hr) or after several hours at work. Review of material safety data sheets (MSDSS) is essential for identifying any agents known to cause OA (3).

If the history is positive for OA, then a test of NSBH (i.e., methacholine or histamine provocation) should be performed at work or within 2 hr after the workshift. Results of this test are usually reported as PC_{20} measurements (provocative concentration of methacholine or histamine causing a 20% decrease in FEV_1). A negative methacholine test ($PC_{20} > 15$ mg/mL) would exclude asthma, and no further evaluation would be necessary. A positive methacholine test is consistent with asthma but is nonspecific and does not by itself confirm a diagnosis of OA. In this case, assessment of lung function performed at and away from the workplace is essential for making a diagnosis of OA. If possible, supervised measurements of lung function (i.e., FEV_1) should be made at the actual worksite before and during workshifts for at least 1 week of work exposure. This is referred to as a workplace challenge. Improvement of symptoms and lung function after removal from the workplace with subse-

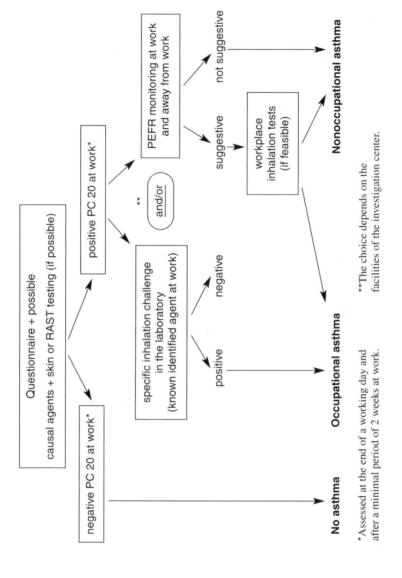

Figure 2 An algorithmic approach for the assessment and diagnosis of occupational asthma. (From Ref. 3.)

quent deterioration after reintroduction into the workplace supports a diagnosis of OA except in the case of RADS (3).

If a workplace challenge cannot be performed, peak expiratory flow rate monitoring should be conducted over 2–3 weeks at work. The worker should measure and record his or her PEFR every 3 hr while awake or at least four times a day (3). Work exposure, symptoms, and medication usage should be recorded over this time. A diurnal variability of greater than 20% at work compared to normal variability at home is consistent with OA (3). Visual analysis of weekly plots of PEFR measurements by a blinded physician is the most reliable method of analysis. A consistent pattern of declining PEFRs at work and improvement away from work confirms a diagnosis of OA. Peak expiratory flow rate measurements should be interpreted with caution in that there could be potential falsification of readings by a worker seeking compensation.

The gold standard for the diagnosis of OA is the specific bronchoprovocation test (SBPT) (3–5). If a specific substance in the workplace is suspected of causing OA and the workplace challenge is equivocal, an SBPT may be necessary. The PC_{20} ascertained by methacholine or histamine testing may be helpful for estimating the initial dose of an occupational agent prior to the specific inhalation challenge test (3,5). Because these tests are very time-consuming and potentially risky, they should be performed only by experienced individuals. An SBPT should not be performed in workers with severe cardiac or pulmonary disease ($FEV_1 < 60\%$) (3). Specific inhalation challenge tests have also been used to document causation of OA by new substances in index cases and for medical or legal purposes in proving or excluding a worker's eligibility for workmen's compensation. As indicated in Figure 2, although specific challenge tests confirm a diagnosis of OA if positive, negative tests do not always exclude the diagnosis in workers who have been removed from the workplace for a period of time during which bronchial sensitivity to the suspected agent may have been lost (3). It is therefore important to perform an SBPT either before or shortly after removing the worker from exposure in the workplace. Another potential problem with specific inhalation challenge testing is the lack of use of standardized methods among different centers. It may also be impossible to reproduce work exposure conditions in the laboratory, as a number of technical factors such as temperature, atmospheric pressure, and concentration must be controlled in order to ensure consistent exposures to chemical agents (e.g., toluene diisocyanate). Ideally, standardized methodologies should be adapted by laboratories that perform inhalational challenges in the future (5).

In addition to lung function assessment, it is important to identify whether the worker is atopic by skin testing with common aeroallergens and other appropriate allergens, especially when HMW substances are suspected of causing OA. These workers can often be skin tested with the actual antigen they are exposed to, such as flour, coffee beans, castor beans, and egg enzymes (Table 3). In vitro assays to measure specific IgE to these proteins can also be performed but are less specific than *in vivo* skin testing. It should be emphasized that the presence of either positive skin prick tests or specific IgE in the serum only indicates IgE-mediated sensitization and does not prove a clinical diagnosis of OA (3).

Immunological testing by RAST or ELISA methods using serum from workers exposed to LMW reactive chemicals is also useful for supporting IgE-mediated respiratory sensitization when present. IgG antibodies may represent markers of exposure to a particular chemical antigen. In vivo skin testing to LMW chemical agents has been less reliable for confirming IgE-mediated sensitization. Other techniques, such a leukocyte histamine release and leukocyte inhibitory factor, have been reserved for research purposes (Table 3) (3,10).

Table 3   Validity of Questionnaires in Various Epidemiological Surveys

Agent workplace	Number of participating/total workers	Number of workers with a history suggestive of OA	Number of workers with OA(%)[a]
Guar gum	162/177	37	3(8%)
Carpet manufacturer			
Snow crab	303/313	64	33(52%)
Snow crab processors			
Spiramycin	51/51	12	3(25%)
Pharmaceutical company			
Psyllium	130/140	39	5(13%)
Pharmaceutical company			
Psyllium	197/252	79	8(10%)
Chronic care nurses			
Isocyanates	48/48	14	6(43%)
Paint shops			

[a]Percent of those with a history suggestive of OA with diagnosis confirmed with specific inhalational challenge and/or serial peak expiratory flow rate monitoring.
Source: Ref. 4.

VII. Treatment

Once the diagnosis of OA has been confirmed, treatment should be directed toward removing the worker from further exposure (3–5). Studies evaluating the clinical course of workers after removal from exposure have found that the persistence of their asthma frequently depended on the duration of symptoms prior to diagnosis. Individuals with OA caused by diisocyanates or western red cedar wood dust had a better prognosis if they were diagnosed early with relatively preserved lung function and a lesser degree of NSBH (7,8,29). By contrast, symptomatic workers who remained in the workplace for longer periods of time experienced deterioration in lung function and chronic persistent asthma with increased medication requirements (4). Use of respirators in the work environment generally does not reduce exposure or prevent clinical deterioration. Some studies have suggested that certain types of respirators such as airstream helmets may offer the worker adequate protection from the offending agent. However, they are generally not considered to be adequate substitutes for absolute avoidance measures (4). Pharmacological treatment of acute or chronic OA is similar to nonoccupational asthma, which involves selective β_2-agonists, theophylline, cromolyn or nedocromil sodium, and inhaled and systemic corticosteroids in various combinations depending on the severity of the worker's symptoms (3,4). In the future, immunotherapy may play a role in the treatment of some forms of OA caused by protein allergens such as laboratory animal proteins, latex proteins, and shellfish (e.g., oysters) (10).

VIII. Prevention

Effective prevention of OA requires cooperation between management and workers in the implementation of good industrial measures aimed at preventing human exposure to agents that have the potential for causing OA. Every attempt should be made to minimize a worker's exposure to potentially problematic agent(s) through the institution of strict handling procedures. Workers should be continually educated about the importance of adhering to those procedures that avoid large chemical spills (3,4). Prescreening of already hired workers for atopy should be considered before assigning employees to jobs that involve inhalational exposure to proteins (e.g., latex, laboratory animal proteins, and enzymes). Comprehensive immunosurveillance programs for detecting and monitoring workers at increased risk for exposure to known inducers of OA need to be implemented in industries that commonly use agents known to cause OA (3,4). Industries that have implemented such comprehensive immunosurveillance programs have been successful in significantly reducing the incidence of OA in the workplace (30).

References

1. Harber P. Decreasing work disability from asthma. WJM 1996; 165(3):142–143.
2. Blane PD, Cisternas M, Smith S, Yelin E. Occupational asthma in a community-based survey of adult asthma. Chest 1996; 109(3):56S–57S.
3. Bernstein DI. Clinical assessment and management of occupational asthma. In: Bernstein IL, Chan-Yeung M, Malo J-L, Bernstein DI, eds. Asthma in the Workplace. New York: Marcel Dekker, 1993:103–123.
4. Bernstein JA, Bernstein DI, Bernstein IL. Occupational asthma. In: Bierman CW, Pearlman DS, Shapiro GG, Busse W, eds. Asthma and Immunology in Infancy to Adulthood. 3rd ed. Philadelphia: WD Saunders, 1996:529–548.
5. Malo J-L, Chan-Yeung M. Population surveys of occupational asthma. In: Bernstein IL, Chan-Yeung M, Malo J-L, Bernstein DI, eds. Asthma in the Workplace. New York: Marcel Dekker, 1993:145–170.
6. Chan H, tech ed. NIOSH Pocket Guide to Chemical Hazards. Washington, DC: US Department of Health & Human Services, 1997.
7. Park H-S, Nahm D-H. Prognostic factors for toluene diisocyanate-induced occupational asthma after removal from exposure. Clin Exp Allergy 1997; 27:1145–1150.
8. Lin FJ, Dimich-Ward H, Chan-Yeung M. Longitudinal decline in lung function in patients with occupational asthma due to western red cedar. Occup Environ Med 1996; 53:753–756.
9. Brooks SM, Bernstein IL. Reactive airways dysfunction syndrome or irritant-induced asthma. In: Bernstein IL, Chan-Yeung M, Malo J-L, Bernstein DI, eds. Asthma in the Workplace. New York: Marcel Dekker, 1993:533.
10. Grammar LC, Patterson R. Immunologic evaluation of occupational asthma. In: Bernstein IL, Chan-Yeung M, Malo J-L, Bernstein DI, eds. Asthma in the Workplace. New York: Marcel Dekker, 1993:125–143.
11. Pepys J, Pickering CA, Hughes EG. Asthma due to inhaled chemical agents: complex salts of platinum. Clin Allergy 1972; 2:391–396.
12. Feinberg SM, Watrous RM. Atopy to simple compounds: sulfonechloramides. J Allergy 1945; 16:209–220.
13. Biagini RE, Bernstein IL, Gallagher JS, Moorman WJ, Brooks S, Gann PH. The diversity of reaginic immune responses to platinum and palladium metallic. J Allergy Clin Immunol 1985; 76:794.
14. Lushniak BD, Reh CM, Gallagher JS, et al. Indirect assessment of exposure to MDI by evaluation of specific immune responses to MDI-HSA in foam workers. J Allergy Clin Immunol 1990; 85:251.

15. Biagini RE, Klincewicz SL, Henningsen GM, MacKenzie BA, Gallagher JS, Bernstein DI, Bernstein IL. Antibodies to morphine in workers exposed to opiates at a narcotics manufacturing facility and evidence for similar antibodies in heroin abusers. Life Sci 1990; 47(10):897–908.

16. Zeiss CR, Patterson R, Pruzansky JJ, Miller MM, Rosenberg M, Levitz D. Trimellitic anhydride-induced airway syndrome: clinical and immunologic studies. J Allergy Clin Immunol 1997; 60:96–103.

17. Sarlo K, Carl ED, Ryan CA, Bernstein DI. ELISA for human IgE antibody to subtilisin A (Alcalase): correlation with RAST and skin test results with occupationally exposed individuals. J Allergy Clin Immunol 1990; 86:393–399.

18. Venables KM, Topping MD, Nunn AJ, Howe W, Newman-Taylor AJ. Immunological and function consequences of clinical tetrachlorophthalic anhydride induced asthma after four years of avoidance of exposure. J Allergy Clin Immunol 1987; 80:212–218.

19. Malo JL, Cartier A, Ghezzo H, Lafrance M, Mccants M, Lehrer SB. Patterns of improvement on spirometry, bronchial hyperresponsiveness and specific IgE antibody levels after cessation of exposure in occupational asthma caused by snow-crab processing. Am Rev Respir Dis 1988; 138:807–812.

20. Enarson DA, Chan-Yeung M. Determinants of FEV_1 changes over a workshift. Br J Ind Med 1985; 42:202–204.

21. Cote J, Kennedy S, Chan-Yeung M. Sensitivity and specificity of PC_{20} and peak expiratory flow rate in cedar asthma. J Allergy Clin Immunol 1990; 85:592–598.

22. Perrin B, Malo JL, L'Archeveque J, Ghezzo H, Lagier F, Cartier A. Comparison of monitoring of peak expiratory flow rates and bronchial responsiveness with specific inhalation challenges in occupational asthma. Am Rev Respir Dis 1990; 141:A79.

23. Cartier A, Malo JL, Forest F, Lafrance M, Pineau L, St.-Aubin JJ, Dubois JY. Occupational asthma in snow crab-processing workers. J Allergy Clin Immunol 1984; 74:261–269.

24. Malo JL, Cartier A, L'Archeveque J, Ghezzo H, Lagier F, Trudeau C, Dolovich J. Prevalence of occupational asthma and immunological sensitization to psyllium among health personnel in chronic care hospitals. Am Rev Respir Dis 1990; 142:1359–1366.

25. Cockcroft D, Ruffin R, Frith P, Cartier A, Juniper EF, Dolovich J, Hargreave FE. Determinants of allergen-induced asthma: dose of allergen, circulating IgE antibody concentration, and bronchial responsiveness to inhaled histamine. Am Rev Respir Dis 1979; 120:1053–1058.

26. Bernstein JA. Overview of diisocyanate occupational asthma. Toxicology 1996; 111:181–189.

27. Brooks S, Weiss MA, Bernstein IL. Reactive airways dysfunction syndrome: persistent asthma syndrome after high-level irritant exposure. Chest 1985; 88:376–384.

28. Brooks SM, Bernstein IL. Reactive airways dysfunction syndrome or irritant-

induced asthma. In: Bernstein IL, Chan-Yeung M, Malo J-L, Bernstein DI, eds. Asthma in the Workplace. New York: Marcel Dekker, 1993:533–549.

29.   Lemiere C, Cartier A, Dolovich J, Chan-Yeung M, Grammar L, Ghezzo M, L'Archeveque J, Malo JL. Outcome of specific bronchial responsiveness to occupational agents after removal from exposure. Am J Respir Crit Care Med 1996; 154:329–333.

30.   Bernstein DI, Korbee L, Stauder T, Bernstein JA, Scinto J, Herd ZL, Bernstein IL. The low prevalence of occupational asthma and antibody-dependent sensitization to diphenylmethane diisocyanate in a plant engineered for minimal exposure to diisocyanates. J Allergy Clin Immunol 1993; 92:387–396.

14

Specific Immunotherapy in Asthma

PASCAL DEMOLY, FRANÇOIS-BERNARD MICHEL, and JEAN BOUSQUET

University Medical School and
Hôpital Arnaud de Villeneuve
Montpellier, France

I. Introduction

Asthma and allergies are among the most common chronic diseases. Allergen immunotherapy is the practice of administering gradually increasing quantities of an allergen extract to an allergic subject to ameliorate the symptoms associated with the subsequent exposure to the causative allergen (1). Allergen immunotherapy was introduced to treat allergic rhinitis by Noon in 1911 (2). Since then, immunotherapy has been used to treat allergic diseases caused by inhalant allergens.

The role of inhalant allergens has been clearly demonstrated in the pathogenesis of asthma (3,4), but the importance of specific immunotherapy (SIT) in its treatment is still controversial (5,6) despite a meta-analysis by Abramson et al. (7). Guidelines and indications for immunotherapy with inhalant allergens have been published within the past decade (8–14). A WHO position paper on SIT published in 1998 (1) defines indications for asthma.

II. Objectives of Immunotherapy

Asthma is a multifactorial and complex disease in which allergenic factors and nonallergenic triggers interact and result in bronchial obstruction and inflammation. The inhalation of allergens leads to a complex activation of various types of cells and the release of proinflammatory mediators; however, two different situations seem to exist. Although very few pollen grains can reach the lower airways, these allergens carried on submicrometric particles frequently induce asthma via an IgE-mediated mechanism. Pollen-induced allergic reactions occurring over several days almost always lead to nonspecific bronchial hyperreactivity (BHR). This BHR is usually transient in patients allergic only to pollens and generally lasts from a few weeks to a few months after the end of the pollen season. On the other hand, house dust mites and other perennial allergens induce a long-sustained inflammation of the bronchi leading to a variable degree of nonspecific bronchial hyperreactivity (BHR) and symptoms. It has been shown that patients with chronic asthma present airways remodeling (15). Inflammation and airways remodeling may be involved in the "accelerated decline" of the pulmonary function characterized by a poorly reversible bronchial obstruction appearing after some decades of ongoing chronic asthma (16) as well as permanent bronchial wall alterations as shown by CT scans. It is therefore proposed that immunological and anti-inflammatory treatments should be associated, but after a long course of the disease, inflammation becomes the major cause of symptoms, suggesting that the immunological treatment should then be replaced by anti-inflammatory drugs. However, the airways remodeling in asthma may differ according to the etiology of the disease. It has been shown that patients with intrinsic asthma have a steeper rate of decline of the pulmonary function than those with extrinsic asthma (17).

The natural history of asthma in children is not completely known, but a large proportion of children with episodic mild asthma will outgrow their symptoms within several years, whereas in those with a more severe form of the disease, asthma will persist later in life (18).

These considerations suggest that (1) SIT may be more rapidly effective in patients allergic to grass pollen than in those sensitized to perennial allergens, (2) after a long course of the disease, patients with perennial asthma may have permanent airways abnormalities that cannot be reversed by SIT, and (3) grass pollen allergy may be an adequate model to study the effects of SIT in patients with normal bronchi whereas SIT in mite allergy may be used to examine the effects of the treatment in patients with a variable degree of bronchial inflammation and damage.

The major objectives of immunological treatment are, in the short term, to reduce the allergic triggers precipitating symptoms and, in the long term, to decrease bronchial inflammation and BHR when it is not too severe and when bronchial damage is not prominent. Moreover, at present, SIT appears to be the only treatment that might modify the course of the disease either by preventing the development of new sensitivities or by altering the natural history of asthma.

III. Mechanisms of SIT in Asthma

Recent studies have provided insight into the mechanisms of this form of treatment. Whereas earlier work focused on circulating antibody and effector cells, recent studies suggest that these changes may be secondary to an influence of SIT on T-cell response to allergen. Most work has examined allergen injection immunotherapy rather than SIT by alternative routes. Mechanisms are likely to be heterogeneous depending on the nature of the allergen; the site of allergy; the route, dose, and duration of immunotherapy; the use of different adjuvants; and, not least, the genetic background of the host.

A. Modification of Serum Immunoglobulins

During SIT, one frequently observes an initial rise of specific serum IgE levels followed, after several months or even years of treatment, by a reduction, rarely lower than the starting levels (except during SIT to *Hymenoptera* venom) and a blockage of pollen season induced elevation of specific IgE titers (20).

During SIT, one also frequently observes a rise in specific IgG levels, the so-called IgG blocking antibodies reported to "capture" allergens before they reach the mast cell bound IgE (13,21).

This theory has led to attempts to explain the efficacy of desensitization by the development of subtypes of IgG (22) or via increases in IgA or IgG secretion, but to date no precise correlation has been found (23). IgG may, however, modulate the immune reaction via an intermediary of the network idiotype–anti-idiotype (24).

These immunoglobulin variations certainly do not explain the benefits of SIT for subjects with allergy to inhaled allergens.

B. Reduction of Inflammation and Immunotherapy in Cells and Tissues

When effective, SIT is accompanied by a reduction in cutaneous (25,26), bronchial (27,28), nasal (28–30), and ocular reactivity to the allergen provocation tests, with an increased quantity of allergen necessary to provoke a reaction in the target organ and a reduction in inflammatory mediator release (31,32) and in cellular recruitment (33,34).

Tissue hyposensitization appears rapidly when the dose is sufficient, disappears after a period of several months or a few years when SIT is stopped, does not correlate with levels of allergen-specific serum immunoglobulins (IgE or IgG) (35), but often correlates with clinical improvements (36).

Moreover, a reduction in cellular reactivity to the allergen has been shown during SIT for blood basophils, platelets (37), eosinophils (38–40), and blood mononuclear cells, among them T cells (41–43). In patients who have not received SIT, one observes an increase in the levels of eosinophil cationic protein (ECP) in the serum (38) as well as a chemotactic activity toward eosinophils (40), the appearance of these two substances being blocked in desensitized subjects. The same author also demonstrated the reduction of pulmonary inflammation during desensitization to extracts of birch pollen (41).

The mechanisms underlying this cellular and tissue hyposensitization are, however, poorly understood at present, possibly involving cytokines and histamine-releasing factors (42) and T-cell subclass modulation.

C. Modulation of the Lymphocyte Subclass

The synthesis of IgE is governed by the powerful action of T cells (helper and suppressor) on the B lymphocytes carrying the membrane IgE. Over the past few years, cytokines have radically changed our understanding of the synthesis of IgE. The interleukins IL-4, IL-13, and IL-5 facilitate the synthesis of IgE, while the interferons IFN-γ and IFN-α inhibit it. At the same time, there is a modulation of proinflammatory cytokines released by T cells and also by mast cells and basophils.

Studies of allergen-induced late responses in the skin (44) and nose (45) have indicated that SIT results in a reduction in local eosinophilia as well as in CD4[+] cell recruitment. These changes were accompanied by increases in a subpopulation of Th1 CD4[+] cells expressing IFN-γ mRNA transcripts after allergen provocation, whereas cells expressing mRNA for IL-4 and IL-5 remained unchanged, which closely correlated with the clinical response to SIT (45). Studies of late cutaneous biopsies suggested that these responses may be amplified or sustained by local production of IL-12, a potent inducer of Th1 responses. The cell source of IL-12 was identified as the tissue macrophage (CD68[+]) (46). An alternative explanation for these observed increases in IFN-γ+ cells may be the generation of allergen-specific CD8[+] T cells (47,48), inasmuch as increases in CD8[+] cells have been observed in both peripheral blood (47) and tissue (44) following conventional SIT.

Studies of T-cell lines (allergen-specific polyclonal T cells) and clones provide further support for a shift in T-cell responses, following SIT with a decrease in IL-4 and increase in IFN-γ in grass- and mite-desensitized patients (51,52).

The mechanisms of this cytokine switch is still a matter of debate. It seems likely that allergen SIT acts by modifying T-cell responses either by immune deviation (increase in Th0/Th1) (49) or T-cell anergy (decrease in Th2/Th0) (53,54), or more likely both, depending on a number of factors including the nature of the allergen, the allergen dose (52), adjuvants used, etc. Nevertheless, further studies are required, in particular to identify more "targeted" strategies, which are both more efficacious and safe.

Studies in tissues suggest that immune deviation may be more relevant (43–45). CD28 expression by blood mononuclear cells following venom SIT is not downregulated as it should be if anergy had occurred, again consistent with immune deviation (55). However, Akdis et al. (56,57) demonstrated a decrease in allergen (phospholipase A_2) specific proliferation and reduced production of both IFN-γ and IL-4 in vitro by T-cell lines following venom SIT. These responses were allergen-specific and reversible by addition of either IL-2 or IL-15, providing the first evidence for "anergy" following SIT in humans, although its mechanism in nonatopic subjects may be different from that involved for inhalant allergens in atopic patients.

IV. Allergenic Preparations

Allergenic extracts (vaccines) and products have been defined. "Allergenic extract" means a preparation of an allergen obtained by extraction of the active constituents from animal or vegetable substances with a suitable menstruum. "Allergenic product" means a biological product, including allergenic extracts and others, that is administered to humans for diagnosis, prevention, and treatment of allergy and allergenic diseases (58). In the European Pharmacopoeia (59).

> Allergen products are pharmaceutical preparations which are derived from extracts of naturally occurring source materials containing allergens, which are substances that cause and/or provoke allergic (hypersensitivity) disease. The allergenic components are most often of a proteinaceous nature. Allergen products are intended for in vivo diagnosis and/or treatment of allergic hypersensitivity diseases attributed to these allergens.

Successful immunotherapy is dependent on the production of high quality allergen extract vaccines that are properly standardized and can be manufactured with consistency. The WHO recommendation on allergen standardization was adapted largely for the recently approved position statements of the

EAACI (60) and AAAAI (61). Both European and U.S. recommendations require measurements of total allergenic potency and biological activity as well as encouraging major allergen measurements and the gradual adoption of mass units for allergens.

The rapid development of new technologies for both DNA and protein analysis offers opportunities for improved standardization. Many important allergens from pollen, dust mites, animal danders, insects, and foods have now been cloned and are being expressed as homogeneous recombinant proteins that, in several cases, have comparable allergenic activity to the natural protein allergen (for review see Ref. 62). With these new technologies, an allergen extract can be characterized in terms of major allergen content (in nanograms or micrograms), and the consistency of each lot can be accurately monitored. Such measurements will facilitate objective comparisons of allergen extracts (63–66). Measurements of allergens in mass units is favored by the recent WHO position paper on SIT (1).

Standardized allergens are often available in a lyophilized form that is very stable and represents a marked advance in allergology (67). The standard allergens are certainly high quality products; however, if they are inappropriately used they may cause secondary systemic reactions that can be very severe.

Nonstandardized allergens in aqueous solutions have been used for decades, require frequent injections, and run the risk of causing unforeseen systemic reactions that are sometimes violent. It is strongly recommended that the dose of allergen administered be reduced when material is taken from a new vial. In about 1955, the use of so-called delayed forms of allergens, prepared either by absorption of the extract on aluminum then calcium salts or by modifying the extraction of the allergen by pyridine, for example, was suggested to address two of the principal defects of nonstandardized aqueous allergens. The use of allergens absorbed on aluminum or calcium phosphate is still proposed, and they are now often prepared from standardized extracts. They are efficient, but a desorption of allergens from aluminum exists and is not controlled. These extracts are therefore not completely safe.

Allergen extract vaccines should be distributed, provided their potency, composition, and stability have been documented as (1)

1. Extracts from a single source material.
2. Mixtures of related cross-reacting allergen extracts such as grass pollen extracts, deciduous tree pollen extracts, related ragweed allergen extracts, and related mite allergen extracts.

3. Mixtures of other allergen extracts provided that stability data and data on clinical efficacy are available. Where mixtures are marketed, the relative amount of each component of the mixture should be indicated.

V. Efficacy and Safety of Subcutaneous SIT

Studies used to assess the efficacy of immunotherapy should fulfill the following criteria (1)

1. Double-blind, placebo-controlled randomized study.
2. Study published in English as a full paper in a peer-reviewed journal.
3. Patients selected according to well-defined clinical criteria and a specific allergy diagnosis.
4. Allergen extract vaccines defined. If possible, the extract should be standardized and the dose(s) or major allergen defined. This latter requirement is not available for most studies carried out before 1990. It was observed for grass pollen immunotherapy that the extract should contain all the active proteins, not only major allergens (68). However, for ragweed pollen immunotherapy, a single major allergen, Amb a1, was found to be equally as effective as the whole ragweed pollen extract (69).
5. An optimal maintenance dose. It has been shown that low-dose immunotherapy is ineffective (70–72) and that high doses of allergen extract vaccines were inducing a high and unacceptable rate of systemic reactions. Thus, optimal doses using extracts labeled either in biological units (73,74) or in mass of major allergens (75) have been proposed. The optimal dose may be defined as the dose of allergen extract vaccine that induces a clinically relevant effect in the majority of patients without causing unacceptable side effects (76,77). The optimal dose should be targeted for maintenance for all patients (73), because it has been shown that a dose of 5–20 µg of major allergen is required for domestic mites (73,77,78), cat dander (79,80), ragweed pollen (81–83), or *Hymenoptera* venoms (84,85). However, systemic side effects in some patients will require adjustment of the goal. The majority of patients with allergic diseases can reach this target without difficulty. In selected individuals who have experienced reactions during their buildup phase, a slower schedule or a

lower dose may be necessary. As with any therapeutic approach, the benefit-to-risk ratio must be carefully weighed in order to determine whether immunotherapy should be maintained.

6. A sufficient duration of treatment. The magnitude of efficacy was related to the duration of the treatment in some studies (86,87), although efficacy was demonstrated during the first year of treatment in many others (88,89).

7. Statistical analysis and reported data of the clinical efficacy.

Immunotherapy is specific to the antigen administered (90,91) and requires a complete allergy diagnosis before it is started.

Since allergens interact with nasal, bronchial and ocular mucosa, it seems appropriate to consider the efficacy of immunotherapy by allergen species rather than by allergic disease.

A. Pollen Asthma

Efficacy

Only a few controlled studies have investigated the efficacy of SIT in grass pollen asthma. Some studies have consistently demonstrated that patients receiving SIT had an improvement of the $PD_{20}FEV_1$ (provocative dose inducing a 20% decrease in FEV_1) to allergen (92–94). Most recent studies carried out during the pollen season using aqueous or standardized extracts or formaldehyde allergoids have shown that SIT has a beneficial effect on bronchial symptoms, but only when optimal conditions are used (32,68,95–106). These conclusions were restricted to grass, mountain cedar, *Parietaria,* and birch pollen allergy, but similar favorable results were more recently observed for ragweed pollen asthma in the NIH collaborative study.

During the pollen season, patients with asthma often present an increased BHR. The effect of SIT on bronchial reactivity measured by methacholine was investigated in patients with birch pollen asthma (104). Untreated patients had a decreased $PD_{20}FEV_1$ to methacholine, whereas those who received SIT did not present a significant decrease of $PD_{20}FEV_1$. This study also showed that eosinophilic inflammation was decreased in subjects receiving SIT.

Sensitization of the Patients

The benefits of SIT are specific for the allergen(s) used in treatment, and some studies have shown that SIT with a single extract provides incomplete relief of

Table 1 Safety of Immunotherapy with Pollen Extracts

Author	Species	Patient N°	Extract	Dose schedule	Systemic reactions, % patients
Bousquet et al. (89)	Grass	15	Alum-pyridine	Classical	13.3
	Grass	23	Standardized	Rush	40
Bousquet et al. (36)	Grass	15	Standardized	Rush	36.8
	Grass	19	Formald. allergoid	Rush	20
Bousquet et al. (96)	Grass	18	Standardized	Rush	11
	Grass	15	Formald. allergoid	Clustered	20
	Grass	13	HMW allergoid	Clustered	0
Bousquet et al. (32)	Grass	16	Standardized	Rush	18.7
Hejjaoui et al. (111)	Grass	74	Standardized	Rush	31.1
	Grass	102	Standardized, premedication	Rush	14.7
	Grass	200	Standardized, premed-precaution	Rush	7.5
	Grass	78	Standardized step	Step	2.6
Machiels et al. (99)	Grass	37	Ag-Ab complexes	Classical	0
Østerballe (68)	Grass	20	Standardized alum	Classical	40
	Grass	20	Fraction 19–25 alum	Classical	70
Pastorello et al. (101)	Grass	10	Formald. allergoid alum	Classical	10 (late)
Varney et al. (24)	Grass	20	Standardized, alum	Classical	10
Grammer et al. (113)	Ragweed	19	Polymerized glutaraldehyde	Classical	0
Iliopoulos et al. (34)	Ragweed	21	Standardized	Conventional	28.6
Van-Metre et al. (70)	Ragweed	15	Aqueous	Classical	46.6
Van-Metre et al. (82)	Ragweed	17	Aqueous	Classical	46.8
	Ragweed	18	Aqueous	Clustered	55.5
Norman et al. (69)	Ragweed	27	Aqueous whole rw	Classical	33
	Ragweed	16	Ag E	Classical	9.5
Norman and Lichtenstein (90)	Ragweed	16	Formald. allergoid	Cluster	22.7
	Ragweed	20	Aqueous	Classical	36.2
Bousquet et al. (32)	Multiple species	16	Standardized	Rush	18.7

HWM: high molecular weight; Ag-Ab: antigen–antibody.
Source: Adapted from Ref. 1.

symptoms (68). This may be due to failure to immunize with the relevant allergens, as many patients have multiple sensitivities, but it has also been shown that these polysensitized patients appear to present an IgE immune response different from that of monosensitized patients. Patients sensitized to a single allergen species have significantly lower total serum IgE than those allergic to multiple allergen species (107). The lymphocyte reactivity of these two groups of patients is also different, as the cells of the monosensitized group release significantly lower levels of IgE, IL-4, and CD23 than cells from the polysensitized group. On the other hand, the production of IFN-γ is similar in both groups (108). This study suggests that mono- and polysensitized subjects are different in terms of IgE immune response and regulation. A double-blind placebo-controlled study compared the efficacy of SIT in these two groups of patients (32). Grass pollen allergic patients were treated with an optimal maintenance dose of a standardized orchard grass pollen extract, whereas those allergic to multiple pollen species received the same biologically equivalent dose of all standardized allergens to which they were sensitized. The results of the study indicated that grass pollen allergic patients were significantly protected but polysensitized patients were not. Using a higher allergen dose it might be possible to show efficacy in the polysensitized group, but the rate of systemic reactions using standardized extracts would have been unacceptable with the rush protocol used.

Safety

Pollen extract vaccines are usually potent extracts, and systemic reactions are not rare (109,110) (Table 1). The rate and severity of systemic reactions vary according to the extract used and the schedule of administration of SIT. Premedication was shown to be an effective approach to reduce the rate and severity of systemic reactions (111,112).

Duration

Duration of the effects of SIT after its cessation is another matter of debate, and there are no available data for pollen asthma, but it is suggested that a long-term treatment, lasting at least 3 years, is required. For nasal symptoms, it is suggested that the effects of grass pollen SIT last for several years after its cessation (113,114), but relevant controlled studies have yet to be performed, so no definite conclusion can be reached.

B. House Dust Mite Asthma

Efficacy

Bronchial challenges with mite extracts showed that the threshold dose eliciting an immediate bronchial obstruction was increased in many studies after treatment and that the late-phase reaction was inhibited in most (27,28,87, 115–119) but not all studies (120). These studies suggest that SIT is effective and may decrease inflammation because the late-phase reaction was decreased.

The review of the literature available indicates that SIT with mites is more effective than SIT with house dust. Although very few studies have been conclusive (121), SIT with house dust extracts should no longer be used owing to the great heterogeneity of house dust and the impossibility of appropriately standardizing house dust extracts (9–11).

Using aqueous or standardized *Dermatophagoides pteronyssinus* and/or *D. farinae* extracts, many studies found a significant effect of SIT. However, the results are not always impressive and, especially in adults, are sometimes negative. With other extracts, results are even more variable (27,77,116,122– 127). Haugaard et al. (77) examined the dose of allergen required to induce a significant clinical effect. With a maximal dose of 7 μg of Der p 1, patients presented a significant improvement in $PD_{20}FEV_1$, but the maximal effect was observed for a dose of 21 μg of Der p1. It appears that patients with severe asthma (FEV_1 under 70% of predicted values after optimal pharmacological treatment) present less improvement that those with milder asthma (128).

Studies examining the evolution of BHR in patients undergoing mite SIT are still inconclusive; some have found an improvement of BHR (116,127), whereas others have not (129). Although controlled studies using bronchial biopsies and bronchial challenge are still missing from the literature, indirect indices of inflammation have been studied. It has been shown that blood eosinophils are decreased in asthmatic patients who had effective SIT with standardized mite extracts.

Safety

The safety of mite SIT is critical, since many, if not most, of the patients who have died from an allergen injection were asthmatic, and in most cases their death was caused by an irreversible bronchial obstruction (109,130). Some investigators suggest that SIT is indicated in patients with severe forms of the disease (131). Controlled studies have been carried out with different types of allergen extract vaccines. As for pollen SIT, standardized extracts expose patients to a higher risk of unwanted reactions because of their potency (116, 122,125,132,133). Uncontrolled asthma or an FEV_1 under 70% of predicted values are risk factors for developing a bronchial reaction (83,132). Moreover, patients with asthma tend to have more severe bronchial reactions than non-asthmatic individuals.

Duration

The duration of SIT with mite extracts is still a subject of debate. Price et al. (134) stopped SIT after a year of treatment in half of the children enrolled in a double-blind, placebo-controlled study and noticed that most children who stopped SIT presented a relapse within a year.

Availability of Suitable Extracts

Dermatophagoides pteronyssinus is widely available. In many countries standardized extracts from *Dermatophagoides pteronyssinus* and *D. farinae* are available. These extracts are usually in lyophilized or aqueous form, but in Europe they are often adsorbed on alum.

C. Allergy to Animal Proteins

Clinical Efficacy

A number of studies have demonstrated significant improvement in bronchial sensitivity in patients with cat allergic asthma following cat vaccine immunotherapy (79,135–145). Three studies have confirmed the clinical efficacy of cat immunotherapy, showing improvement in symptoms (80,140, 146,147) and reduction of medication needs (80) in patients who kept their animal at home.

Safety

In animal dander SIT, the rate of systemic reactions was highly variable, ranging from none to 80% of patients (82,135–137,140,141), and many of these reactions were severe. Most studies were carried out with standardized extracts. However, the number of patients treated is low, and this high rate of adverse reactions may have been observed because the maximal tolerated dose had been used.

Availability of Suitable Extracts

In many countries standardized extracts of cat and dog allergens are available. They are sometimes labeled in weight or units of major allergen.

D. Allergy to Molds

Clinical Efficacy

Mold allergens often cause rhinitis and asthma. Multiple mold allergy is often present. The quality of mold vaccines available in the past was often poor (148). However, immunotherapy with standardized *Cladosporium* and *Alternaria* vaccines was found to be highly effective in rhinitis and/or asthma in two studies (149,150) although less effective in another (151).

Safety

Immunotherapy with mold extracts may also expose subjects to systemic reactions. In studies using a standardized *Cladosporium* extract, most patients developed systemic reactions (150,151); whereas in another using a standardized *Alternaria* extract, none of the patients had any systemic reaction (149). In this study the optimal dose of the standardized *Alternaria* extract was calculated before any injection by means of parallel line bioassay using skin tests. The long-term safety of mold SIT with unstandardized extracts has been questioned (152).

Availability of Suitable Extracts

Cladosporium and *Alternaria* standardized extracts are available in some countries. However, other extracts are not standardized, and usually their quality is poor, seriously limiting the use of SIT in asthma due to molds.

E. Immunotherapy with Other Allergen Extracts

Efficacy of house dust vaccine immunotherapy is doubtful, and the characterization of these vaccines is poor. Double-blind, placebo-controlled studies of immunotherapy with bacterial vaccines for treatment of rhinitis and/or asthma did not show efficacy (for review see Ref. 153). There is no study of immunotherapy with *Candida albicans* or *Trichophyton,* and the characterization of the vaccines is usually poor.

F. Meta-Analysis of Efficacy of Immunotherapy in Asthma

A meta-analysis of clinical trials of allergen immunotherapy was undertaken to assess the efficacy of this form of therapy in asthma (7). A computerized bibliographic search revealed 20 randomized placebo-controlled double-blind trials of allergen immunotherapy for treatment of asthma. Criteria analyzed included asthmatic symptoms, medication requirements, and measurement of lung function and bronchial hyperreactivity (BHR). Categorical outcomes were expressed as odds ratios and continuous outcomes as effect sizes. The combined odds of symptomatic improvement from immunotherapy with any allergen were 3.2 (95% CI 2.2–4.9). The odds for reduction in medication after mite immunotherapy were 4.2 (95% CI 2.2–7.9). The combined odds for reduction in BHR were 6.8 (95% CI 3.8–12.0). The mean effect size for any allergen immunotherapy on all continuous outcomes was 0.71 (95% CI 0.43–1.00), which would correspond to a mean 7.1% predicted improvement in FEV_1 from immunotherapy. Although the benefits of allergen immunotherapy could be overestimated because of unpublished negative studies, an additional 33 such studies would be necessary to overturn these results.

G. Immunotherapy with Mixtures of Allergen Vaccines in Unselected Allergic Asthmatic Children

A study reported a controlled trial of immunotherapy for treatment of mild to severe asthma in a nonselected population of allergic children (6). The children were closely supervised and given optimal medical therapy. The results showed no significant difference between the placebo and active treatment groups. However, several methodological factors may have led to the negative results. Among them, the study was carried out using mixtures of allergens including mold vaccines, some important allergens such as cockroaches were not used, and the population of asthmatic children was nonselected, whereas guidelines have indicated that only selected asthmatic patients should receive immunotherapy (10–12).

VI. Other Routes for Allergen Administration

Parenteral allergen injection has been the principal approach for the application of immunotherapy in the treatment of allergic respiratory airway diseases. However, the inconvenience of frequent injection visits, the discomfort associated with injections, and the possibility of adverse reactions have led to the investigation of alternative routes of delivery of effective doses of allergen extracts. Local administration of allergens can also have the advantage of stimulating the local immune system where the allergic reaction occurs. Moreover, it has been shown that local application of allergens has a systemic effect.

The first attempts at local immunotherapy were made early in the century, and local immunotherapy has been used in clinical practice without rigorous controls for decades. Interest in local immunotherapy was renewed in 1980 after reports appeared concerning fatalities due to immunotherapy. However, this form of therapy is still a matter of debate in many countries. Several noninjective routes of specific immunotherapy have been proposed. These include (1)

1. The *oral route,* in which the extract (prepared as drops, capsules, or tablets) is immediately swallowed. Clinical efficacy is therefore not demonstrated, and further studies are needed before this form of therapy can be recommended for clinical practice (1). Significant adverse reactions (urticaria) related to the treatment were observed in only two studies that employed very high doses of extract (154,155).
2. *Sublingual-swallow SIT,* in which the extract has to be held sublingually for 1–2 min and then swallowed. Five studies (156–159) demonstrated the clinical effectiveness of sublingual immunotherapy with grass, *Parietaria,* and mite extracts. A reduction in target organ sensitivity (nasal or bronchial challenge) was described. No systemic side effects have been reported in adults, and in most of these studies there was no difference between the placebo and the active treatment in the side effect profile. However, in one study performed in children, systemic side effects (urticaria and/or asthma) were reported (158). Sublingual administration of very low dose allergenic solutions including both food and inhalant allergen extracts have been prescribed by some physicians, particularly those identified as "clinical ecologists" to treat patients with both typical allergic symptoms and a variety of other undefined symptoms that are not allergic in nature. There are no data that show that this type of therapy is effective.
3. *Sublingual-spit SIT* in which the extract is held in the mouth sublingually for 1–2 min and then spit out. The only double-blind, placebo-controlled study on sublingual-spit was carried out in cat-allergic patients (160) and cannot be analyzed due to methodological problems, specifically that in this challenge study, the cat room exposure levels were highly variable.
4. The *nasal route* in which the extract (aqueous or powdered) is delivered in the nose by proper devices. No studies in asthma have been published (1).

5. The *bronchial route* in which the extract (aqueous or powdered) is delivered in the bronchi by proper devices. Several bronchial reactions have been reported with this route of administration (161,162).

VII. Pediatric Issues in Immunotherapy

The use of allergen immunotherapy in children requires specialist assessment, because there are special problems and questions among this age group. Immunotherapy started early in the disease process should modify the spontaneous long-term progress of the allergic inflammation and disease (10,163). Some pediatricians recommend treatment in children at 1–2 years of age (10), but it is desirable to evaluate more closely in controlled studies the benefits of immunotherapy in patients below 5 years of age. Usually immunotherapy is started after the age of 5 years. At the moment it is not known whether immunotherapy should be administered to very young children.

Specific allergy diagnosis forms the basis for the selection of patients and of allergen extracts for immunotherapy. The diagnosis of allergic rhinoconjunctivitis in children under the age of 4–5, however, is usually difficult. They may show sensitization in allergy testing, but this does not necessarily prove allergic disease. In this age group the frequency of acute viral respiratory infections is high, and the differential diagnosis of hay fever and acute viral infection is not clear. The clinical diagnosis of allergy is always based on the combination of clinical evaluation (clinical history, monitoring of symptoms, use of drugs) and the results of the diagnostic tests. The considerations for diagnosis and treatment listed for adults also apply to children (1).

VIII. Can Immunotherapy Alter the Course of Asthma?

A. Prevention of Asthma

One of the major goals in the next few years will be to determine whether early administration of SIT in patients with rhinitis may prevent the onset of asthma. However, there are no data from a controlled study available yet, although a large multicentric study has been started in Europe (preventive allergy treatment).

B. Prevention of the Development of New Sensitivities

It has been proposed in the past that SIT with one allergen may prevent the development of new sensitivities. If this were the case, SIT should be started very early in life, as soon as an allergic sensitization has developed. Recently, it has been shown that about 50% of young children (aged 2–6 years) sensitized to a single allergen species and who received SIT did not develop new allergenic sensitivities over a period of 3 years, whereas all those who did not receive SIT did during the same period of time. This study requires further confirmation but suggests that SIT can alter the natural course of allergy (164).

IX. Indications and Contraindications of Immunotherapy in Asthma According to Recent International Guidelines

A. General Considerations

Specific immunotherapy should be prescribed by specialists and administered by physicians who are trained to use emergency techniques if anaphylaxis occurs. Before starting immunotherapy each patient should be informed of the risks, duration, and effectiveness of this treatment, and cooperation and compliance to the treatment are absolute requirements before starting it. Pharmacological treatment acts specifically on allergic inflammation and its symptoms, while immunotherapy affects the immunological and inflammatory response and is aimed at modifying the natural history of the disease (1).

It is essential to carefully select the patients and consider several factors in order to appreciate the value of SIT in comparison with other available therapeutic methods including allergen avoidance and pharmacotherapy:

1. Potential severity of the affection to be treated
2. Efficacy of available treatments
3. Optimal use of SIT using standardized extracts, high quality modified extracts, or purified components of known composition and efficacy
4. Cost and duration of each type of treatment
5. Risk incurred by the patient due to the allergic disease and the treatment
6. Modification of the course of the disease by each type of treatment

The indications of immunotherapy in asthma and rhinitis have been separated in some guidelines (11,12), and this artificial separation has led to unresolved discussions (165,166), possibly because the IgE-mediated reaction has not been considered as a multiorgan involvement. It is therefore important to consider immunotherapy from the point of view of the allergen sensitization rather than of the disease itself (1).

The indication of SIT should be carefully considered for highly selected patients (167) (Table 2). Doctors should always discuss the length and cost of

Table 2   Considerations for Initiating Immunotherapy

1. Presence of a demonstrated IgE-mediated disease
   a.   Positive skin tests and/or serum-specific IgE

2. Documentation that specific sensitivity is involved in asthma symptoms
   a.   Exposure to the allergen(s) determined by allergy testing related to appearance of symptoms
   b.   If required, bronchial challenge with the relevant allergen(s)

3. Characterization of other triggers that may be involved in asthma symptoms

4. Severity and duration of asthma symptoms
   a.   Subjective symptoms
   b.   Objective parameters, e.g., work loss, school absenteeism
   c.   Pulmonary function (essential): EXCLUDE patients with severe asthma
   d.   Monitoring of the pulmonary function by peak flow

5. Response of asthma symptoms to nonimmunological treatment
   a.   Response to allergen avoidance
   b.   Response to pharmacotherapy

6. Availability of standardized or high quality extracts

7. Age of the patient. Consider other treatment in
   a.   Children under 5
   b.   Adults over 50

8. Contraindications
   a.   Treatment with β-blocker
   b.   Other immunological disease
   c.   Inability of patients to comply

9. Sociological factors
   a.   Cost
   b.   Occupation of candidate
   c.   Asthma impairing quality of life despite adequate pharmacological treatment

10. Objective evidence of efficacy of immunotherapy for the selected patient (availability of controlled clinical studies)

Source: Adapted from Ref. 167.

Table 3 Recommendations to Minimize Risk and Improve Efficacy of SIT in Asthma

1. Specific immunotherapy must be prescribed by specialists and administered by physicians trained to manage systemic reactions if anaphylaxis occurs.
2. Patients with multiple sensitivities and/or nonallergic triggers may not benefit from specific immunotherapy.
3. Specific immunotherapy is more effective in children and young adults than later in life.
4. It is essential for safety reasons that patients be asymptomatic at the time of the injections because lethal adverse reactions are more often found in asthma patients with severe airway obstruction.
5. FEV_1 with pharmacological treatment should reach at least 70% of the predicted values for both efficacy and safety reasons.

Source: Ref. 11

the treatment with their patients, as compliance with antiasthmatic treatments and SIT is often poor (168). To minimize risk and improve efficacy, SIT needs to be prescribed by specialists and administered by or under the close supervision of physicians trained to manage acute systemic reactions if anaphylaxis occurs (11) (Table 3) Absolute contraindications include patients with other serious immunopathological conditions, malignancies, poor compliance, severe psychological disorders, and/or treatment with beta-blocking agents, even when administered topically.

Before initiating SIT, avoidance of exposure to the allergen(s) causing asthma should always be attempted. Except in the case of animal dander, most common aeroallergens cannot be avoided completely, and this is particularly true for patients allergic to house dust mites and those who are allergic to multiple allergens.

B. Pollen Allergy

The indication for immunotherapy in pollen-induced allergic diseases is based on the severity of the disease and the duration of symptoms according to the criteria set above. Moreover, it is commonly accepted that immunotherapy is indicated if the season is prolonged or in some polysensitized patients exposed to several subsequent pollen seasons (i.e., tree and grass pollen sensitivity) (8,10).

Since rhinoconjunctivitis is present in most if not all patients suffering from pollen allergy, and asthma occurs generally in the most severely affected patients, it is impossible to propose indications without considering all symptoms (105). It also appears that immunotherapy is indicated when asthma during the pollen season complicates rhinoconjunctivitis. British recommendations have proposed that patients with asthma should be specifically excluded (169), but this is the only guideline that has made this recommendation.

C. Domestic Mite Allergy

House dust must not be used to treat allergic patients (10). Patients allergic to mites are candidates for immunotherapy if they have a relevant exposure to domestic mites and if mite avoidance measures are not completely effective. Patients who are sensitized to mites but in whom symptoms are caused to only a minor degree by exposure to mites are not candidates for immunotherapy. The indication for immunotherapy in rhinitis and asthma is based on the severity of the disease and the duration of symptoms according to the criteria set above.

D. Immunotherapy with Animal Dander Allergens

Avoidance is the treatment of choice for animal-induced allergic diseases. However, complete avoidance is often impossible due to exposure to animal allergens in environments in which animals are not present (170). Immunotherapy to cat may be prescribed for patients in whom avoidance of animal allergens is incompletely effective, in animal-induced occupational allergic diseases, and in some patients who refuse to evict an animal from their home.

E. Immunotherapy with Molds

Avoidance where possible of indoor mold allergens is the treatment of choice. Certain studies have demonstrated clinical improvement when well-characterized extracts of *Cladosporium* or *Alternaria* have been used in the treatment of mold-induced allergy. Patients with positive skin tests who have symptoms to other relevant mold allergens may be considered for immunotherapy.

F. Immunotherapy with Other Allergens

Immunotherapy with extracts of undefined allergens (house dust, bacteria, *Candida albicans, Trichophyton,* etc.) should not be used (10).

G. Other Routes for Allergen Administration

The usual route of administration of immunotherapy is the subcutaneous one, but oral, sublingual, nasal, and bronchial routes have been proposed. A workshop of the European Academy of Allergy and Clinical Immunology was convened in Portofino, Italy, September 28, 1996 to assess the efficacy and safety of local route immunotherapy. The following recommendations of the workshop are proposed.

> Sublingual (swallow) immunotherapy has shown some efficacy in four double-blind, placebo-controlled studies in patients suffering from rhinitis using pollen extracts and domestic mites. The overall safety has likewise been documented in adults. The treatment is currently not recommended in children except as part of a controlled study. Further studies with standardized extracts are needed to fully designate the indication of sublingual immunotherapy.
> Bronchial and oral immunotherapy, due to insufficient documentation of efficacy and a risk of severe side effects (bronchial immunotherapy), are not recommended except as part of a controlled study.

H. Monitoring of Immunotherapy

The monitoring of immunotherapy with inhalant allergens can be based only on the evolution of clinical symptoms and the reduction of pharmacotherapy for optimal control of the allergic disease. There is to date no in vitro marker that can be used.

I. Contraindications to Immunotherapy

Contraindications for venom immunotherapy and immunotherapy with inhalant allergens are similar (10) and may be absolute or relative:

1. Presence of serious immunopathological disease.
2. Malignancies.
3. Severe psychological disorders.
4. Treatment with beta-blockers (171), even when administered topically.
5. Poor compliance with treatment.
6. Severe asthma uncontrolled by pharmacotherapy and patients with irreversible airways obstruction (FEV_1 consistently under 70% of predicted after an adequate pharmacological treatment) (12).
7. Presence of significant cardiovascular disease, making epinephrine injection possibly dangerous.
8. Except for *Hymenoptera* venoms, allergen injections represent a relative contraindication in children under 5 years of age.

Pregnancy is not considered a contraindication for continuation of immunotherapy, but, in general, treatment should not be started during pregnancy (172).

X. Future Trends

The introduction of recombinant DNA technology has been a milestone in the
characterization and large-scale production of allergens. This technology offers
the possibility of producing recombinant allergens (RAs) in high quality and
unlimited quantities for use not only as diagnostic agents but also as therapeutic
agents (173). RAs may be added to commonly used natural extracts to certify
standardized quality. In addition, RAs allow the application of tailor-made
preparations. Although this type of vaccine seems to be very expensive, it is of
particular interest because during traditional immunotherapy patients receive
large quantities of proteins to which they are not allergic. Furthermore, although
local immunotherapy—oral, sublingual, nasal, or bronchial route—has been
used for decades, evidence of the efficacy of this therapy could not be fully
established. Using a pure RA as whole or partial molecules, a reevaluation of
this type of therapy seems to be possible. Recombinant allergens may be especially useful here because very large doses can be easily produced and specific
delivery systems may help to target the allergen on the mucosa-associated lym-
phoid tissue thought to be important in the generation of immunotolerance (1).

A. Administration

The future of SIT could follow several different paths. First of all, the methods
of administering treatment could be improved, whether by using a sublingual
route, by using oral administration (with the addition of immunomodulators
that could enhance the efficacy of the therapy), or by turning to new technologies that will permit the use of fewer, widely spaced injections.

B. Specific Immunotherapy

Use of specific epitopes from T-lymphocyte receptors (174) could enable peptide fragments with 8–10 amino acids to be obtained that could immunize the
subject without the risk of secondary reactions, since IgE essentially recog-
nizes conformational allergens (175,176). Therapeutic trials using Fel d1
(major "cat" allergen) and Amb a1 (major allergen of *Ambrosia* pollen) peptides have been carried out (177,178). Unfortunately, due to the occurrence of
delayed systemic reactions, this form of treatment has been stopped.

Other methods such as the injection of anti-idiotype antibodies (24,179) or the injection of immune allergen–antibody complexes have been suggested. Several studies have been undertaken using these immune allergen–antibody complexes, and the results seem remarkable (99,100). It would be prudent, however, to be cautious in advocating the more widespread use of this method.

C. Nonspecific Immunotherapy

Immunomodulators can modify both the immune and inflammatory responses in an allergic subject and induce a more rapid and longer lasting therapeutic effect. On the other hand, many groups are attempting to modify IgE response in both animals and humans, either on the basis of cytokines (180,181) or by modulation of IgE (182–184) or their receptors (185). These approaches are certainly interesting; however, some, applied to humans, have been disappointing. In the main, they are theoretical and require a very progressive and ethical approach.

XI. Conclusions

Although the importance of specific immunotherapy was seriously disputed in 1990, this form of therapy should still represent one of the treatments of allergic asthma. However, its indications must be restricted to highly selected cases.

New scenarios for the development of immunotherapy are enough to suggest that immunotherapy can be thought of as a therapy for the future.

References

1. Bousquet J, Lockey R, Malling H. WHO position paper. Allergen immunotherapy: therapeutic vaccines for allergic diseases. Allergy 1998; 53(suppl):1–42.
2. Noon L. Prophylactic inoculation against hay fever. Lancet 1911; i:1572–1573.
3. Platts-Mills TA, Sporik RB, Chapman MD, Heymann PW. The role of domestic allergens. Ciba Found Symp 1997; 206:173–185.
4. Reid MJ, Moss RB, Hsu YP, Kwasnicki JM, Commerford TM, Nelson BL. Seasonal asthma in northern California: allergic causes and efficacy of immunotherapy. J Allergy Clin Immunol 1986; 78:590–600.
5. Bousquet J, Hejjaoui A, Michel FB. Specific immunotherapy in asthma. J Allergy Clin Immunol 1990; 86:292–305.
6. Adkinson N Jr, Eggleston PA, Eney D, et al. A controlled trial of immunotherapy for asthma in allergic children. N Engl J Med 1997; 336:324–331.
7. Abramson MJ, Puy RM, Weiner JM. Is allergen immunotherapy effective in asthma? A meta-analysis of randomized controlled trials [see comments]. Am J Respir Crit Care Med 1995; 151:969–974.

8. WHO. The current status of allergen immunotherapy (hyposensitisation). Report of a WHO/IUIS working group. Allergy 1989; 44:369–379.
9. WHO. Current status of allergen immunotherapy. Shortened version of a World Health Organisation/International Union of Immunological Societies Working Group Report. Lancet 1989; 1:259–261.
10. Malling H, Weeke B. Immunotherapy. Position Paper of the European Academy of Allergy and Clinical Immunology. Allergy 1993; 48(suppl 14):9–35.
11. International Consensus Report on Diagnosis and Management of Asthma. International Asthma Management Project. Allergy 1992; 47:1–61.
12. WHO. Global strategy for asthma management and prevention. WHO/NHLBI workshop report. In: National Institutes of Health, National Heart, Lung and Blood Institute Pub 95–3659, 1995.
13. Frew AJ. Injection immunotherapy. British Society for Allergy and Clinical Immunology Working Party. Brit Med J 1993; 307:919–923.
14. Nicklas R, Bernstein I, Blessing-Moore J, et al. Practice parameters for allergen immunotherapy. J Allergy Clin Immunol 1996; 6:1001–1011.
15. Bousquet J, Chanez P, Lacoste JY, et al. Asthma: a disease remodeling the airways. Allergy 1992; 47:3–11.
16. Peat JK, Woolcock AJ, Cullen K. Rate of decline of lung function in subjects with asthma. Eur J Respir Dis 1987; 70:171–179.
17. Ulrik CS, Backer V, Dirksen A. A 10 year follow up of 180 adults with bronchial asthma: factors important for the decline in lung function. Thorax 1992; 47:14–18.
18. Gerritsen J, Koeter GH, Postma DS, Schouten JP, Knol K. Prognosis of asthma from childhood to adulthood. Am Rev Respir Dis 1989; 140:1325–1330.
19. Lichtenstein L, Norman P, Kagey-Sobotka A, Adkinson N Jr, Golden D. The immunologic basis for the efficacy of immunotherapy. In: Kerr J, Ganderton M, eds. Proceedings of the XI Congress of Allergology and Clinical Immunology. Chester, UK: Macmillan, 1983:285–288.
20. Gleich GJ, Zimmermann EM, Henderson LL, Yunginger JW. Effect of immunotherapy on immunoglobulin E and immunoglobulin G antibodies to ragweed antigens: a six-year prospective study. J Allergy Clin Immunol 1982; 70:261–271.
21. Leynadier F, Abuaf N, Halpern GM, Murrieta M, Garcia-Duarte C, Dry J. Blocking IgG antibodies after rush immunotherapy with mites. Ann Allergy 1986; 57: 325–329.
22. Djurup R, Osterballe O. IgG subclass antibody response in grass pollen-allergic patients undergoing specific immunotherapy. Prognostic value of serum IgG subclass antibody levels early in immunotherapy. Allergy 1984; 39:433–441.
23. Xiao SF, Okuda M, Ohnishi M, Okubo K. Specific IgA and IgG antibodies to house dust mite Dermatophagoides farinae in nasal secretions. Arerugi 1994; 43: 634–644.
24. Hebert J, Bernier D, Mourad W. Detection of auto-anti-idiotypic antibodies to Lol p I (rye I) IgE antibodies in human sera by the use of murine idiotypes: levels in atopic and non-atopic subjects and effects of immunotherapy. Clin Exp Immunol 1990; 80:413–419.

25. Bousquet J, Guerin B, Dotte A, et al. Comparison between rush immunotherapy with a standardized allergen and an alum adjuved pyridine extracted material in grass pollen allergy. Clin Allergy 1985; 15:179–193.

26. Van-Metre TE J, Marsh DG, Adkinson N Jr, et al. Immunotherapy decreases skin sensitivity to cat extract. J Allergy Clin Immunol 1989; 83:888–899.

27. Warner JO, Price JF, Soothill JF, Hey EN. Controlled trial of hyposensitisation to Dermatophagoides pteronyssinus in children with asthma. Lancet 1978; 2:912–915.

28. Bousquet J, Calvayrac P, Guerin B, et al. Immunotherapy with a standardized Dermatophaoides pteronyssinus extract. I. In vivo and in vitro parameters after a short course of treatment. J Allergy Clin Immunol 1985; 76:734–744.

29. Bousquet J, Lebel B, Dhivert H, Bataille Y, Martinot B, Michel FB. Nasal challenge with pollen grains, skin-prick tests and specific IgE in patients with grass pollen allergy. Clin Allergy 1987; 17:529–536.

30. Frostad AB, Grimmer O, Sandvik L, Aas K. Hyposensitization. Comparing a purified (refined) allergen preparation and a crude aqueous extract from timothy pollen. Allergy 1980; 35:81–95.

31. Creticos PS, Adkinson N Jr, Kagey-Sobotka A, et al. Nasal challenge with ragweed pollen in hay fever patients. Effect of immunotherapy. J Clin Invest 1985; 76:2247–2253.

32. Bousquet J, Becker WM, Hejjaoui A, et al. Differences in clinical and immunologic reactivity of patients allergic to grass pollens and to multiple-pollen species. II. Efficacy of a double-blind, placebo-controlled, specific immunotherapy with standardized extracts. J Allergy Clin Immunol 1991; 88:43–53.

33. Furin MJ, Norman PS, Creticos PS, et al. Immunotherapy decreases antigen-induced eosinophil cell migration into the nasal cavity. J Allergy Clin Immunol 1991; 88:27–32.

34. Iliopoulos O, Proud D, Adkinson N Jr, et al. Effects of immunotherapy on the early, late, and rechallenge nasal reaction to provocation with allergen: changes in inflammatory mediators and cells. J Allergy Clin Immunol 1991; 87:855–866.

35. Hedlin G, Silber G, Schieken L, et al. Attenuation of allergen sensitivity early in the course of ragweed immunotherapy. J Allergy Clin Immunol 1989; 84:390–399.

36. Bousquet J, Maasch H, Martinot B, Hejjaoui A, Wahl R, Michel FB. Double-blind, placebo-controlled immunotherapy with mixed grass-pollen allergoids. II. Comparison between parameters assessing the efficacy of immunotherapy. J Allergy Clin Immunol 1988; 82:439–446.

37. Tsicopoulos A, Tonnel AB, Wallaert B, Joseph M, Ramon P, Capron A. A circulating suppressive factor of platelet cytotoxic functions after rush immunotherapy in Hymenoptera venom hypersensitivity. J Immunol 1989; 142:2683–2688.

38. Rak S, Lowhagen O, Venge P. The effect of immunotherapy on bronchial hyperresponsiveness and eosinophil cationic protein in pollen-allergic patients. J Allergy Clin Immunol 1988; 82:470–480.

39. Nagata M, Shibasaki M, Sakamoto Y, et al. Specific immunotherapy reduces the

antigen-dependent production of eosinophil chemotactic activity from mononuclear cells in patients with atopic asthma. J Allergy Clin Immunol 1994; 94:160–166.

40. Rak S, Bjornson A, Hakanson L, Sorenson S, Venge P. The effect of immunotherapy on eosinophil accumulation and production of eosinophil chemotactic activity in the lung of subjects with asthma during natural pollen exposure. J Allergy Clin Immunol 1991; 88:878–888.

41. Rak S, Hallden G, Sorenson S, Margari V, Scheynius A. The effect of immunotherapy on T-cell subsets in peripheral blood and bronchoalveolar lavage fluid in pollen-allergic patients. Allergy 1993; 48:460–465.

42. Kuna P, Alam R, Kuzminska B, Rozniecki J. The effect of preseasonal immunotherapy on the production of histamine-releasing factor (HRF) by mononuclear cells from patients with seasonal asthma: results of a double-blind, placebo-controlled, randomized study. J Allergy Clin Immunol 1989; 83:816–824.

43. Durham S, Varney V, Gaga M, Frew A, Jacobson M, Kay A. Immunotherapy and allergic inflammation. Clin Exp Allergy 1991; 21(suppl 1):206–210.

44. Varney VA, Hamid QA, Gaga M, et al. Influence of grass pollen immunotherapy on cellular infiltration and cytokine mRNA expression during allergen-induced late-phase cutaneous responses. J Clin Invest 1993; 92:644–651.

45. Durham SR, Ying S, Varney VA, et al. Grass pollen immunotherapy inhibits allergen-induced infiltration of CD4+ T lymphocytes and eosinophils in the nasal mucosa and increases the number of cells expressing messenger RNA for interferon-gamma. J Allergy Clin Immunol 1996; 97:1356–1365.

46. Hamid Q, Schotman E, Jacobson M, Walker S, Durham S. Increases in interleukin-12 (IL-12) messenger RNA+ (mRNA+) cells accompany inhibition of allergen induced late skin responses following successful grass pollen immunotherapy. J Allergy Clin Immunol 1997; 99:254–260.

47. Rocklin RE, Sheffer AL, Greineder DK, Melmon KL. Generation of antigen-specific suppressor cells during allergy desensitization. N Engl J Med 1980; 302:1213–1219.

48. Renz H, Lack G, Saloga J, et al. Inhibition of IgE production and normalization of airways responsiveness by sensitized CD8 T cells in a mouse model of allergen-induced sensitization. J Immunol 1994; 152:351–360.

49. Jutel M, Pichler WJ, Skrbic D, Urwyler A, Dahinden C, Muller UR. Bee venom immunotherapy results in decrease of IL-4 and IL-5 and increase of IFN-gamma secretion in specific allergen-stimulated T cell cultures. J Immunol 1995; 154:4187–4194.

50. McHugh SM, Deighton J, Stewart AG, Lachmann PJ, Ewan PW. Bee venom immunotherapy induces a shift in cytokine responses from a TH-2 to a TH-1 dominant pattern: comparison of rush and conventional immunotherapy. Clin Exp Allergy 1995; 25:828–838.

51. Secrist H, Chelen CJ, Wen Y, Marshall JD, Umetsu DT. Allergen immunotherapy decreases interleukin 4 production in CD4+ T cells from allergic individuals. J Exp Med 1993; 178:2123–2130.

52. Secrist H, DeKruyff RH, Umetsu DT. Interleukin 4 production by CD4+ T cells from allergic individuals is modulated by antigen concentration and antigen-presenting cell type. J Exp Med 1995; 181:1081–1089.
53. Lamb JR, Skidmore BJ, Green N, Chiller JM, Feldmann M. Induction of tolerance in influenza virus-immune T lymphocyte clones with synthetic peptides of influenza hemagglutinin. J Exp Med 1983; 157:1434–1447.
54. Fasler S, Aversa G, Terr A, Thestrup-Pedersen K, de-Vries JE, Yssel H. Peptide-induced anergy in allergen-specific human Th2 cells results in lack of cytokine production and B cell help for IgE synthesis. Reversal by IL-2, not by IL-4 or IL-13. J Immunol 1995; 155:4199–4206.
55. Tsicopoulos A, Labalette M, Akoum H, et al. CD28 expression is increased in venom allergic patients but is not modified by specific immunotherapy. Clin Exp Allergy 1996; 26:1119–1124.
56. Akdis CA, Blesken T, Akdis M, et al. Induction and differential regulation of bee venom phospholipase A2-specific human IgE and IgG4 antibodies in vitro requires allergen-specific and nonspecific activation of T and B cells. J Allergy Clin Immunol 1997; 99:345–353.
57. Akdis CA, Akdis M, Blesken T, et al. Epitope-specific T cell tolerance to phospholipase A2 in bee venom immunotherapy and recovery by IL-2 and IL-15 in vitro. J Clin Invest 1996; 98:1676–1683.
58. Fed Reg. Biological products: allergenic extracts: implementation of efficacy review. Federal Register, Food and Drug Administration 1985; 21 CRF Parts 600, 610 and 680 [Docket No. 81N-0096].
59. Practice Parameters for Allergen Immunotherapy. Joint Task Force on Practice Parameters (American Academy of Allergy, Asthma and Immunology, the American College of Allergy, Asthma and Immunology, the Joint Council of Allergy, Asthma and Immunology). J Allergy Clin Immunol 1996; 98:1001–1011.
60. Dreborg S, Frew A. Allergen standardization and skin tests. EAACI position paper. Allergy 1993; 48(suppl 14).
61. Chapman N. Allergen standardization. Academy News, AAAAI Position Statement, August/September 1996.
62. Scheiner O, Kraft D. Basic and practical aspects of recombinant allergens. Allergy 1995; 50:384–392.
63. Platts-Mills TA, Chapman MD. Allergen standardization. J Allergy Clin Immunol 1991; 87:621–625.
64. Liu DT. Regulation of allergenic products in the USA; CBER initiatives. Arb Paul Ehrlich Inst Bundesamt Sera Impfstoffe Frankf A M 1994; 87:8–12.
65. Norman PS. WHO-IUIS International Standards: advantages of these extracts. Arb Paul Ehrlich Inst Bundesamt Sera Impfstoffe Frankf A M 1994; 87:59–64.
66. Chapman M. Monoclonal antibody immunoassays: quantitative methods for allergen standardization. Arb Paul Ehrlich Inst Bundesamt Sera Impfstoffe Frankf A M 1994; 87:120–124.
67. Reed CE, Yunginger JW, Evans R. Quality assurance and standardization of allergy extracts in allergy practice. J Allergy Clin Immunol 1989; 84:4–8.

68. Osterballe O. Immunotherapy in hay fever with two major allergens 19, 25 and partially purified extract of timothy grass pollen. A controlled double blind study. In vivo variables, season I. Allergy 1980; 35:473–489.
69. Norman P, Winkenwerder W, Lichtenstein L. Immunotherapy of hay fever with ragweed antigen E: comparisons with whole extracts and placebo. J Allergy 1968; 42:93–108.
70. Van-Metre TEJ, Adkinson N Jr, Lichtenstein LM, et al. A controlled study of the effectiveness of the Rinkel method of immunotherapy for ragweed pollen hay fever. J Allergy Clin Immunol 1980; 65:288–297.
71. Hirsch SR, Kalbfleisch JH, Golbert TM, et al. Rinkel injection therapy: a multi-center controlled study. J Allergy Clin Immunol 1981; 68:133–155.
72. Hirsch SR, Kalbfleisch JH, Cohen SH. Comparison of Rinkel injection therapy with standard immunotherapy. J Allergy Clin Immunol 1982; 70:183–190.
73. Bousquet J, Des-Roches A, Paradis L, Dhivert H, Michel FB. Specific immuno-therapy in house dust mite allergy. Clin Rev Allergy Immunol 1995; 13: 151–159.
74. Turkeltaub PC, Campbell G, Mosimann JE. Comparative safety and efficacy of short ragweed extracts differing in potency and composition in the treatment of fall hay fever. Use of allergenically bioequivalent doses by parallel line bioassay to evaluate comparative safety and efficacy. Allergy 1990; 45:528–546.
75. Carreira J, Lombardero M, Ventas P. New developments in in vitro methods. Quantification of clinically relevant allergens in mass units. Arb Paul Ehrlich Inst Bundesamt Sera Impfstoffe Frankf A M 1994; 87:155–164.
76. Creticos PS, Van-Metre TE, Mardiney MR, Rosenberg GL, Norman PS, Adkin-son N Jr. Dose response of IgE and IgG antibodies during ragweed immunother-apy. J Allergy Clin Immunol 1984; 73:94–104.
77. Haugaard L, Dahl R, Jacobsen L. A controlled dose–response study of immuno-therapy with standardized, partially purified extract of house dust mite: clinical efficacy and side effects. J Allergy Clin Immunol 1993; 91:709–722.
78. Olaguibel J, Tabar A, Garcia-Figueroa B, Cortes C. Immunotherapy with stan-dardized extract of Dermatophagoides pteronyssinus in bronchial asthma: a dose–titration study. Allergy 1997; 52:168–178.
79. Van-Metre TE J, Marsh DG, Adkinson N Jr, et al. Immunotherapy for cat asthma. J Allergy Clin Immunol 1988; 82:1055–1068.
80. Alvarez-Cuesta E, Cuesta-Herranz J, Puyana-Ruiz J, Cuesta-Herranz C, Blanco-Quiros A. Monoclonal antibody-standardized cat extract immunotherapy: risk-benefit effects from a double-blind placebo study. J Allergy Clin Immunol 1994; 93:556–566.
81. Creticos PS, Marsh DG, Proud D, et al. Responses to ragweed-pollen nasal chal-lenge before and after immunotherapy. J Allergy Clin Immunol 1989; 84:197–205.
82. Van-Metre TE J, Adkinson N Jr, Amodio FJ, et al. A comparison of immunother-apy schedules for injection treatment of ragweed pollen hay fever. J Allergy Clin Immunol 1982; 69:181–193.

83. Creticos PS, Reed CE, Norman PS, et al. Ragweed immunotherapy in adult asthma [see comments]. N Engl J Med 1996; 334:501–506.

84. Hunt KJ, Valentine MD, Sobotka AK, Benton AW, Amodio FJ, Lichtenstein LM. A controlled trial of immunotherapy in insect hypersensitivity. N Engl J Med 1978; 299:157–161.

85. Muller U, Mosbech H. Position paper: immunotherapy with Hymenoptera venoms. Allergy 1993; 48(suppl 14):37–46.

86. Dolz I, Martinez-Cocera C, Bartolome J, Cimarra M. Placebo-controlled study of immunotherapy with grass pollen extract Alutard SQ during a 3 year period with initial rush immunotherapy. Allergy 1996; 1996:489–500.

87. Van-Bever HP, Stevens WJ. Evolution of the late asthmatic reaction during immunotherapy and after stopping immunotherapy. J Allergy Clin Immunol 1990; 86:141–146.

88. Lichtenstein L, Norman P, Winkenwerder L. A single year of immunotherapy in ragweed hay fever. Am J Med 1971; 44:514–524.

89. Bousquet J, Hejjaoui A, Skassa-Brociek W, et al. Double-blind, placebo-controlled immunotherapy with mixed grass-pollen allergoids. I. Rush immunotherapy with allergoids and standardized orchard grass-pollen extract. J Allergy Clin Immunol 1987; 80:591–598.

90. Norman PS, Lichtenstein LM. The clinical and immunologic specificity of immunotherapy. J Allergy Clin Immunol 1978; 61:370–377.

91. Frostad AB, Grimmer O, Sandvik L, Moxnes A, Aas K. Clinical effects of hyposensitization using a purified allergen preparation from timothy pollen as compared to crude aqueous extracts from timothy pollen and a four-grass pollen mixture respectively. Clin Allergy 1983; 13:337–357.

92. McAllen M. Hyposensitization in grass pollen hay fever. Acta Allergol 1969; 24: 421–431.

93. Ortolani C, Pastorello E, Moss RB, et al. Grass pollen immunotherapy: a single year double-blind, placebo-controlled study in patients with grass pollen-induced asthma and rhinitis. J Allergy Clin Immunol 1984; 73:283–290.

94. Citron K, Frankland A, Sinclair J. Inhalation tests of bronchial hypersensitivity in pollen asthma. Thorax 1958; 13:229–232.

95. Armentia-Medina A, Blanco-Quiros A, Martin-Santos JM, et al. Rush immunotherapy with a standardized Bermuda grass pollen extract. Ann Allergy 1989; 63:127–135.

96. Bousquet J, Maasch HJ, Hejjaoui A, et al. Double-blind, placebo-controlled immunotherapy with mixed grass-pollen allergoids. III. Efficacy and safety of unfractionated and high-molecular-weight preparations in rhinoconjunctivitis and asthma. J Allergy Clin Immunol 1989; 84:546–556.

97. Frankland A, Augustin R. Prophylaxis of summer hay fever and asthma: a controlled trial comparing crude grass pollen extract with the isolated main protein components. Lancet 1954; 1:1055–1058.

98. Hill DJ, Hosking CS, Shelton MJ, Turner MW. Failure of hyposensitisation in treatment of children with grass-pollen asthma. Br Med J Clin Res 1982; 284: 306–309.

99. Machiels JJ, Buche M, Somville MA, Jacquemin MG, Saint-Remy JM. Complexes of grass pollen allergens and specific antibodies reduce allergic symptoms and inhibit the seasonal increase of IgE antibody. Clin Exp Allergy 1990; 20:653–660.

100. Machiels JJ, Somville MA, Jacquemin MG, Saint-Remy JM. Allergen-antibody complexes can efficiently prevent seasonal rhinitis and asthma in grass pollen hypersensitive patients. Allergen–antibody complex immunotherapy. Allergy 1991; 46:335–348.

101. Pastorello EA, Pravettoni V, Incorvaia C, et al. Clinical and immunological effects of immunotherapy with alum-absorbed grass allergoid in grass-pollen-induced hay fever. Allergy 1992; 47:281–290.

102. D'Amato G, Kordash TR, Liccardi G, Lobefalo G, Cazzola M, Freshwater LL. Immunotherapy with Alpare in patients with respiratory allergy to Parietaria pollen: a two year double-blind placebo-controlled study. Clin Exp Allergy 1995; 25:149–158.

103. Pence H, Mitchell D, Greenly R, Updegraft B, Selfridge H. Immunotherapy for mountain cedar pollinosis. A double-blind controlled study. J Allergy Clin Immunol 1976; 58:39–50.

104. Rak S, Hakansson L, Venge P. Eosinophil chemotactic activity in allergic patients during the birch pollen season: the effect of immunotherapy. Int Arch Allergy Appl Immunol 1987; 82:349–350.

105. Varney VA, Gaga M, Frew AJ, Aber VR, Kay AB, Durham SR. Usefulness of immunotherapy in patients with severe summer hay fever uncontrolled by antiallergic drugs. Brit Med J 1991; 302:265–269.

106. Creticos P, Reed C, Norman P, Subcenter Investigators of the NIAIAD Study. The NIAIAD cooperative study of the role of ???immunotherapy in seasonal ragweed-induced adult asthma. J Allergy Clin Immunol 1993; 91:226 (abstract).

107. Bousquet J, Hejjaoui A, Becker WM, et al. Clinical and immunologic reactivity of patients allergic to grass pollens and to multiple pollen species. I. Clinical and immunologic characteristics. J Allergy Clin Immunol 1991; 87:737–746.

108. Pene J, Rivier A, Lagier B, Becker WM, Michel FB, Bousquet J. Differences in IL-4 release by PBMC are related with heterogeneity of atopy. Immunology 1994; 81:58–64.

109. Lockey RF, Benedict LM, Turkeltaub PC, Bukantz SC. Fatalities from immunotherapy (IT) and skin testing (ST). J Allergy Clin Immunol 1987; 79:660–677.

110. Bousquet J, Michel FB. Safety considerations in assessing the role of immunotherapy in allergic disorders. Drug Safety 1994; 10:5–17.

111. Hejjaoui A, Ferrando R, Dhivert H, Michel FB, Bousquet J. Systemic reactions occurring during immunotherapy with standardized pollen extracts. J Allergy Clin Immunol 1992; 89:925–933.

112. Jarisch R, Gotz M, Aberer W, et al. Reduction of side effects of specific immuno-therapy by premedication with antihistaminics and reduction of maximal dosage to 50,000 SQ-U/ml. Arb Paul Ehrlich Inst Bundesamt Sera Impfstoffe Frankf A M 1988; 82:163–175.

113. Grammer LC, Shaughnessy MA, Suszko IM, Shaughnessy JJ, Patterson R. Persistence of efficacy after a brief course of polymerized ragweed allergen: a controlled study. J Allergy Clin Immunol 1984; 73:484–489.

114. Mosbech H, Osterballe O. Does the effect of immunotherapy last after termination of treatment? Follow-up study in patients with grass pollen rhinitis. Allergy 1988; 43:523–529.

115. McAllen M, Assem E, Maunsell K. House-dust mite asthma. Results of challenge tests on five criteria with Dermatophagoides pteronyssinus. Brit Med J 1970; 2: 501–504.

116. Machiels JJ, Somville MA, Lebrun PM, Lebecque SJ, Jacquemin MG, Saint-Remy JM. Allergic bronchial asthma due to Dermatophagoides pteronyssinus hypersensitivity can be efficiently treated by inoculation of allergen-antibody complexes. J Clin Invest 1990; 85:1024–1035.

117. Van-Bever HP, Stevens WJ. Effect of hyposensitization upon the immediate and late asthmatic reaction and upon histamine reactivity in patients allergic to house dust mite (Dermatophagoides pteronyssinus). Eur Respir J 1992; 5:318–322.

118. Garcia-Ortega P, Merelo A, Marrugat J, Richart C. Decrease of skin and bronchial sensitization following short-intensive scheduled immunotherapy in mite-allergic asthma. Chest 1993; 103:183–187.

119. Wahn U, Schweter C, Lind P, Lowenstein H. Prospective study on immunologic changes induced by two different Dermatophagoides pteronyssinus extracts prepared from whole mite culture and mite bodies. J Allergy Clin Immunol 1988; 82:360–370.

120. Mosbech H, Dreborg S, Frolund L, et al. Hyposensitization in asthmatics with mPEG modified and unmodified house dust mite extract. II. Effect evaluated by challenges with allergen and histamine. Allergy 1989; 44:499–509.

121. Aas K. Hyposensitization in house dust allergy asthma. Acta Paediatr Scand 1971; 60:264–268.

122. D'Souza M, Pepys J, Wells I, et al. Hyposensitization with Dermatophagoides pteronyssinus in house dust allergy: a controlled study of clinical and immunological effects. Clin Allergy 1973; 3:177–193.

123. Gaddie J, Skinner C, Palmer K. Hyposensitization with house dust mite vaccine in bronchial asthma. Brit Med J 1976; 2:561–562.

124. Amaral-Marques R, Avila R. Results of a clinical trial with a Dermatophagoides pteronyssinus tyrosine adsorbed vaccine. Allergol Immunopathol Madr 1978; 6: 231–235.

125. Pauli G, Bessot JC, Bigot H, et al. Clinical and immunologic evaluation of tyrosine-adsorbed Dermatophagoides pteronyssinus extract: a double-blind placebo-controlled trial. J Allergy Clin Immunol 1984; 74:524–535.

126. Newton D, Maberley D, Wilson R. House dust mite hyposensitization. Br J Dis Chest 1978; 72:21–28.

127. Machiels JJ, Lebrun PM, Jacquemin MG, Saint-Remy JM. Significant reduction of nonspecific bronchial reactivity in patients with Dermatophagoides pteronyssinus-sensitive allergic asthma under therapy with allergen-antibody complexes. Am Rev Respir Dis 1993; 147:1407–1412.

128. Bousquet J, Hejjaoui A, Clauzel AM, et al. Specific immunotherapy with a standardized Dermatophagoides pteronyssinus extract. II. Prediction of efficacy of immunotherapy. J Allergy Clin Immunol 1988; 82:971–977.

129. Murray AB, Ferguson AC, Morrison BJ. Non-allergic bronchial hyperreactivity in asthmatic children decreases with age and increases with mite immunotherapy. Ann Allergy 1985; 54:541–544.

130. Committee on Safety of Medicines. Desensitizing vaccines. Brit Med J 1986; 293:948.

131. Mosbech H. Who will benefit from hyposensitization? Predictive parameters in house dust mite allergic asthmatics. Allergy 1990; 45:209–212.

132. Bousquet J, Hejjaoui A, Dhivert H, Clauzel AM, Michel FB. Immunotherapy with a standardized Dermatophagoides pteronyssinus extract. III. Systemic reactions during the rush protocol in patients suffering from asthma. J Allergy Clin Immunol 1989; 83:797–802.

133. Hejjaoui A, Dhivert H, Michel FB, Bousquet J. Immunotherapy with a standardized Dermatophagoides pteronyssinus extract. IV. Systemic reactions according to the immunotherapy schedule. J Allergy Clin Immunol 1990; 85:473–479.

134. Price JF, Warner JO, Hey EN, Turner MW, Soothill JF. A controlled trial of hyposensitization with adsorbed tyrosine Dermatophagoides pteronyssinus antigen in childhood asthma: in vivo aspects. Clin Allergy 1984; 14:209–219.

135. Bertelsen A, Andersen JB, Christensen J, Ingemann L, Kristensen T, Ostergaard PA. Immunotherapy with dog and cat extracts in children. Allergy 1989; 44:330–335.

136. Bucur J, Dreborg S, Einarsson R, Ljungstedt-Pahlman I, Nilsson JE, Persson G. Immunotherapy with dog and cat allergen preparations in dog-sensitive and cat-sensitive asthmatics. Ann Allergy 1989; 62:355–361.

137. Hedlin G, Graff-Lonnevig V, Heilborn H, et al. Immunotherapy with cat- and dog-dander extracts. II. In vivo and in vitro immunologic effects observed in a 1-year double-blind placebo study. J Allergy Clin Immunol 1986; 77:488–496.

138. Hedlin G, Graff-Lonnevig V, Heilborn H, et al. Immunotherapy with cat- and dog-dander extracts. V. Effects of 3 years of treatment. J Allergy Clin Immunol 1991; 87:955–964.

139. Lilja G, Sundin B, Graff-Lonnevig V, et al. Immunotherapy with cat- and dog-dander extracts. IV. Effects of 2 years of treatment. J Allergy Clin Immunol 1989; 83:37–44.

140. Ohman J Jr, Findlay SR, Leitermann KM. Immunotherapy in cat-induced asthma.

Double-blind trial with evaluation of in vivo and in vitro responses. J Allergy Clin Immunol 1984; 74:230–239.

141. Rohatgi N, Dunn K, Chai H. Cat- or dog-induced immediate and late asthmatic responses before and after immunotherapy. J Allergy Clin Immunol 1988; 82: 389–397.

142. Sundin B, Lilja G, Graff-Lonnevig V, et al. Immunotherapy with partially purified and standardized animal dander extracts. I. Clinical results from a double-blind study on patients with animal dander asthma. J Allergy Clin Immunol 1986; 77: 478–487.

143. Taylor WW, Ohman J Jr, Lowell FC. Immunotherapy in cat-induced asthma. Double-blind trial with evaluation of bronchial responses to cat allergen and histamine. J Allergy Clin Immunol 1978; 61:283–287.

144. Valovirta E, Viander M, Koivikko A, Vanto T, Ingeman L. Immunotherapy in allergy to dog. Immunologic and clinical findings of a double-blind study. Ann Allergy 1986; 57:173–179.

145. Valovirta E, Koivikko A, Vanto T, Viander M, Ingeman L. Immunotherapy in allergy to dog: a double-blind clinical study. Ann Allergy 1984; 53:85–88.

146. Haugaard L, Dahl R. Immunotherapy in patients allergic to cat and dog dander. I. Clinical results. Allergy 1992; 47:249–254.

147. Varney V, Edwards J, Tabbah K, Brewster H, Marvroleon G, Frew A. Clinical efficacy of specific immunotherapy to cat dander: a double-blind placebo-controlled trial. Clin Exp Allergy 1997; 27:860–867.

148. Salvaggio J, Aukrust L. Postgraduate course presentations. Mold-induced asthma. J Allergy Clin Immunol 1981; 68:327–346.

149. Horst M, Hejjaoui A, Horst V, Michel FB, Bousquet J. Double-blind, placebo-controlled rush immunotherapy with a standardized Alternaria extract. J Allergy Clin Immunol 1990; 85:460–472.

150. Malling HJ, Dreborg S, Weeke B. Diagnosis and immunotherapy of mould allergy. V. Clinical efficacy and side effects of immunotherapy with Cladosporium herbarum. Allergy 1986; 41:507–519.

151. Dreborg S, Agrell B, Foucard T, Kjellman NI, Koivikko A, Nilsson S. A double-blind, multicenter immunotherapy trial in children, using a purified and standardized Cladosporium herbarum preparation. I. Clinical results. Allergy 1986; 41:131–140.

152. Kaad PH, Ostergaard PA. The hazard of mould hyposensitization in children with asthma. Clin Allergy 1982; 12:317–320.

153. Allergenic extracts made from bacteria. Federal Register, 42 FR 58266, 44 FR 1544 1979.

154. Taudorf E, Laursen LC, Lanner A, et al. Oral immunotherapy in birch pollen hay fever. J Allergy Clin Immunol 1987; 80:153–161.

155. Mosbech H, Dreborg S, Madsen F, et al. High dose grass pollen tablets used for

hyposensitization in hay fever patients. A one-year double blind placebo-controlled study. Allergy 1987; 42:451–455.

156. Feliziani V, Lattuada G, Parmiani S, Dall'Aglio PP. Safety and efficacy of sublingual rush immunotherapy with grass allergen extracts. A double blind study. Allergol Immunopathol Madr 1995; 23:224–230.

157. Sabbah A, Hassoun S, Le-Sellin J, Andre C, Sicard H. A double-blind, placebo-controlled trial by the sublingual route of immunotherapy with a standardized grass pollen extract. Allergy 1994; 49:309–313.

158. Tari MG, Mancino M, Monti G. Efficacy of sublingual immunotherapy in patients with rhinitis and asthma due to house dust mite. A double-blind study. Allergol Immunopathol Madr 1990; 18:277–284.

159. Troise C, Voltolini S, Canessa A, Pecora S, Negrini AC. Sublingual immunotherapy in Parietaria pollen-induced rhinitis: a double-blind study. J Invest Allergol Clin Immunol 1995; 5:25–30.

160. Nelson HS, Oppenheimer J, Vatsia GA, Buchmeier A. A double-blind, placebo-controlled evaluation of sublingual immunotherapy with standardized cat extract. J Allergy Clin Immunol 1993; 92:229–236.

161. Crimi E, Voltolini S, Troise C, et al. Local immunotherapy with Dermatophagoides extract in asthma. J Allergy Clin Immunol 1991; 87:721–728.

162. Tari MG, Mancino M, Monti G. Immunotherapy by inhalation of allergen in powder in house dust allergic asthma: a double-blind study. J Invest Allergol Clin Immunol 1992; 2:59–67.

163. Ownby DR, Adinoff AD. The appropriate use of skin testing and allergen immunotherapy in young children. J Allergy Clin Immunol 1994; 94:662–665.

164. Des-Roches A, Paradis L, Ménardo J-L, Bouges S, Daurès J-P, Bousquet J. Immunotherapy with a standardized Dermatophagoides pteronyssinus extract. VI. Specific immunotherapy prevents the onset of new sensitizations in children. J Allergy Clin Immunol 1997; 99:450–453.

165. Norman P. Is there a role for immunotherapy in the treatment of asthma? Yes. Am J Respir Crit Care Med 1996; 154:1225–1226.

166. Barnes P. Is there a role for immunotherapy in the treatment of asthma? No. Am J Respir Crit Care Med 1996; 154:1227–1228.

167. Bush R, Huftel M, Busse W. Patient selection. In: Lockey R, Bukantz S, eds. Allergen Immunotherapy. New York: Marcel Dekker, 1991:25–49.

168. Cohn JR, Pizzi A. Determinants of patient compliance with allergen immunotherapy. J Allergy Clin Immunol 1993; 91:734–737.

169. Position paper on allergen immunotherapy. Report of a BSACI working party. January-October 1992. Clin Exp Allergy 1993; 3:1–44.

170. Munir AK, Bjorksten B, Einarsson R, et al. Cat (Fel d I), dog (Can f I), and cockroach allergens in homes of asthmatic children from three climatic zones in Sweden. Allergy 1994; 49:508–516.

171. Kaplan AP, Anderson JA, Valentine MD, et al. Beta-adrenergic blockers, immu-

notherapy, and skin testing. American Academy of Allergy and Immunology. J Allergy Clin Immunol 1989; 84:129–130.

172. Schwartz HJ, Golden DB, Lockey RF. Venom immunotherapy in the Hymenoptera-allergic pregnant patient. J Allergy Clin Immunol 1990; 85:709–712.

173. Valenta R, Kraft D. Recombinant allergens for diagnosis and therapy of allergic diseases. Curr Opin Immunol 1995; 7:751–756.

174. O'Hehir RE, Lamb JR. Human in vitro experimental model for CD4+ T cell targeted immunotherapy to house dust mite. Ann Allergy 1993; 71:317–321.

175. Schad VC, Garman RD, Greenstein JL. The potential use of T cell epitopes to alter the immune response. Semin Immunol 1991; 3:217–224.

176. Bousquet J, Breitenbach M, Dreborg S, Kenimer M, Løwenstein S, Norman P. Diagnosis and specific immunotherapy using recombinant allergens and epitopes. In: Kraft D, Sehon A, eds. Molecular Biology and Immunology of Allergens. Boca Raton: CRC Press, 1993:311–320.

177. Wallner BP, Gefter ML. Immunotherapy with T-cell-reactive peptides derived from allergens. Allergy 1994; 49:302–308.

178. Norman P, Ohman J Jr, Long A, et al. Treatment of cat allergy with T-cell reactive peptides. Am J Respir Crit Care Med 1996; 154:1623–1628.

179. Hebert J, Bernier D, Boutin Y, Jobin M, Mourad W. Generation of anti-idiotypic and anti-anti-idiotypic monoclonal antibodies in the same fusion. Support of Jerne's network theory. J Immunol 1990; 144:4256–4261.

180. Li JT, Yunginger JW, Reed CE, Jaffe HS, Nelson DR, Gleich GJ. Lack of suppression of IgE production by recombinant interferon gamma: a controlled trial in patients with allergic rhinitis. J Allergy Clin Immunol 1990; 85:934–940.

181. Cooper KD. Atopic dermatitis: recent trends in pathogenesis and therapy. J Invest Dermatol 1994; 102:128–137.

182. Presta LG, Lahr SJ, Shields RL, et al. Humanization of an antibody directed against IgE. J Immunol 1993; 151:2623–2632.

183. Davis FM, Gossett LA, Pinkston KL, et al. Can anti-IgE be used to treat allergy? Springer Semin Immunopathol 1993; 15:51–73.

184. Haak-Frendscho M, Ridgway J, Shields R, Robbins K, Gorman C, Jardieu P. Human IgE receptor alpha-chain IgG chimera blocks passive cutaneous anaphylaxis reaction in vivo. J Immunol 1993; 151:351–358.

185. Dombrowicz D, Flamand V, Brigman KK, Koller BH, Kinet JP. Abolition of anaphylaxis by targeted disruption of the high affinity immunoglobulin E receptor alpha chain gene. Cell 1993; 75:969–976.

15

Future Directions

ROBERT K. BUSH

University of Wisconsin–Madison Medical School and
William S. Middleton Memorial Veterans Hospital
Madison, Wisconsin

I. Introduction

The role of the environment in the pathogenesis of asthma and its perpetuation have become increasingly evident in the past several years. The disturbingly increasing prevalence in asthma mortality may be attributable in part to environmental influences. This has been well demonstrated by the identification of cockroach allergens as a risk factor for asthma affecting children residing in inner city environments. Although physicians are currently well armed with a variety of effective treatments for asthma, preventive measures, which include environmental controls, will be important in curbing the increasing prevalence and reducing the risk of asthma mortality. The identification of major allergens has been an important advance leading to the discovery of risk factors for asthma and of means of controlling them. However, much work is needed in the future to improve our current state of knowledge and translate it into appropriate treatment recommendations.

II. Immune Mechanisms in Asthma

Although considerable insight has been gained into the immune mechanisms involved in the pathogenesis of asthma, much remains to be learned. Studies of the immune mechanisms involved in asthma are important for development of potential ways for its disruption. In allergic asthma, the central role of IgE antibodies has been well understood. However, the mechanisms that lead to the allergic response are still not completely defined. Cytokines such as IL-5, which is necessary for the generation and survival of eosinophils; IL-4, which plays a key role in the generation of IgE antibodies; and IL-10, which is important as an inflammatory modulator, are centrally involved in the pathogenesis of asthma (1). Indeed, studies are being conducted with the use of anti-IL-5 and anti-IL-4 treatments to counteract or abolish the allergic response and eosinophilic inflammation.

Likewise, protein molecules such as ICAM and VCAM are important in the adhesion of inflammatory cells and their transmigration into tissues. VCAM is especially important in the adhesion of eosinophils to endothelial cells, and its central role has been demonstrated by a number of studies. Anti-VCAM therapy may also prove to be beneficial in treating asthma in the future.

Clearly, environmental influences can activate a number of cytokines and adhesion molecules through both immunological and nonimmunological mechanisms. The role of environmental influences and their potential to initiate these responses remains to be fully elucidated.

III. Risk Factors

Genetic factors clearly have a pivotal role in the development of asthma. It has long been known that asthma, along with other atopic diseases, is a familial disease. Currently, much work is being done to identify candidate genes that are involved in the production of IgE antibody, regulation of cytokines, beta-adrenergic receptors, and the generation of inflammatory mediators such as leukotrienes. The keys to understanding the pathogenesis of asthma and its management will be gleamed from these studies. It may be possible in the future to evaluate individuals for the presence of genetic markers that would indicate the specific therapies that are most likely to be effective.

It is clearly known that allergens play a major role as risk factors in the development of asthma. Primarily, these have been indoor allergens as discussed in this work. House dust mites, animal danders, cockroaches, and fungi such as *Alternaria* have been well established as important risk factors. These allergens share a common characteristic in that they are in the patient's environment throughout much of the year. This is in contrast to pollens, which may appear for brief periods of time. Clearly, symptoms can be attributable to pollen exposure but they have not been defined as clear risk factors as have indoor allergens (2).

Both indoor and outdoor pollutants are contributing factors to asthma symptoms. Their central role in the pathogenesis of asthma is not well established; however, it is clear that maternal smoking is a major factor in the development of childhood asthma.

The role of viral infections in asthma also is important. Studies have indicated that allergen sensitization may require the presence of a viral infection (1). The viruses involved in these responses and their timing in concert with allergen exposure are under investigation.

Questions to be answered in the future regarding risk factors include whether or not exposure to multiple allergens and the interaction of pollutants and allergens act synergistically. Recent evidence suggests that diesel exhaust particles when combined with allergens enhance the allergic response to the allergen. Other factors that may be involved in these responses include the presence of volatile organic compounds that occur in fungus-contaminated environments. Likewise, endotoxins and damp environments may be potential catalysts for the development of sensitization to allergens such as the house dust mite. Clearly, environmental tobacco smoke is another factor that has been well studied and has been shown to increase serum IgE levels and perhaps the risk of allergen sensitization.

Further questions to be explored include, At what age is exposure to allergens critical for the development of sensitization? In most studies of children below the age of 2, those with wheezing episodes have these attacks due to viral respiratory infections. However, environmental exposure to allergens is occurring during this time, although sensitization does not usually appear until approximately age 2 and above.

IV. Population Studies

In order to clearly appreciate the role of environmental influences on the development and exacerbations of asthma, susceptible populations need to be evaluated. Furthermore, measurable health outcomes need to be included (3). Objective measurements of lung function and evidence of sensitization through the measurement of serum-specific IgE antibodies or by appropriate skin testing need to be conducted. Assessment of airway hyperresponsiveness may also be included in these studies.

To establish the diagnosis of allergic asthma or to determine the presence of specific IgE antibodies, standardized diagnostic allergenic reagents need to be produced. At the present time house dust mite extracts, cat allergen extracts, and grass and ragweed pollen extracts are standardized in the United States. However, other materials that are used for diagnostic purposes that may be important in assessing indoor exposure such as dog dander extracts and fungal extracts have not yet been standardized.

V. Need for Identification and Purification of Allergens

Improvement of the quality of diagnostic reagents and the development of immunoassays and other methods to assess exposure to allergens will require the identification and purification of major allergens. Molecular biological techniques have allowed great strides in this area in the past few years. The major allergens from a number of sources have been molecularly cloned, and monoclonal antibodies have been produced against the proteins. These sources include house dust mite, cat, cockroach, and a few fungal species. However, for many allergies the principal allergens have not yet been identified or purified.

VI. Exposure Assessment

The identification of major allergens has also led to our ability to assess exposure to these allergens and to accumulate information regarding threshold levels that lead to sensitization and to asthma symptoms. This has been particularly useful in the study of house dust mite allergy, and data have been accumulated for cat and cockroach allergens. However, in the case of fungi much work needs to be done.

The studies of damp homes or those with reported mold growth indicated that there may be a role for indoor fungal exposure in the development of the symptoms of asthma. However, quantitative methods for fungal allergen exposure have not yet been developed. Currently, it is recommended (3) that duplicate cultures of air samples be prepared at different times in one season and during different seasons. Also, in addition to cultures, airborne samples should be microscopically examined for spores.

Other techniques include the use of biomarkers to assess allergen exposure indirectly by the measurement of fungal products such as $(1 \rightarrow 3)\beta$-glucan, extracellular polysaccharides, and ergosterol. Relationships between these biomarkers and other more traditional methods of assessing fungal allergen exposure such as spore counts or culture techniques have not been determined.

The recent identification of major fungal allergens by the use of biotechnology will improve our ability to assess allergenic exposure to these important fungal allergens. Immunoassays that measure Alt a 1 have been developed. With the identification of a number of *Aspergillus fumigatus, Cladosporium,* and *Penicillium* allergens, these proteins may also be amenable to quantitation in environmental samples.

For many exposures, however, the threshold levels leading to sensitization and the development of asthma symptoms remain to be elucidated.

VII. Do Control Measures Work?

Although threshold levels for some allergen exposures that lead to sensitization have been promulgated (4), questions remain as to whether or not avoiding allergens or reducing them to low levels may be preventive (5). Questions remain as to whether primary prevention of sensitization and asthma can be achieved by avoidance of one major allergen, such as house dust mite. Will this protect against sensitization in asthma when other allergen exposures are not controlled (6)? Further questions that remain to be answered include, In which local environment or populations can allergen avoidance be effective?

Once sensitization has occurred and asthma symptoms have developed, the question remains, Can allergen avoidance measures prevent relapse of symptoms and airway inflammation or reduce airway hyperresponsiveness?

The practical aspects of allergen control measures still require controlled prospective studies (7). Although some evidence has accumulated that the use of mattress covers and scrupulous reduction in house dust mite exposure can be effective, this approach has been questioned. It has been demonstrated that removal of sensitized individuals from house dust mite environments does lead to improved symptom control, improvement in lung function, and reduction in medication use. However, once the individual returns to an environment where exposure is present, the symptoms return.

In addition to the overall evaluation of environmental control measures, which individual elements of allergen control contribute to the overall efficacy and health benefits? Furthermore, are the recommendations, such as carpet removal and humidity control, truly cost-effective?

VIII. Immunotherapy

Immunotherapy for the treatment of allergic asthma remains controversial. While a number of studies and meta-analysis of accumulated data suggest that allergen immunotherapy can be useful as an adjunct to the management of allergic asthma, other studies have not supported its use. In part this may be due to the lack of standardized allergenic vaccines. A number of studies have demonstrated that when appropriate materials are utilized, the chances of successful treatment increase.

Most immunotherapy studies have taken place in patients with established asthma, where the benefits of treatment may be less successful. A current study based in Europe is looking at early intervention in allergic rhinitis with immunotherapy to determine if this will prevent the subsequent development of asthma. Preliminary indications suggest that early use of immunotherapy for childhood allergic rhinitis may actually prevent many children from subsequently developing asthma.

Much interest is focused on the peptides that initiate the T-cell response to allergens. Indeed, a few studies of peptide-based vaccines have been conducted to determine their effectiveness in the treatment of allergic rhinitis in asthma. While animal models indicate that this approach may be successful, human trials have not been as convincing. Nonetheless, the use of modified T-cell epitope therapy using peptides recognized by T cells may be an important new addition in our armamentarium as further studies are conducted.

Another rationale for molecular biological studies of allergens is the identification of the DNA sequences that encode for the allergenic protein. Recent evidence indicates that DNA-based vaccines may counteract IgE responses by driving the immune mechanisms toward a Th1 response. This offers a new and potentially practical approach to treatment of IgE-mediated asthma. Such studies, however, are very preliminary at the present time and require further study.

IX. Conclusion

The human respiratory system is subjected to a variety of environmental pollutants and allergens. In susceptible individuals, these factors alone or in combination may lead to the development of the condition known as asthma. Tools are available for the diagnosis and recognition of allergic asthma. The role of pollutants is also important although not as thoroughly studied. Identification and purification of major allergens have been key steps in the discovery of methods for assessing exposure and establishing threshold dose–response relationships. These investigations have led to the development of appropriate control measures for reducing allergen exposure in the indoor as well as outdoor environments. In the management of the asthmatic patient it is important to recognize the environmental factors and to deal with them appropriately. Further studies may allow us to reduce the prevalence and mortality of asthma by appropriate interventions.

References

1. Busse WW. Current research and future needs in allergic rhinitis and asthma. J Allergy Clin Immunol 1998; 100:S424–S426.
2. Peat JK, Li J. Reversing the trend: reducing the prevalence of asthma. J Allergy Clin Immunol 1999; 103:1–10.
3. Verhoeff AP, Burge HA. Health risk assessment of fungi in home environments. Am Allergy Asthma Immunol 1997; 78:544–554.
4. Platts-Mills TAE, Vervloet D, Thomas WR, Aalberse RC, Chapman MD. Indoor allergens and asthma: report of the Third International Workshop. J Allergy Clin Immunol 1997; 100:S2–S24.
5. Munir AKM, Kjellman M, Björkstén B. Exposure to indoor allergens in early infancy and sensitization. J Allergy Clin Immunol 1997; 100:177–181.
6. Peat J, Björkstén B. Primary and secondary prevention of allergic asthma. Eur Respir J 1998; 12(suppl 27): 28s–34s.
7. Custovic A, Simpson A, Chapman MD, Woodcock A. Allergen avoidance in the treatment of asthma and atopic disorders. Thorax 1998; 53:63–72.

AUTHOR INDEX

Italic numbers give the page on which the complete reference is listed.

SUBJECT INDEX

A

Acid aerosols (*see* Sulfur dioxide)
  bronchospasm and sulfur dioxide,
    121–122
  sulfur dioxide, 120–121
Airborne pollens, 91–112
  exposure, 94–95
  release and dispersion, 93–94
  structure and function, 92–93
Air pollutants, 8, 119–139
  indoor air, 8, 141–164, 170–171
  outdoor air, 8, 119–139, 171–173
Airway inflammation, 13–14
  eosinophilic, 13–14
Airway remodeling, 23–25
Animal allergens, 5–6, 53–63
  control measures, 5–6, 60–62
  domestic animals, 53
  farm animals, 53
  laboratory animals, 53, 59–60
  particle size, 5
  threshold for sensitization, 6
Antigen-presenting cells (APCs), 14
Antigen sensitization, 14–18, 42
Arterial blood gases, 195–196
Asthma
  allergen exposure and, 40–43
  population studies, 323–324
  prevalence, 1–2
  risk factors, 322–323

B

Building-related illness, 144–145

C

Cat allergens, 54–55, 58–59
  distribution, 56–57
  Fel d 1, 54–55
Cigarette smoke, 8
Cockroach allergens, 6–7, 169–170
  control measures, 7
  threshold for sensitization, 7

D

Dendritic cells, 14
Dermatophagoides pteronyssinus (*see
  also* House dust mites), 35, 170
Dermatophagoides farinae (*see also*
  House dust mites), 35
Diagnostic approaches, 3–4, 183–204
Diesel exhaust particles, 8, 128–129
Differential diagnosis of asthma,
  184–185
DNA-based vaccines, 10
Dog allergens, 54–55, 58–59
  Can f 1, 54–55
  distribution of, 56–57
Dust samples, 36
  mite counts and dust samples, 36
  processing, 36